Current Clinical Psychiatry

Series Editor
Jerrold F. Rosenbaum, MD
Chief of Psychiatry, Massachusetts General Hospital, Boston, MA

For further volumes:
http://www.springer.com/series/7634

Lee Baer · Mark A. Blais
Editors

Handbook of Clinical Rating Scales and Assessment in Psychiatry and Mental Health

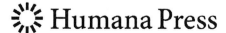 Humana Press

Editors

Lee Baer
Department of Psychiatry
Massachusetts General Hospital
Harvard Medical School
One Bowdoin Square
Boston MA 02114
USA
lbaer@partners.org

Mark A. Blais
Department of Psychiatry
Massachusetts General Hospital
Harvard Medical School
One Bowdoin Square
Boston MA 02114
USA
mblais@partners.org

ISBN 978-1-58829-966-6   e-ISBN 978-1-59745-387-5
DOI 10.1007/978-1-59745-387-5

Library of Congress Control Number: 2009933281

Printed on acid-free paper

springer.com

L. B.: Dedicated to Carole Ann, Emily, David, and Bernice Baer.

M. A. B.: Dedicated to Earlene Shannon Blais "The best mom a boy like me could ever have."

Preface

Our intention in preparing this handbook was to provide the busy psychiatric clinician (psychiatrist, psychologist, social worker, psychiatric nurse or counselor) with a truly easy-to-use and practical guide to using focused assessments for improving the care of their patients. We hope we have come close to realizing this goal, and that you will find, as we have, that integrating a few select scales, like those included in this volume, into your routine clinical practice will benefit you and your patients.

To accomplish our goal of making this a clinically useful book, we have invited our chapter authors (who are primarily members of specialty clinical and clinical research programs at our hospital, Massachusetts General Hospital in Boston): (1) to identify the "gold-standard" scales they routinely use to assess patients in their own clinics, (2) to provide ready-to-copy versions of these scales (when copyrights permit), and (3) to provide practical information about the clinical use of the scales (i.e., when to administer, how to score, how to interpret results, and how to use to measure clinical change in patients). In addition, we asked each author to include the latest information available about the psychometric characteristics of the scales, such as reliability, validity, and sensitivity to change (these concepts are reviewed in Chapter 1), as well as alternative or supplementary scales that are available for assessing patients with that particular disorder.

Before describing the organization of the chapters, we first want to address a basic question: Why should psychiatric clinicians routinely use rating scales with their patients?

In our experience, most clinicians do not use rating scales routinely as part of their standard delivery of care. This appears to us to be true regardless of the psychotherapy orientation of the clinician, or whether or not they prescribe medications as part of their treatment (the only exception may be clinicians who were trained in cognitive-behavior therapy [CBT] where outcome measures are more often used, although far from universally).

Why don't more clinicians use rating scales? Some reasons we have heard include the following: time pressure, not knowing which scales to use, the cost of commercially available scales, worrying whether quantitative rating scales can capture the truly important aspects of improvement in their patients, and believing that rating scales are useful only in research settings. We hope that the following chapters will address all of these issues.

The last few years have witnessed a substantial increase in our understanding of the benefit offered by integrating measurement into routine clinical care. For example, studies such as STAR*D [1] and STEP-BD [2] have shown that integrating measurement into clinical care helps produce real world treatment effects similar to those of efficacy studies. In psychotherapy, when measurement data are routinely evaluated to assess progress treatment failure rates are reduced [3]. What are the compelling reasons to use rating scales that we believe far outweigh these perceived negatives? Here are a few:

1. *Rating scales will help you and your patient determine if, and how well, your treatment is working.* For example, patients are often unaware of gradual improvements in their symptoms or their functioning. By having a "baseline" measure of their functioning before treatment, and repeated ratings thereafter (say, every 2 weeks), you can point out to your patient that they improved by, say 15% on the targeted rating scale so far, thus all their hard work is beginning to bear fruit, even if gradually. On the other hand if, after months of treatment, your patient's score has not budged from its baseline level, or has worsened, this should be a clear signal to both of you that the current treatment should be reviewed and changes be considered. The joint review of rating scale information helps improve treatment collaboration and maintain the patient's active involvement in their care.

2. *Rating scales will help you to better link your clinical work to the growing empirical literature, and to better use it to guide your treatments.* It would be nearly impossible for any treatment outcome paper to be published in a psychiatric journal today without at least one objective rating scale having been used to both characterize the patients eligible for the study, and to assess the degree of improvement with treatment. Imagine that you pick up your favorite psychiatric journal and read a paper reporting that a new treatment for obsessive-compulsive disorder (OCD) was effective for patients with an average baseline score of 17 on the Yale-Brown Obsessive-Compulsive Scale (YBOCS) rating scale, with response defined as a 25% improvement on this same scale. Now, when you sit across from a new patient with OCD, unless you routinely use the YBOCS scale, how can you know whether she is similar in severity to the subjects in the research report, and furthermore, how can you tell her how much improvement she can reasonably expect from your planned treatment? Of course, a clinical practice is very different from a research program, and your patients cannot sit through a battery of tests with an interviewer prior to every session with you. However, one carefully selected scale (chosen from this volume) that is accepted as a gold standard in the field, can either be completed by your patient in the waiting room before a visit, or administered by you in 5 minutes during the visit.

3. *Rating scales provide clinicians with a systematic method for asking about key symptoms on a regular schedule*: For example, a rating scale like the Hamilton or Beck depression scales will remind us to ask our patients about their eating, sleep, energy, sexual interest, and suicidal ideation at nearly every visit, some questions which might otherwise slip our minds if not volunteered by our

patients. Likewise, administering a rating scale asking about quality of life will remind us to focus on how our patients are functioning in their daily lives, which is as, or more important, as their symptom level.

4. *Using Rating Scales Can Facilitate Collaboration with Third-Party Payers*: Imagine you work for an insurance company that authorizes and pays for mental-health visits for their customers. One day, a provider calls you requesting an additional 10 visits for her patient, and gives you the following justification: "Mrs. Jones' depressive symptoms have begun to respond to treatment as shown by her 35% improvement on the Hamilton Depression Scale, and we will need an additional 10 sessions to continue to further reduce them to a remission level, which has been shown to greatly reduce her risk of future relapse." Would you deny the additional requested visits? And, if so, how would you justify your decision to your supervisor when it is appealed, and probably, reversed?

5. *Using Screening Questionnaires Can Identify "Hidden" Comorbid Problems*: The screening questionnaires included in this handbook can be used to rapidly screen your patients for common problems (such as personality disorders or alcohol abuse), information which patients typically do not volunteer unless specifically asked. As with rating scales, using such scales with your patients can help ensure that you do not miss a condition that can complicate the treatment of the patients' presenting problem, but that can be controlled with proper treatment.

The bottom line: we recommend that you choose a few rating scales from the following chapters that are most appropriate for your particular patient mix, and then use them routinely until they become part of your everyday clinical practice.

In Chapter 2, Dr. Cusin et al. consider rating scales used to assess patients with depression (specifically, unipolar, non-psychotic depression). The gold-standard scales they describe are the Hamilton Depression Inventory (administered by the clinician), and the Beck Depression Inventory (a self-report questionnaire). They also consider several other depression scales, including the MADRAS, IDS, and Zung scales.

In Chapter 3, Dr. Marques et al. consider assessment instruments used for a variety of common anxiety disorder diagnoses. For panic disorder and agoraphobia, they recommend the Panic Disorder Severity Scale as the gold standard, and also describe the Anxiety Sensitivity Index and the Agoraphobia Cognitions Questionnaire as additional, adjunctive measures. For social anxiety disorder (also known as social phobia), they recommend the Liebowitz Social Anxiety Scale as the gold standard measure, along with several alternatives. For generalized anxiety disorder (GAD), they suggest the Hamilton Anxiety Scale as the gold-standard measure, and also discuss several alternatives. For obsessive compulsive disorder (OCD), the gold-standard scale is the Yale-Brown Obsessive Compulsive Scale. For post-traumatic stress disorder (PTSD), the gold-standard scale they recommend is the Short PTSD Rating Interview.

In Chapter 4, Dr. Perlis considers rating scales for bipolar disorder. This is one of several chapters in which different scales must be considered for different aspects, or dimensions of a particular disorder, because no single scale exists for a single overall assessment. So, when assessing the depressive symptoms of bipolar disorder, Dr. Perlis considers many of the same instruments as described in Chapter 2 (Depression). However, when considering rating scales for manic or mixed symptoms, he recommends the Young Mania Rating Scale as the gold standard. He goes on to describe instruments used to assess psychotic symptoms in bipolar disorder (the Brief Psychiatric Rating Scale, which is also considered in Chapter 10 on Schizophrenia). Finally, he describes a new, integrated symptom assessment approach developed and used at Massachusetts General Hospital, and he ends by considering diagnostic scales for bipolar disorder.

In Chapter 5, Dr. Yeterian et al. present the main assessment scales used in alcohol and nicotine dependence. They consider both screening scales and outcome rating scales used for these addictive disorders.

In Chapter 6, Dr. Siefert offers several scales used for screening patients for the presence of personality disorders and for dysfunctional interpersonal styles. Personality disorders are often underdetected in clinical practice and can have a negative impact on treatment response. To help address this clinical problem, the focus of Dr. Siefert's chapter is on screening for potential comorbid personality disorders and he outlines a brief but sophisticated screen approach.

In Chapter 7, Dr. Derenne et al. consider the complex area of eating disorders and provide an outstanding review of multiple screening and assessment strategies. In addition to offering practical information on specific screening instruments, the chapter contains links to helpful websites with additional measurement information and materials.

In Chapter 8, Dr. White et al. outline the use of rating scales in clinical work with children. The chapter presents some of the important lessons learned by their group as they implemented a large scale program-wide outcomes measurement program for child mental-health service. The chapter also provides a concise review of a number of potential child outcomes instruments and specific information on using the Brief Psychiatric Rating Scale – Child Version.

In Chapter 9, Drs. Knouse and Safren discuss the use of rating scales in attention-deficit hyperactivity disorder, and include a copy of the Adult ADHD Self-Report Scale. Identifying ADD/ADHD in adults is an increasingly important but still evolving area of practice, the information provided in their chapter will help clinicians approach this condition in a more systematic manner.

In Chapter 10, Dr. Gottlieb et al. consider rating scales used in schizophrenia treatment. Like bipolar disorder, there is an array of scales used to assess the various dimensions of this complex disorder: for assessing the general symptoms of schizophrenia, they recommend the Positive and Negative Syndrome Scale as the gold standard (although they note that specialized training is needed in the use of this scale). For assessing psychotic symptoms in schizophrenia, they recommend the Psychotic Symptom Rating Scale as the gold standard. They also consider scales to assess other important dimensions of schizophrenia, including quality of life, cognitive functioning, attitudes toward taking antipsychotic medication, medication side effects, and assessments for comorbid depression or drug abuse.

In Chapter 11, Dr. Baity considers the use of brief assessments of cognitive and neuropsychological status for patients with a primary psychiatric illness. Cognitive impairment is increasingly being recognized as a significant problem associated with many common (depression and anxiety) as well as severe (psychosis and bipolar illness) psychiatric conditions. Dr. Baity reviews a number of simple but effective instruments capable of identifying moderate cognitive impairment in psychiatric patients.

In Chapter 12, Drs. Owen and Immel discuss the efficient use of rating scales in psychotherapy practice and how to employ these scales in the treatment of individual psychotherapy patients. Through their chapter, Drs. Owen and Immel demonstrate how brief scales can be integrated into the psychotherapy process (frame) and how data from these scales can enhance treatment.

In Chapter 13, Drs. Sinclair and LoCicero discuss assessment of a new problem, worry about terrorism. Relevant to the unfortunate events of our modern age, this chapter presents an overview of a new clinical concept Terrorism Fear, an evolving anxiety related disorder. The chapter also contains a recently developed scale, Terrorism Catastrophizing Scale, designed to measure this fear along with a conceptual approach to treating the condition.

In Chapter 14, Dr. Smith et al. discuss the benefits of comprehensive psychological and neuropsychological assessment as aids to diagnosis and treatment planning. They also offer recommendations for locating assessment psychologists, and how to pose an effective referral question for psychological assessment of your patients.

Finally, in Chapter 15, Drs. Wiechers and Weiss offer an informative overview of the rapidly changing field of quality improvement with a particular emphasis on the role of outcomes measurement in documenting and monitoring treatment quality. The information presented in this chapter will help program managers and practitioners in group practices think more clearly about aggregate outcomes measurement and service evaluation.

References

1. Trivedi, M., Rush, A., Wisniewski, S., et al. Evaluation of outcomes with citalopram for depression using measurement-based care in STAR*D: Implications for clinical practice, Am J Psychiatry, 163:1, 28–40, 2006.
2. Nierenberg, A., Ostacher, M., Borrelli, D., et al. The integration of measurement and management for the treatment of bipolar disorder: A STEP-BD model of collaborative care in psychiatry, J Clin Psychiatry, 67 (suppl 11), 3–6, 2006.
3. Lambert, M. Presidential address: What we have learned from a decade of research aimed at improving psychotherapy outcomes. Psychother Res, 17(1): 1–14, 2007.

                                                                              Lee Baer, PhD
Boston, Massachusetts   Mark Blais, PsyD

Contents

Contributors

Lee Baer, Ph.D. Department of Psychiatry, Massachusetts General Hospital and Harvard Medical School, Boston, MA, USA

Matthew R. Baity, Ph.D. Department of Psychiatry, Massachusetts General Hospital and Harvard Medical School, Boston, MA, 02114, USA, mbaity@partners.org

Christina W. Baker, Ph.D. Department of Psychiatry, Massachusetts General Hospital and Harvard Medical School, Boston, MA, USA

Anne E. Becker, M.D., Ph.D., Sc.M. Department of Psychiatry, Massachusetts General Hospital and Harvard Medical School, Boston, MA, USA

Mark A. Blais, Psy.D. Department of Psychiatry, Massachusetts General Hospital and Harvard Medical School, Boston, MA, USA, mblais@partners.org

Anne Chosak, Ph.D. Department of Psychiatry, Massachusetts General Hospital and Harvard Medical School, Boston, MA 02114, USA

Cristina Cusin, M.D. Department of Psychiatry, Massachusetts General Hospital and Harvard Medical School, Boston, MA 02114, USA, ccusin@partners.org

Sherrie S. Delinsky, Ph.D. Department of Psychiatry, Massachusetts General Hospital and Harvard Medical School, Boston, MA 02114, USA

Jennifer L. Derenne, M.D. Division of Child and Adolescent Psychiatry, Medical College of Wisconsin, Milwaukee, WI, USA

A. Eden Evins, M.D. Department of Psychiatry, Massachusetts General Hospital and Harvard Medical School, Boston, MA 02114, USA

Xiaoduo Fan, M.D. Department of Psychiatry, Massachusetts General Hospital and Harvard Medical School, Boston, MA 02115, USA

Maurizio Fava, M.D. Department of Psychiatry, Massachusetts General Hospital and Harvard Medical School, Boston, MA 02114, USA

Donald C. Goff, M.D. Freedom Trail Clinic, Schizophrenia Program of the Massachusetts General Hospital, Boston, MA 02114, USA, goff@psych.mgh.harvard.edu

Jennifer D. Gottlieb, Ph.D. Department of Psychiatry and Massachusetts General Hospital, Dartmouth Medical School, Concord, NH 03301, USA

Zac Imel University of Wisconsin-Madison, Wisconsin, WI, USA

Michael S. Jellinek, M.D. Department of Psychiatry, Massachusetts General Hospital and Harvard Medical School, Boston, MA 02114, USA; Newton Wellesley Hospital, Newton, MA, USA

John F. Kelly, Ph.D. Department of Psychiatry, Massachusetts General Hospital and Harvard Medical School, Boston, MA 02114, USA, jkelly11@partners.org

Laura E. Knouse, Ph.D. Department of Psychiatry, Massachusetts General Hospital and Harvard Medical School, Boston, MA 02115, USA

Jessica A. Little, Ph.D. Department of Psychiatry, Massachusetts General Hospital and Harvard Medical School, Graduate School of Education, University of California, Santa Barbara, CA, USA, jalittle@partners.org

Alice LoCicero, Ph.D., A.B.P.P., M.B.A. Department of Psychology, Suffolk University, Boston, MA 02114, USA; Center for Multicultural Mental Health, Boston University, Boston, MA, USA

Luana Marques, Ph.D. Department of Psychiatry, Massachusetts General Hospital and Harvard Medical School, Boston, MA 02114, USA

J. Michael Murphy, Ed.D. Department of Psychiatry, Massachusetts General Hospital and Harvard Medical School, Boston, MA 02114, USA, mmurphy6@partners.org

Lisa A. Nowinski, Ph.D. Department of Psychology, University of California, Santa Barbara, CA, USA, lnowinski@partners.org

Jesse Owen, Ph.D. Counseling Psychology Program, Psychology Department, Gannon University, Erie, PA, 16541, USA, owen002@gannon.edu

Gladys Pachas Department of Psychiatry, Massachusetts General Hospital, Boston, MA 02114, USA

Roy H. Perlis, MD, MSc Department of Psychiatry, Massachusetts General Hospital and Harvard Medical School, Boston, MA 02114, USA, rperlis@partners.org

Dieu-My Phan, B.A. Department of Psychiatry, Massachusetts General Hospital and Harvard Medical School, Boston, MA 02114, USA

Mark Pollack, M.D. Department of Psychiatry, Massachusetts General Hospital and Harvard Medical School, Boston, MA 02114, USA

Steven Safren, Ph.D. Department of Psychiatry, Massachusetts General Hospital and Harvard Medical School, Boston, MA 02115, USA, ssafren@partners.org

Caleb J. Siefert, Ph.D. Department of Psychiatry, Massachusetts General Hospital and Harvard Medical School, Boston, MA 02115, USA, csiefert@partners.org

Naomi M. Simon, M.D. Department of Psychiatry, Massachusetts General Hospital and Harvard Medical School, Boston, MA 02114, USA

Samuel J. Sinclair, Ph.D. Department of Psychiatry, Massachusetts General Hospital and Harvard Medical School, Boston, MA 02114, USA; Department of Psychology, Suffolk University, Boston, MA 02114, USA, jsincl@post.harvard.edu

Steven R. Smith, Ph.D. The Gervitz School, Graduate School of Education, University of California, Santa Barbara, CA, USA, ssmith@education.ucsb.edu

Sara J. Walker, Ph.D. Graduate School of Education, University of California, Santa Barbara, CA, USA, swalker@education.ucsb.edu

Anthony Weiss, MD, MSc Department of Psychiatry, Massachusetts General Hospital and Harvard Medical School, Boston, MA 02114, USA, aweiss@partners.org

Gwyne W. White Department of Psychiatry, Massachusetts General Hospital and Harvard Medical School, Boston, MA 02114, USA

Ilse R. Wiechers, MD, MPP Department of Psychiatry, Massachusetts General Hospital and Harvard Medical School, Boston, MA, USA

Sabine Wilhelm, Ph.D. Department of Psychiatry, Massachusetts General Hospital and Harvard Medical School, Boston, MA 02114, USA, wilhelm@psych.mgh.harvard.edu

Huaiyu Yang, M.D. Department of Psychiatry, Massachusetts General Hospital and Harvard Medical School, Boston, MA 02114, USA

Julie D. Yeterian, B.A. Department of Psychiatry, Massachusetts General Hospital, Boston, MA 02114, USA

Albert Yeung, M.D. Department of Psychiatry, Massachusetts General Hospital and Harvard Medical School, Boston, MA 02114, USA

Table of All Rating Scales Contained in This Handbook

Scale name	Short name	Indication	Type of scale	Administration method	Page
Hamilton Depression Rating Scale – 17-item version	*HAMD-17 or HDRS*	Depression	Rating scale	Clinician administered	25
Montgomery Asberg Depression Rating Scale	*MADRS*	Depression	Rating scale	Clinician administered	28
Quick Inventory of Depressive Symptomatology (16-item, self-report version)	*QIDS-SR*	Depression	Rating scale	Self-report	30
Zung Self-Rated Depression Scale	*Zung*	Depression	Rating scale or screening test	Self-report	33
Panic Disorder Severity Scale	PDSS	Anxiety (panic)	Rating scale	Clinician administered	56
Liebowitz Social Anxiety Scale		Anxiety (social anxiety)	Rating scale	Clinician administered	60
Hamilton Anxiety Rating Scale	*HAM-A*	Anxiety	Rating scale	Clinician administered	62
Yale-Brown Obsessive Compulsive Scale	*YBOCS*	Anxiety (OCD)	Rating scale	Either	67
Short PTSD Rating Scale	SPRINT	Anxiety (PTSD)	Rating scale	Clinician administered	72
Hamilton Depression Rating Scale – 31-item version	*HAMD-31*	Depression (Bipolar disorder)	Rating scale	Clinician administered	78
Young Mania Rating Scale	YMRS	Bipolar disorder (Mania)	Rating scale	Clinician administered	82
Internal State Scale	ISS	Bipolar disorder	Rating scale	Self-report	84
Clinical Monitoring Form		Bipolar disorder	Questionnaire	Either	85
Alcohol Use Disorders Identification Test	*AUDIT*	Alcohol	Screening test	Either	108

(continuned)

Scale name	Short name	Indication	Type of scale	Administration method	Page
Questionnaire for Frequency of Alcohol Use		Alcohol	Questionnaire	Either	110
Leeds Dependence Questionnaire	LDQ	Any substance dependence	Rating scale	Self-report	111
Clinical Institute Withdrawal Assessment for Alcohol	CIWA	Alcohol withdrawal	Rating scale	Clinician administered	112
Short Index of Problems	SIP	Alcohol-related consequences	Rating scale	Self-report	114
Assessment of Warning Signs of Relapse Scale	AWARE	Alcohol relapse risk	Rating scale	Self-report	116
Fagerstrom Test for Nicotine Dependence	FTND	Nicotine	Rating scale	Self-report	123
Five Factor Model Rating Form	FFMRF	Personality dimensions	Screening test	Rating scale and screen	140
Inventory of Interpersonal Problems	IIP-PD-25	Personality disorder	Screening test	Clinician administered	141
Standardized Assessment of Personality – Abbreviated Scale	SAPAS	Personality disorder	Screening test	Clinician administered	144
Eating Attitudes Test	EAT	Eating disorders	Screening test	Self-report	171
Body Shape Questionnaire	BSQ	Eating disorders (Body image disturbance)	Rating scale	Self-report	172
Eating Disorders Diagnostic Scale	EDDS	Eating disorders	Screening test	Self-report	174
Brief Psychiatric Clinical Rating Scale for Children	BPRS -C	Children (any disorder)	Rating scale	Clinician administered	192
Adult ADHD Self-Report Scale	ASRS	ADHD	Screening test	Self-report	206
Psychotic Symptoms Rating Scale	PSYRATS	Schizophrenia (Psychotic symptoms)	Rating scale	Clinician administered	222
Quality of Life Scale		Schizophrenia (Quality of life, social functioning)	Rating scale	Clinician administered	225
Abnormal Involuntary Movements Scale	AIMS	Schizophrenia (Medication side effects)	Rating scale	Clinician administered	237
Brief Psychiatric Rating Scale	BPRS	Schizophrenia	Rating scale	Clinician administered	238

(continued)

Scale name	Short name	Indication	Type of scale	Administration method	Page
Draw a Clock Test	*DCT*	Cognitive functioning	Rating scale	Clinician administered	250
Trail Making Test	*TMT*	Cognitive functioning	Rating scale	Clinician administered	252
Schwartz Outcome Scale	*SOS-10*	Psychotherapy practice (Quality of life & psychological well-being)	Rating scale	Self-report	268
Outcome Rating Scale	ORS	Psychotherapy practice	Rating scale	Self-report	269
Session Rating Scale (Version 3.0)	*SRS v3.0*	Psychotherapy practice	Rating scale	Self-report	270
Terrorism Catastrophizing Scale	TCS	Fear of terrorism	Rating scale	Self-report	285

Chapter 1
Understanding Rating Scales and Assessment Instruments

Mark Blais and Lee Baer

Abstract The successful integration of screening tests and brief rating scales into clinical practice requires an adequate understanding of a few basic psychometric and statistical concepts. This chapter provides an overview of such concepts as reliability, validity, diagnostic accuracy and sensitivity to change. In addition we attempt to demonstrate how these concepts relate to clinical care. We believe that a solid understanding of these concepts will increase the utility and benefit patients and clinicians obtain through the integration of brief measurement tools into their practice.

Keywords Rating scales · Questionnaires · Psychometrics · Assessment · Psychiatry

It is only in the past 60 years that measurement has become a routine part of healthcare practice and research. In psychiatry and psychology, many of the characteristics we are most interested in, such as quality of life, depression, anxiety, or personality style, are not physical entities like body weight or heart rate. Rather they are subjective experiences or theoretical constructs that cannot be directly measured, but are instead inferred from observable patterns of behavior, such as responses to a rating scale. Self-report instruments and clinician-administered rating scales can aid clinicians in identifying, quantifying, and tracking change in these important but not directly observable variables. The overarching goal of this handbook is to provide you, as a mental health clinician, with the knowledge and tools necessary to integrate measurement into your ongoing clinical practice.

M. Blais (✉)
Department of Psychiatry, Massachusetts General Hospital and Harvard Medical School, Boston, MA, USA
e-mail: mblais@partners.org

L. Baer, M.A. Blais (eds.), *Handbook of Clinical Rating Scales and Assessment in Psychiatry and Mental Health*, Current Clinical Psychiatry, DOI 10.1007/978-1-59745-387-5_1,
© Humana Press, a part of Springer Science+Business Media, LLC 2010

Types of Rating Scales Presented in This Handbook

Measurement tools can take many different forms and serve a variety of important functions. The following chapters focus primarily on two types of measurement instruments: screening tests and symptom- or disorder-specific rating scales. See the table in the front of this handbook (page xix) for a listing of all rating scales reproduced in this handbook; the fourth column of this table describes what type of rating scale each represents.

Screening tests are assessment tools designed to identify the presence or absence of a target disorder (such as ADHD or OCD) or condition (such as personality disorder or cognitive impairment). Clinicians typically administer screening tests to rule out the presence of important co-morbid conditions, such as alcohol abuse in patients with attention deficit disorder, at the initiation of care. Thus, screening tests are similar to diagnostic instruments like structured diagnostic interviews (such as the SCID), but are briefer and typically less precise.

Symptom- or disorder-specific rating scales are designed to quantify the severity of a disorder after the presence of the disorder has been established (quantifying the severity of depressive symptoms for patients treated in a depression clinic). Symptom or disorder rating scales can be administered at anytime during treatment to help quantify the severity of the disorder. Information provided by these scales can inform treatment planning (such as helping establish the appropriate level of care or frequency of sessions) and monitor patients' progress over the course of treatment. Both types of scales can be either patient rated (self-report) or clinician rated (clinician-administered).

Basic Statistical Concepts

The branch of statistics known as psychometrics is concerned with the scientific properties of measurement instruments, such as those described in the following chapters. Some of the questions addressed by psychometrics are as follows: (1) how reproducible is our patients' score on a particular rating scale (reliability), (2) how well is the rating scale measuring the intended construct (construct validity and dimensionality), and (3) how useful is the scale for tracking a patient's progress across the course of treatment (sensitivity to change). Questionnaires that are simply for information gathering and whose responses are not combined into a total score are generally not assessed using psychometric methods (these instruments are noted as "Questionnaire" in the fourth column of the Table of Rating Scales on p. xix).

Reliability and validity are generally presented in the form of a correlation coefficient with absolute values ranging from 0.00 to 1.00. A coefficient of 0.00 represents no reliability (or validity), while a coefficient of 1.00 indicates perfect reliability (or validity). But measurement is never perfect. Anytime we measure a characteristic of a person or object, the value we obtain contains some degree of error.

Reliability

Reliability statistics provide a means for quantifying this degree of error contained in our measurement and indicating the consistency and stability of the score. Reliability is a necessary, but not a sufficient, quality of useful rating scales. The more reliable an instrument is, the more consistent a patient's score will be over time or across different raters (in the case of self-report scales and clinician-administered scales, respectively, as shown in Table 1.1). Important reliability concepts include internal consistency, test–retest reliability, and inter-rater agreement.

Table 1.1 Psychometric considerations for various types of rating scales

	Types of scale			
	Screening		Rating scale	
	Self-report	Clinician-administered	Self-report	Clinician-administered
Reliability[a]				
Test–retest	X		X	
Inter-rater		X		X
Internal consistency	X	X	X	X
Validity[b]				
Sensitivity	X	X		
Specificity	X	X		
Positive predictive value	X	X		
Convergent validity			X	X
Divergent validity			X	X
Face validity	X	X	X	X

[a]Test–retest and inter-rater reliabilities assess the average reproducibility of a score on a particular scale, over time and with different raters, respectively. Internal consistency reliability assesses the degree to which a particular scale is measuring a single concept (such as depression or reading ability).

[b]Validity statistics assess the usefulness of a scale for a particular purpose. Sensitivity and specificity are related to the rates of false negatives and false positives, respectively, for a given screening or diagnostic test. Positive predictive value is related to the meaning of a positive test, given the base rate of the particular disorder. Convergent and divergent validity is the degree to which a scale is more closely related (correlated) to scales measuring the same construct than it is to scales measuring different or unrelated constructs. Face validity is not assessed statistically, but refers to the degree to which a test seems to the test-taker to be measuring what it is intended to measure.

Internal Consistency

Internal consistency reflects the degree to which items in a scale measure a single property or dimension. Typically, instruments that are used clinically should have internal consistency coefficients (often expressed as "Coefficient Alpha") of 0.80 or higher (often closer to 0.90). Scale length affects measures of internal consistency, so that briefer scales (10 items or less) often have lower internal consistency coefficients simply due to having fewer items.

Test–Retest Reliability

Test–retest reliability reflects the stability of scores over repeated testings (across time) and is often slightly lower than internal consistency (stability coefficients between 0.75 and 0.85 would be considered acceptable). Knowing the test–retest time period is important when assessing a stability coefficient. A time interval of 2–3 weeks may be adequate for a test of depression (a state condition), while an interval of a few months would be appropriate for a measure of narcissistic personality (a trait condition).

Inter-rater Reliability

For clinician-rated scales it is important to know the extent to which different clinicians agree when assigning ratings; this is referred to as inter-rater agreement. Inter-rater agreement is typically reported as either a Kappa coefficient (for outcomes with two or three categories) or an intra-class correlation coefficient (for continuous outcomes). Kappa coefficients are often weighted to correct for chance agreement (i.e., given as "weighted Kappa"). Although there are no firm rules for interpreting Kappa values, Kappa coefficients ≤ 0.40 are usually considered "poor," values between 0.60 and 0.70 are considered "good," and coefficients > 0.70 are considered "excellent." Kappa values can be affected by (1) the number of choices raters are required to make (e.g., "present or absent" versus "mild, moderate, or severe") or (2) the base rate (prevalence) of the target condition.

Validity

Validity is a more complicated topic than reliability. Validity refers to the degree of correspondence between a test score and the construct (e.g., "hopelessness") or diagnosis (e.g., "panic disorder") that it was designed to measure. The absence of true gold standards for measuring psychiatric condition makes assessing validity even more difficult in our field. It may be best to think of validity as indicating the accuracy of a score. Basic forms of validity include content validity, criterion validity, and construct validity.

Content Validity

Content validity refers to the extent to which a scale adequately covers the important features of a condition or construct. For example an anxiety scale that did not contain a "worry" item may have questionable content validity. Evaluations of content validity tend to be rational and not empirically based.

Criterion Validity

Criterion validity is measured by a correlation coefficient (like a reliability coefficient) showing the correspondence between the test score and known or accepted markers of the target condition (for a new depression scale this might include scores on an existing measure of depression or receiving an independent diagnosis of major depressive disorder).

Construct Validity

Construct validity represents the most comprehensive and complex assessment of score validity. Construct validity is the accumulated weight of evidence indicating that a measurement tool (1) adequately covers the full range of the target construct, (2) does so across a variety of clinical situations (inpatient and outpatient settings), and (3) does so across a wide range of subjects (e.g., young adults as well as older adults). There is no single measure of construct validity.

Diagnostic Accuracy

Statistics assessing diagnostic accuracy are useful for evaluating tests that are designed to screen for (predict) DSM-IV disorders. Chief among these statistics are sensitivity and specificity. These are often thought of as additional types of validity measures.

Sensitivity and Specificity

Sensitivity is the probability (ranging from 0.00 to 1.00) that a subject who screens positive actually has the condition. *Specificity* is the probability that a subject who screened negative does not have the condition. For example, using a depression screening test with sensitivity of .80, you would expect that 8 out of 10 subjects who are actually depressed would score positive on the screening test; if the specificity of the same test were .70, you would expect that 7 out of 10 subjects who are not actually depressed would score negative on the screening test. The appropriate balance of sensitivity and specificity for a given screening test depends in part on the base rate of the condition to be detected. If the base rate is high, then the specificity should be high, while if the base rate is low, then the sensitivity should be increased. A caveat: although diagnostic accuracy statistics provide helpful information, they require a presumed standard (typically a structured interview diagnosis) against which to judge the screening test.

Sensitivity to Treatment-Induced Change

Sensitivity to treatment-induced change is an important quality for any scale that is used to track clinical outcomes. Sensitivity to change is the degree to which a baseline score on a rating scale changes (for better or worse) as a result of active treatment. Scales that are valid for the purpose of identifying a condition like fear of panic attack are not all equal in their ability to track changes in the condition. Sensitivity to change is often expressed as a treatment effect size (ES, which reflects the mean pre-post change score of a group of treated patients, expressed in standard deviation units). The most common ES measure is Cohen's *d*. A Cohen's *d* of 0.40 higher is generally considered an adequate indication of a scale's sensitivity to change (interpreting Cohen's *d*: 0.00–0.19 as "no effect," 0.20–0.39 as "a small effect," 0.40–0.69 as "a medium effect," and 0.70 and higher as "a large effect").

Table 1.1 summarizes how these psychometric concerns relate to the types of rating scales contained in this handbook. Keep these points in mind to assess how useful a particular scale is for your purpose. Remember, reliability is a necessary but not sufficient characteristic of your particular rating scale. The scale must also be valid for the particular purpose for which you are using it.

Summary

You do not need to become an expert in psychometrics to effectively use the rating scales described in this handbook. However, developing a basic understanding of reliability, validity, and a few other key psychometric concepts will help you to recognize the strengths and limitations of the scales that you choose for use with your patients.

Chapter 2
Rating Scales for Depression

**Cristina Cusin, Huaiyu Yang, Albert Yeung,
and Maurizio Fava**

Abstract Over the past few decades, a number of clinician-rated and patient-rated instruments have been developed as primary efficacy measures in depression clinical trials. All those scales have relative strengths and weaknesses and some of them have been more successful than others, and have become the gold standards for depression clinical research. With all these measures available and with the evidence of their variable performance in clinical trials, it is becoming increasingly important to select primary efficacy measures that are reliable, valid, and that fit well within the aims of depression clinical trials. This article will review the main considerations that investigators need to make when choosing a primary efficacy measure for major depressive disorder (MDD). There is a clear need for a thorough discussion of the methodological issues concerning the use of these scales, as suggested also by Demyttenaere and De Fruyt in a recent review [1], because clinical trials researchers in depression continue to struggle with the ability to detect signals of the efficacy of antidepressant agents.

Keywords Depression · Rating scales · Questionnaires · Assessment · Mood · Psychiatry

Gold Standard Rating Scales

- The Hamilton Rating Scale for Depression (HAM-D or HRSD) [2] (clinician-administered)
- The Beck Depression Inventory (BDI) [27] (patient-rated)
- Inventory of Depressive Symptomatology (IDS or QIDS) [35] (patient-rated or clinician administered)

C. Cusin (✉)
Department of Psychiatry, Massachusetts General Hospital and Harvard Medical School, Wang Ambulatory Care Center 812, 15 Parkman Street, Boston, MA 02114, USA
e-mail: ccusin@partners.org

L. Baer, M.A. Blais (eds.), *Handbook of Clinical Rating Scales and Assessment in Psychiatry and Mental Health*, Current Clinical Psychiatry, DOI 10.1007/978-1-59745-387-5_2,
© Humana Press, a part of Springer Science+Business Media, LLC 2010

Hamilton Rating Scale for Depression (HAM-D or HRSD)

This is one of the earliest scales to be developed for depression, and is a clinician-rated scale aimed at assessing depression severity among patients. The original HAM-D included 21 items, but Hamilton pointed out that the last four items (diurnal variation, depersonalization/derealization, paranoid symptoms, and obsessive-compulsive symptoms) should not be counted toward the total score because these symptoms are either uncommon or do not reflect depression severity [2].

Therefore, the 17-item version of the HAM-D (reproduced in the appendix to this chapter) has become the standard for clinical trials and, over the years, the most widely used scale for controlled clinical trials in depression (we found in a recent Medline search that more than 500 studies have used the HAM-D as primary efficacy measure). Its widespread use, however, has not prevented investigators from recognizing the limitations of this instrument and from trying to improve it. The main limitations of the original 17-item version of the HAM-D were recognized to be (1) the failure to include all symptom domains of major depressive disorder (MDD), in particular, reverse neurovegetative symptoms, (2) the presence of items measuring different constructs (e.g., irritability and anxiety, loss of interest and hopelessness), and (3) the uneven weight attributed to different symptom domains (e.g., insomnia may be rated up to 6 points, while fatigue only up to 2).

Application of Scale

Method of Administration

The scale is widely used in clinical trials and in clinical practice, and in general is administered weekly. To improve inter-rater reliability, a structured interview guide for the HAM-D was developed in 1988 by Janet Williams (SIGH-D) [3, 4] and her guide soon became the gold standard for training and for clinical studies (see for example: http://www.ids-qids.org/translations/english/SIGHD-IDSCEnglish-USA.pdf.). We recommend using the interview guide to improve inter-rater reliability.

Timing of Administration

Considering the busy schedule of both patients and health professionals, the time needed to administer a scale could represent a significant burden. Our research has found that the average duration of the HAM-D interviews was 12 minutes. However, our estimations of the length of those interviews are underestimates and features of depression such as psychomotor retardation may significantly increase their duration. It is noteworthy that in our simulation, using a structured interview did not seem to considerably increase the duration of the administration of the scale.

Because of its widespread use over the course of decades, the HAM-D is the most popular depression severity measure in the history of MDD trials, and is very familiar to most clinical researchers in the area of depression.

Reliability and Internal Consistency

The HAM-D is a multidimensional scale, and this implies that the score of a specific item cannot be considered a good predictor of the total score [5]. It also means that identical total scores from two different patients may have different clinical meanings (i.e., a very high rating on few items can yield the same score as a moderate rating on many items) [6]. A number of studies have shown the internal consistency of different versions of HAM-D to range widely from 0.48 to 0.92. Higher coefficient alpha values were reached with the use of a structured interview (see [7] for more details). A recent study reported internal consistency coefficients of 0.83 for HAM-D-17 and 0.88 for HAM-D-24 [8]. A complete review of the psychometric properties of the HAM-D has been published recently. In this paper, the authors reviewed 70 studies on psychometric properties of the HAM-D, published since 1979, and showed that the majority of HAM-D items have adequate reliability [9].

Inter-rater Reliability

Inter-rater reliability has been reported to be very high for HAM-D total scores (0.80–0.98), even if it is poor for some of its items. All items showed adequate reliability when the scale was administered with interview guidelines [10]. A sufficiently high inter-rater reliability (>0.60) was reported for most of the HAM-D items and the total score (0.57–0.73) in a study on inter-rater reliability in 21 psychiatric novices who had negligible previous experience with the HAM-D [11]. This score appears to be improved greatly with the use of appropriate training and structured interview [12].

Test–Retest Reliability

Test–retest reliability for the HAM-D using the Structured Interview Guide has been reported to be as high as 0.81, even among minimally trained raters from multiple disciplines [4, 13, 14].

Validity

Validity of the HAM-D has been reported to range from 0.65 to 0.90 with global measures of depression severity, and to be highly correlated with clinician-rated measures such as MADRS and IDS-C [7].

Scoring Key

The total score is obtained by summing the score of each item, 0–4 (symptom is absent, mild, moderate, or severe) or 0–2 (absent, slight or trivial, clearly present). For the 17-item version, scores can range from 0 to 54.

Cut-Off Scores

It is accepted by most clinicians that scores between 0 and 6 do not indicate the presence of depression, scores between 7 and 17 indicate mild depression, scores between 18 and 24 indicate moderate depression, and scores over 24 indicate severe depression. A total HAM-D score of 7 or less after treatment is for most raters a typical indicator of remission [15]. A decrease of 50% or more from baseline during the course of the treatment is considered indicator of clinical response, or in other words, a clinically significant change.

Beck Depression Inventory (BDI)

The gold standard of self-rating scales is the Beck Depression Inventory (BDI) [16], which was initially developed to assess the efficacy of psycho-analytically oriented psychotherapy in depressed subjects. The BDI is copy-righted by Harcourt Assessment, Inc., and so is not reproduced in this chapter. Information about purchase of this scale and manual are available from their website at: http://harcourtassessment.com/haiweb/cultures/en-us/productdetail. htm?pid=015-8018-370.

This scale was designed to measure the severity of depressive symptoms that the test taker is experiencing "at that moment." The original BDI included 21 items concerning different symptom domains, with four possible answers describing symptoms of increasing severity associated with a score from 0 to 3. It was later amended to BDI-IA [17], and after the publication of the DSM-IV, to the BDI-second edition (BDI-II) [18]. Four new items (agitation, worthlessness, concentration difficulty, and loss of energy) were added to make the BDI-II more reflective of DSM-IV criteria of MDD, and some BDI-IA items (i.e., weight loss, body image change, work difficulty, and somatic preoccupation) were eliminated because they were considered less indicative of the overall severity of depression. Beck and colleagues also rewrote almost all other BDI-II items for clarity, and the time frame for ratings was extended from 1 to 2 weeks [19, 20].

Self-rating scales, such as the BDI, offer some advantages over clinician-rated scales, as they may take less time, do not require trained personnel, and their administration and scoring process appear more standardized [21]. Self-rating scales also require that individuals are able to read at a minimal reading level, and that they speak the language used in at least one translation of the scale.

Reliability and Validity

Reliability

Internal Consistency

Beck and colleagues in 1988 published a meta-analysis of all the psychometric studies on the BDI from 1961 to June 1986 and found a mean coefficient alpha of 0.86 for psychiatric subjects [22]. In 1996, after the publication of the BDI-II, Beck and coworkers compared the BDI-II and BDI-IA scales in a sample of 140 psychiatric outpatients with various psychiatric disorders and found coefficient alpha for the BDI-II and the BDI-IA of 0.91 and 0.89, respectively [19]. The BDI and the BDI-II were also tested on a larger sample ($n = 500$), where the BDI-II showed improved clinical sensitivity, with reliability (alpha = 0.92) higher than the BDI (alpha=0.86) (Psychological Corporation Website, 2003).

Test–Retest Reliability

With self-administered measures, assessing test–retest reliability may be complicated by the fact that the correlation coefficient may increase spuriously because of practice or because of memory effects. However, in a Spanish study, test–retest reliability for the BDI was between 0.65 and 0.72 [23].

Validity

The convergent validity with the BDI has been reported to be extremely variable, ranging between 0.27 and 0.89 [24]. Beck and colleagues showed that in psychiatric patients, the mean correlations of the BDI were 0.72 with clinical ratings and 0.73 with the HAM-D [22] and 0.57–0.83 with the Zung SDS [25].

Inventory of Depressive Symptomatology

In the 1980s, John Rush and colleagues [35] developed and published the clinician-rated Inventory of Depressive Symptomatology (IDS) (reproduced in the appendix to this chapter), which was intended to "remedy the deficits of the HAM-D and the MADRS" by including all the symptom domains of the DSM-based MDD, as well as both melancholic and atypical (e.g., reversed neurovegetative) features, by scaling each item to allow for the measurement of milder forms of MDD, providing clearer items definition (for example, irritability and anxiety were rated separately) and equivalent weight for each symptom domain. The original IDS had 28 items [35], while an additional two items (leaden paralysis; interpersonal rejection sensitivity) were added later to better capture atypical MDD features [36]. Subsequently, Rush and colleagues selected 16 items from the IDS-30, assessing the DSM-IV diagnostic criteria for MDD, and assembled them in the short version of the IDS, namely the Quick Inventory of Depressive Symptomatology (QIDS) [8]. Dr. Rush and Colleagues created a self-rated version of the 28-item IDS-C in the 1980s, called the IDS-SR-28 [35, 37], then added the two items of atypical MDD features to obtain the 30-item version [36], and shortened it to the 16 items of the DSM-IV diagnostic criteria for the QIDS-SR [8] (reproduced in the appendix to this chapter).

Scoring Key

For all the versions, add the scores of the items to obtain the total score, except for items 11–12 (increased or decreased appetite) and 13–14 (increased or decreased weight) for which the highest of the two has to be included. A description of cut-offs for moderate and severe depression for the different versions is available at the website http://www.ids-qids.org/index2.html#table2.

Reliability

Internal Consistency

Internal consistency of the IDS is high. In a study published in 1999 on 68 patients assessed at admission, after 5, 10, and 28 days of antidepressant treatment, the Cronbach's alpha coefficients reported were 0.75 for the IDS-C and 0.79 for the IDS-SR [38]. Alpha values were reported to vary from 0.67 to 0.82 for subjects with current depression in a very large sample [36]. In another study on 544 outpatients with MDD and 402 outpatients with bipolar disorder, the Cronbach's alpha ranged from 0.81 to 0.94 for all four scales (QIDS-C16, QIDS-SR16, IDS-C30, and IDS-SR30) [39]. Cronbach's alpha ranged from 0.81 to 0.90 for the QIDS-C and was reported to be 0.86 for the QIDS-SR (http://www.ids-qids.org/IDS_Website_Document.pdf).

Inter-rater Reliability

Inter-rater reliability for the IDS-C was reported to be very high (0.96). (http://www.ids-qids.org/IDS_Website_Document.pdf).

Validity

IDS-SR correlation with the HAM-D-24 and BDI have been investigated in a sample of 289 patients with mixed diagnoses and reported to be respectively 0.67 and 0.78, while the IDS-C was highly correlated with the HAM-D ($r = 0.92$) and less with the BDI ($r = 0.61$) in a sample of 82 outpatients [35]. In another very large sample ($n = 596$) of patients treated for chronic non-psychotic MDD, the QIDS-SR total scores were highly correlated with IDS-SR-30 (0.96) and with the HAM-D-24 (0.86) total scores [8]. The QIDS-C and QIDS-SR scores have been reported to be correlated (0.72 or more) with those of the HAM-D-17 (http://www.ids-qids.org/IDS_Website_Document.pdf) and HAM-D-24 [40].

Other Scales Available for Rating Depression

Montgomery–Asberg Depression Rating Scale

The clinician-rated Montgomery and Asberg Depression Rating Scale (MADRS) [reproduced in the Appendix to this chapter] was developed in the late 1970s [26] and this 10-item scale was designed to be sensitive to the effects of antidepressant medications, primarily tricyclic antidepressants (TCAs) [26]. Because this scale was never updated or modified, it does not target reverse neurovegetative symptoms. It is commonly used in clinical studies and in clinical practice, administered weekly. Structured interview guides for the MADRS have been developed by a number of investigators [13, 27–29].

Reliability

Internal Consistency

The MADRS appears to be a unidimensional scale, more focused toward psychological, as opposed to somatic aspects of depression [30]. The internal consistency of the MADRS is considered very high, given the high correlation between all items ($r = 0.95$) [31]. In a recent psychometric re-analysis of primary efficacy measures derived from a trial on citalopram efficacy in maintenance therapy of elderly depressed patients, the internal consistency of the MADRS, was found to be superior to that of the HAM-D-17 [6].

Inter-rater Reliability

One of the original goals of the MADRS was to obtain an instrument that could be used by both psychiatrists and professionals without a specific or with minimal psychiatric training. From the original report of the MADRS, the inter-rater reliability ranged from 0.89 to 0.97 [26]. However, in a German study, significant differences resulted when the same patient was rated by various groups of caregivers (psychiatrists, psychologists, students, and psychiatric nurses) [32].

Validity

Correlation of MADRS has been shown to be generally high or very high with the HAM-D (between 0.80 and 0.90) [7, 33], RDC (0.70) [34], and with IDS-C (0.81) [34].

Cut-Off Scores

A score greater than 30 or 35 on the MADRS indicates severe depression, while a score of 10 or below indicates remission.

Zung Self-Report Depression Scale

The Zung Self-Report Depression Scale (Zung SDS) [41] (reproduced in the appendix to this chapter) was published a few years later than the BDI. It is a 20-item self-report index that covers, in varying degree, a broader spectrum of symptoms than the BDI, including psychological, affective, cognitive, behavioral, and somatic aspects of depression.

Scoring Key

Respondents are instructed to rate each item on a scale ranging from 0 to 4 in terms of "how frequently" they have experienced each symptom, instead of "how severe." The time frame was originally "at the present," but in subsequent version the time frame was extended to one week, therefore recommending weekly administration. A total score is derived by summing the individual item scores (1–4), and ranges from 20 to 80. The items are scored as follows: 1 = a little of the time, through 4 = most of the time, *except* for items 2, 5, 6, 11, 12, 14, 16, 17, 18, and 20 which are scored inversely (4 = a little of the time).

Cut-Off Scores

Most people with depression score between 50 and 69, while a score of 70 and above indicates severe depression. No revision of the scale was made after the original publication and is nowadays less used in clinical practice.

Validity

The correlation between Zung SDS and HAM-D was reported to range between 0.68 and 0.76, being lower with HAM-D at baseline [21]. The best results were observed at mild or moderate severity levels, while the greatest disagreement between Zung and HAM-D was observed for patients with non-endogenous symptom patterns [42].

Other Issues in Assessing Depression

Ability of Depression Rating Scales to Detect Clinical Changes with Treatment

The ability of psychometric instruments to detect changes related to treatment is a concept that has been extensively discussed by Robert Kellner [43]. In his review of the literature, he indicated the importance for a measure of capturing changes over time, particularly in those symptoms characterizing MDD [43]. As Kellner stated, a scale may be valid but have low sensitivity to detect change in the state of the patient. For example, a scale may contain items relatively insensitive to change and therefore may be highly stable and underestimate the effects of a treatment. The BDI measures attitudes and cognitions which are fairly stable over time among depressed patients, and therefore may underestimate the degree of improvement during acute pharmacological treatments. In addition, a scale might have items accurately measuring mild depression, but may be less sensitive to moderate or severe depression, leading to a poor sensitivity to detect improvements in patients with more severe depression at baseline. The scales actually used in clinical trials typically are considered to have a relatively good sensitivity to change, with the exception of the Zung scale, which is considered more sensitive to differences across subgroups of patients, than to change over time [44].

Minimizing Biases in the Assessment of Depression Symptom Domains

A possible bias in measurement of depressive symptoms may be related to the variable emphasis on somatic versus psychological symptoms. For example, since 3 of the 17 items of the HAM-D concern sleep disturbances (insomnia) and contribute up to 11.5% of the total score, it has been hypothesized that the HAM-D may favor sedating antidepressant drugs (i.e., some TCAs or trazodone), which may improve sleep, regardless of "true" antidepressant effects. Similarly, drugs associated with side effects such as sleep disturbances, gastrointestinal (GI) symptoms, agitation, and nervousness, such as the SSRIs and the SNRIs, could be associated with an artificially elevated HAM-D score at endpoint, thereby underestimating improvement.

When considering somatic symptoms, the convention is often that such symptoms should be rated at face value, without trying to distinguish side effects from symptoms. This approach may affect all measures of depression severity, as sleep and appetite disturbances may be side effects and/or symptoms of MDD. However, in the case of the HAM-D, psychological, and somatic symptoms/side effects such as anxiety/agitation, sexual dysfunction, dry mouth, and diarrhea may be affecting the score to a greater degree than other scales [45]. The BDI, MADRS, HAM-D-6, IDS, and QIDS are considered to be relatively insensitive to this well-known bias of the HAM-D [46].

Ability of Depression Rating Scales to Measure Symptoms Across Depressive Subtypes

Since major depressive disorder is not a homogeneous clinical entity, a valid scale must measure symptoms across all subtypes, allowing clinicians to compare treatment efficacy in various depressive populations. In fact, inaccurate assessments across subtypes have been hypothesized to be one of the culprits for the high failure rate of many MDD clinical trials [46, 47]. Due to the differences in historical background and rationale behind each rating scale, the HAM-D, the MADRS, and the IDS/QIDS have different levels of ability to reflect the heterogeneity of MDD and to capture symptoms characteristic of depressive subtypes. The HAM-D-28, the IDS, and the BDI-II cover symptoms of both atypical and melancholic depression, while atypical symptoms are far less relevant in the BDI and the Zung scale, where they represent only 5% of the total score, and in the MADRS where these symptoms are not included at all.

Self- Versus Clinician-Administered Depression Rating Scales

The dilemma between self-administered and clinician-rated scales has led to a number of studies investigating differences and similarities between those two ways of assessing depressive symptoms. Although concordance rates between self ratings and observer ratings are generally acceptable, significantly discordant ratings have been obtained in many studies showing that clinicians and patients rate the depressive symptoms differently [48–50]. Clinicians are thought to measure depressive severity more accurately [37, 51]. In fact, in a study of the two versions of IDS (IDS-C and IDS-SR), where these two scales were administered to 64 inpatients with MDD on day 1, 10, and day 28 after antidepressant treatment, the self-rated version of IDS showed a lesser sensitivity to change over time compared to the clinician-rated version [38]. On the other hand, self-rated scales may be more sensitive to detect changes than clinician-rated scales in milder forms of depression. In fact, a study compared the scores from three different scales, HAM-D, IDS-C, and IDS-SR, across severity subgroups in patients with dysthymic depression, non-endogenous MDD, and endogenous MDD. More symptoms were self-reported by the dysthymic patients and the non-endogenous patients than recorded by the clinician, but for the endogenously depressed patients self-reported and clinician-rated symptoms were comparable [37]. Similarly, a study published in 2000 showed that the discrepancies between BDI and HAM-D-21 scores were increased in patients with younger age, higher educational level, atypical depressive subtype, and neurotic personality features, all those factors being associated with higher BDI scores [52]. Sayer et al. [53] investigated the correlation between the HAM-D-24 and the BDI in 114 severely depressed inpatients, treated with electroconvulsive therapy. Their study showed a relatively poor correlation between the instruments at baseline, due to a specific subgroup of depressive patients who were evaluated by the observer as severely depressed, but rated themselves as less symptomatic. Some clinical features of the subgroup were advanced age, less education, presence of psychosis, lack of insight, and severe hypochondriasis. This same subgroup showed the greatest improvement in HAM-D score and contributed largely to the discrepancy in effect size between HDRS and BDI ratings.

When the effect sizes (calculated as the difference between the proportions of responders taking drug and those taking placebo) derived from patient self-ratings and from clinician ratings were compared by Petkova and colleagues, the result was that the self-rating scales were associated with smaller effect sizes, therefore supporting the hypothesis that they are less likely to differentiate active drug from placebo [54]. However, the self-rating scales in the Petkova study did not include scales, such as the IDS-SR or QIDS-SR, which are reported to show more robust performance in clinical trials compared to the older self-rating scales.

In clinical practice, different clinicians choose what scale to administer according to their level of comfort with a scale and to the time available. Some choose to present self-rating scales (most often used are the BDI, IDS-SR or QIDS-SR) to patients in the waiting room and have them fill out the questionnaires. Other clinicians prefer asking patients directly about symptoms and administer the scale themselves during the visit (HAM-D, MADRS or IDS-C), in particular with complicated patients or patients with comorbidities for which answers about physical symptoms may need clarification. The clinician should be aware of strengths and limitations of at least few of the most commonly used scales, and should be able to choose the most appropriate instrument for the patient.

Assessing Depression Across Age Groups

Depression is very common among elderly patients, whose depressive psychopathology has been shown to be different in some aspects from younger individuals, i.e., increased prevalence of sleep disturbances and hypochondriasis [55]. Elderly depressed are more likely to be affected by medical conditions that complicate their evaluation and their treatment. For example, the presence of somatic symptoms due to concomitant medical illnesses may be misattributed to the depression or vice versa [56]. Linden et al. [57] reported that in depressed patients who were 70 years or older and also suffered from a medical illness, eight items of the HAM-D may be elevated by the concurrent somatic disorder (somatic anxiety, GI symptoms, general somatic symptoms, hypochondriasis, weight loss, middle insomnia, and work). In other cases, older patients with clinically significant depression may underreport their symptoms [58]. In addition, the presence of cognitive symptoms may impair the evaluation of depression, as they might be related to natural cognitive functioning decline, to the onset of dementing disorders, or to depression itself. Nebes et al. [59] measured the working memory, information-processing speed, episodic memory, and attention over a 12-week randomized, double-blind trial with nortriptyline and paroxetine. Compared to the elderly controls, cognitive dysfunction persisted in older depressed patients, even after their depression had responded to antidepressant medications. Cognitive symptoms may affect patients' ability to understand and/or respond appropriately to questions about their depressive symptoms. Finally, items assessing thoughts of death, pessimism, and reduced interest or activity may have a different meaning in a geriatric population compared to younger adults. Scales have been developed with the specific purpose of screening for MDD in the geriatric population, of which the gold standard is the Geriatric Depression Scale (GDS), a self-report scale with different versions containing 30, 15, and 4 items [60, 61]. Other scales are the Brief Assessment Schedule Depression Cards (BASDEC), the Cornell Scale for Depression in Dementia and the Geriatric Mental State Schedule (GMSS) (for a review see [62]). Despite the differences in symptoms between geriatric and adult patients with MDD, the primary outcome measures used for the antidepressant trials in the elderly (age $\geq$ 65 years) are still the scales developed in the adult population such as the HAM-D, the BDI and the MADRS [63–66]. However, further studies are necessary to compare the performance of different scales in this specific population.

Similarly, depressive symptoms may be different in children and adolescents from those of adults, challenging the use in children of scales aimed to assess depression among adults. In addition, scales used for adults often use anchor points that are best suited to capture symptoms in adult populations, and may be less useful for children and adolescents. Furthermore, as Poznanski pointed out, the measure of the non-verbal behavior for children and adolescents was most strongly associated with the diagnosis of depression and was also the best predictor of the severity of depression [67]. Many authors have tried to develop instruments to measure depression in children and adolescents. The Children's Depression Rating Scale (CDRS) and its revised version (CDRS-R) are clinician-rated instruments to measure severity of depression in children [67, 68]. The CDRS has been validated for use in children and adolescents [68] and has been used as a primary outcome measure in clinical trials [70, 71].

Self-rated scales are also commonly used in children and adolescents, such as the Kutcher Adolescent Depression Scale (KADS), the Children's Depression Inventory (CDI) [72], the Child Depression Scale [73–75], and the Beck Youth Inventories of Emotional and Social Impairment [76]. Brooks et al. suggested that the 11-item KADS is a sensitive measure of treatment outcome in adolescents diagnosed with MDD [77].

Assessing Depression Across Different Cultures

Cross-cultural variations in presenting symptoms of depression have been reported [78]. For example, certain symptoms, such as self-blame and guilt, are not common to all cultures [79, 80]. In addition, differences have been observed in the severity of decision-making impairments in depression across cultures [81]. Researchers from our group have also observed higher rates of suicidal ideation among Asian-Americans (24%), participants who report ethnic heritage as "Other" (19.5%) Caucasians (16.9%), and Asian-Indians (14%), compared to Hispanics (7.3%) and African-Americans (6%) in a sample of 707 college students [82]. Psychotic symptoms have also been found to be more prevalent in Hispanic patients with MDD seeking treatment, compared to Caucasians and Portuguese patients, but not when compared to African-American [83].

The most striking and consistent finding of cross-cultural studies on depression is the variation in the somatization domain. After screening approximately 26,000 patients for MDD at 15 primary care centers in 14 countries and 5 continents, Simon and colleagues found that the prevalence of somatic symptoms varied across centers from 45% to 95% [84]. Moreover, not only the frequency, but also the type of somatic complaints may be subject to cultural influences, as shown in a study on inpatients admitted for MDD in Greece ($N = 60$) and in Australia ($N = 56$) [85]. Higher rates of somatization have been also reported in depressed Japanese, Chinese, and Turkish patients compared to their western counterparts diagnosed with MDD [86–88]. Relevant differences have also been observed in self-reported scales. Fugita and colleagues analyzed the Zung SDS scores in students from four different countries. Korean and Philippine students had the highest scores, Caucasian Americans the lowest [89]. The relatively greater depression severity in Asian-American populations was confirmed in a recent study comparing BDI results between a sample of Asian-American ($n = 238$) and Caucasian-American students ($n = 556$) [90]. Cross-cultural comparison studies have typically not used outcome measures such as the HAM-D, the MADRS, the IDS and the QIDS, even though all have translated versions available in more than 20 languages. Because of cross-cultural and cross-ethnic differences in patients with MDD, one may argue that scales that were developed for the assessment of depression among Western European and North American Caucasians may not be culturally sensitive in measuring symptoms across other ethnic and cultural groups. However, there is no good evidence that these scales fail to perform well in clinical trials conducted in different countries.

Assessing Depression Across Different Educational and Comprehension Levels

To effectively assess severity of depressive symptoms through a clinician-administered questionnaire, it is necessary that patients understand the meaning of the questions asked. Although readability is widely used as a proxy for comprehension, it might give a false sense of confidence about comprehensibility. In fact, when respondents lacked not only the cognitive capacity to fully understand a standardized question, but also the motivation to answer it thoughtfully, patients often produce a superficially adequate answer (i.e., choosing the first or last response, choosing a neutral response, choosing a socially desirable response or repeating the previous response) [91]. Finally in situations in which respondents' motivation and/or time are limited, even individuals who could understand a complex instrument may not make the effort to answer questions thoughtfully [92].

Assessing Depression with Psychiatric Comorbidities

Little is known about the ability of scales to measure changes in depressive symptomatology across populations with varying degrees of psychiatric comorbidity. For example, it is well known that comorbid anxiety disorders are very common in MDD and the presence of a comorbid anxiety disorder can influence the anxiety and somatic items and therefore inflate the total score of a multidimensional scale such as the HAM-D. Furthermore, core obsessive–compulsive disorder (OCD) symptoms may heavily affect ratings on items covering guilt feelings (because of aggressive/sexual obsessions), work and activities (reduced if the patients are immersed in their compulsions), and anxiety [92]. When a comorbid eating disorder is not an exclusion criterion, the relative influence of items related to weight change, irregular eating habits, guilt, and GI and somatic symptoms has to be carefully considered. For example in the HAM-D 17, the sum of items covering feeling guilty, weight change, somatic anxiety, and gastrointestinal symptoms, may represent 33.6% of the total score, but only 22.2% and 20% of the QIDS and MADRS scores, respectively.

Assessing Depression with Medical Comorbidities

Assessment of depression in medically ill populations is complicated by the fact that emotional, behavioral, or cognitive symptoms may be caused by the concomitant medical illness and/or by the medications used to treat the illness. Ideally, depression assessments should be restricted to variables and items that avoid confounding by medical illness. Two measures have been designed for assessing depression in the medical patients by excluding somatic items: the Hospital Anxiety Depression Scale (HADS) [93] and the Beck Depression Inventory for Primary Care (BDI-PC); however, most of the depression measures developed for medically ill populations have not been adequately tested as outcome measure in depression trials.

Acknowledgments This work has been funded in whole or in part with Federal funds from the National Institute of Mental Health, National Institutes of Health, under Contract N01MH90003 (STAR*D) and GMO N01MH90003 (NIMH Depression Trials Network). The content of this publication does not necessarily reflect the views or policies of the Department of Health and Human Services, nor does mention of trade names, commercial products, or organizations imply endorsement by the U.S. Government.

The authors thank Dr Janet B.W. Williams, Dr Kenneth Kobak, and Dr John Rush for their contributions to this chapter.

References

1. Demyttenaere K, De Fruyt J: Getting what you ask for: on the selectivity of depression rating scales. Psychother Psychosom 2003; 72:61–70
2. Hamilton M: A rating scale for depression. J Neurol Neurosurg Psychiatry 1960; 23:56–62
3. Williams JBW: Research assessments: to standardize or not to standardize?, in Research Designs and Methods in Psychiatry. Edited by Fava M, Rosenbaum JF, Amsterdam, Elsevier, 1992, pp 31–36
4. Williams JB: A structured interview guide for the Hamilton depression rating scale. Arch Gen Psychiatry 1988; 45:742–7
5. Bech P: Measurement issues., in Textbook of biological psychiatry. Part 1: Basic principles. Edited by D'Haenen H. New York, Wiley, 2002
6. Bech P, Tanghoj P, Andersen HF, Overo K: Citalopram dose-response revisited using an alternative psychometric approach to evaluate clinical effects of four fixed citalopram doses compared to placebo in patients with major depression. Psychopharmacology (Berl) 2002; 163:20–5
7. Hamilton M: Hamilton rating scale for Depression (Ham-D), in Handbook of psychiatric measures. Washington DC, APA, 2000, pp 526–8
8. Rush AJ, Trivedi MH, Ibrahim HM, Carmody TJ, Arnow B, Klein DN, Markowitz JC, Ninan PT, Kornstein S, Manber R, Thase ME, Kocsis JH, Keller MB: The 16-Item Quick Inventory of Depressive Symptomatology (QIDS), clinician rating (QIDS-C), and self-report (QIDS-SR): a psychometric evaluation in patients with chronic major depression. Biol Psychiatry 2003; 54:573–83
9. Bagby RM, Ryder AG, Schuller DR, Marshall MB: The Hamilton depression rating scale: has the gold standard become a lead weight? Am J Psychiatry 2004; 161:2163–77
10. Moberg PJ, Lazarus LW, Mesholam RI, Bilker W, Chuy IL, Neyman I, Markvart V: Comparison of the standard and structured interview guide for the Hamilton Depression Rating Scale in depressed geriatric inpatients. Am J Geriatr Psychiatry 2001; 9:35–40
11. Muller MJ, Dragicevic A: Standardized rater training for the Hamilton Depression Rating Scale (HAMD-17) in psychiatric novices. J Affective Dis 2003; 77:65–9
12. Kobak KA, Lipsitz JD, Feiger A: Development of a standardized training program for the Hamilton Depression Scale using internet-based technologies: results from a pilot study. J Psychiatric Res 2003; 37:509–15

13. Takahashi N, Tomita K, Higuchi T, Inada T: The inter-rater reliability of the Japanese version of the Montgomery-Asberg depression rating scale (MADRS) using a structured interview guide for MADRS (SIGMA). Hum Psychopharmacol 2004; 19:187–92
14. Davidson J, Turnbull CD, Strickland R, Miller R, Graves K: The Montgomery-Asberg Depression Scale: reliability and validity. Acta Psychiatrica Scandinavica 1986; 73:544–8
15. Frank E, Prien RF, Jarrett RB, Keller MB, Kupfer DJ, Lavori PW, Rush AJ, Weissman MM: Conceptualization and rationale for consensus definitions of terms in major depressive disorder. Remission, recovery, relapse, and recurrence. Arch Gen Psychiatry 1991; 48:851–5
16. Beck AT, Ward CH, Mendelson M, Mock J, Erbaugh J: An inventory for measuring depression. Arch Gen Psychiatry 1961; 4:561–71
17. Beck AT, Steer RA: Manual for the Beck Depression Inventory. San Antonio, TX, 1993
18. Beck AT, Steer RA, Brown GK: Manual for the Beck Depression Inventory, 2nd ed. San Antonio, TX, 1996
19. Beck AT, Steer RA, Ball R, Ranieri W: Comparison of Beck Depression Inventories -IA and -II in psychiatric outpatients. J Pers Assess 1996; 67:588–97
20. Steer RA, Clark DA, Beck AT, Ranieri WF: Common and specific dimensions of self-reported anxiety and depression: the BDI-II versus the BDI-IA. Behav Res Ther 1999; 37:183–90
21. Biggs JT, Wylie LT, Ziegler VE: Validity of the Zung Self-rating Depression Scale. Br J Psychiatry 1978; 132:381–5
22. Beck AT, Steer RA, Carbin M: Psychometric properties of the Beck depression inventory: Twenty-five years of evaluation. Clin Psychol Rev 1988; 8:77–100
23. Vazquez C, Sanz J: Fiabilidad y validez factorial de la versión española del inventario de depresión de Beck., in III Congreso de Evaluación Psicológica. Barcelona, 1991
24. Richter P, Werner J, Heerlein A, Kraus A, Sauer H: On the validity of the Beck depression inventory. A review. Psychopathology 1998; 31:160–8
25. Zung WWK: Zung Self-rating Depression Scale (Zung SDS), in Handbook of psychiatric measures. Washington, DC, APA, 2000, pp 534–537
26. Montgomery SA, Asberg M: A new depression scale designed to be sensitive to change. Br J Psychiatry 1979; 134:382–9
27. Lobo A, Chamorro L, Luque A, Dal-Re R, Badia X, Baro E: Validation of the Spanish versions of the Montgomery-Asberg depression and Hamilton anxiety rating scales. Med Clin (Barc) 2002; 118:493–9
28. Fleck MP, Guelfi JD, Poirier-Littre MF, Loo H: Application of a structured interview guide adapted to 4 depression scales. Encephale 1994; 20:479–86
29. Williams JB: Structured Interview Guide for the Montgomery Asberg Depression Rating Scale (SIG-MA). Biometrics Research Department, 1996
30. Fava M: Somatic symptoms, depression, and antidepressant treatment. J Clin Psychiatry 2002; 63:305–7
31. Galinowski A, Lehert P: Structural validity of MADRS during antidepressant treatment. Int Clin Psychopharmacol 1995; 10:157–61
32. Schmidtke A, Fleckenstein P, Moises W, Beckmann H: Untersuchungen zur Reliabilitat und Validitat einer deutschen Version der Montgomery-Asberg Depression-Rating Scale (MADRS). Schweizer Archiv fur Neurologie und Psychiatrie 1988; 139:51–65
33. Muller MJ, Himmerich H, Kienzle B, Szegedi A: Differentiating moderate and severe depression using the Montgomery-Asberg depression rating scale (MADRS). J Affective Dis 2003; 77:255–60
34. Montgomery SA, Asberg M: Mongomery-Asberg depression rating scale, in Handbook of psychiatric measures. Washington, DC, APA, 2000, pp 531–33
35. Rush AJ, Giles DE, Schlesser MA, Fulton CL, Weissenburger J, Burns C: The Inventory for Depressive Symptomatology (IDS): preliminary findings. Psychiatry Res 1986; 18:65–87
36. Rush AJ, Gullion CM, Basco MR, Jarrett RB, Trivedi MH: The inventory of depressive symptomatology (IDS): psychometric properties. Psychol Med 1996; 26:477–86

37. Rush AJ, Hiser W, Giles DE: A comparison of self-reported versus clinician-related symptoms in depression. J Clin Psychiatry 1987; 48:246–8
38. Corruble E, Legrand JM, Duret C, Charles G, Guelfi JD: IDS-C and IDS-sr: psychometric properties in depressed in-patients. J Affect Dis 1999; 56:95–101
39. Trivedi MH, Rush AJ, Ibrahim HM, Carmody TJ, Biggs MM, Suppes T, Crismon ML, Shores-Wilson K, Toprac MG, Dennehy EB, Witte B, Kashner TM: The inventory of depressive symptomatology, clinician rating (IDS-C) and self-report (IDS-SR), and the quick inventory of depressive symptomatology, clinician rating (QIDS-C) and self-report (QIDS-SR) in public sector patients with mood disorders: a psychometric evaluation. Psychol Med 2004; 34:73–82
40. Rush AJ, Trivedi MH, Carmody TJ, Ibrahim HM, Markowitz JC, Keitner GI, Kornstein SG, Arnow B, Klein DN, Manber R, Dunner DL, Gelenberg AJ, Kocsis JH, Nemeroff CB, Fawcett J, Thase ME, Russell JM, Jody DN, Borian FE, Keller MB: Self-reported depressive symptom measures: sensitivity to detecting change in a randomized, controlled trial of chronically depressed, nonpsychotic outpatients. Neuropsychopharmacology 2005; 30:405–16
41. Zung WW: A self-rating depression scale. Arch Gen Psychiatry 1965; 12:63–70
42. White J, White K, Razani J: Effects of endogenicity and severity on consistency of standard depression rating scales. J Clin Psychiatry 1984; 45:260–1
43. Kellner R: The development of sensitive scales for research in therapeutics, in Research designs and methods in Psychiatry., vol 9. Edited by Fava M, Rosenbaum JF. Amsterdam, The Netherlands, Elsevier, 1992, pp 213–222
44. Moran P, Lambert MJ: Measurement methods in affective disorders: consistency with DSM-III diagnosis., in The Assessment of Psychotherapy Outcome. Edited by Lambert MJ, DeJulio SS, Christensen ER. New York, Wiley- Interscience, 1983, pp 263–303
45. Maier W, Philipp M: Improving the assessment of severity of depressive states: a reduction of the Hamilton Depression Rating Scale. Pharmacopsychiatry 1985; 18
46. Moller HJ: Methodological aspects in the assessment of severity of depression by the Hamilton Depression Scale. Eur Arch Psychiatry Clin Neurosci 2001; 251 Suppl 2:II13–20
47. Williams JB: Standardizing the Hamilton depression rating scale: past, present, and future. Eur Arch Psychiatry Clin Neurosci 2001; 251 Suppl 2:II6–12
48. Bailey J, Coppen A: A comparison between the Hamilton Rating Scale and the Beck Inventory in the measurement of depression. Br J Psychiatry 1976; 128:486–9
49. Domken M, Scott J, Kelly P: What factors predict discrepancies between self and observer ratings of depression? J Affective Dis 1994; 31:253–9
50. Prusoff BA, Klerman GL, Paykel ES: Concordance between clinical assessments and patients' self-report in depression. Archives of General Psychiatry 1972; 26:546 52
51. Berrios GE, Chen EY: Recognising psychiatric symptoms. Relevance to the diagnostic process. Br J Psychiatry 1993; 163:308–14
52. Enns MW, Larsen DK, Cox BJ: Discrepancies between self and observer ratings of depression. The relationship to demographic, clinical and personality variables. J Affective Dis 2000; 60:33–41
53. Sayer NA, Sackeim HA, Moeller JR, Prudic J, Devanand DP, Coleman EA, Kierksky JE: The relations between observer-rating and self-report of depressive symptomatology. Psychol Assess 1993; 5:350–360
54. Petkova E, Quitkin FM, McGrath PJ, Stewart JW, Klein DF: A method to quantify rater bias in antidepressant trials. Neuropsychopharmacology 2000; 22:559–65
55. Koenig HG, Cohen HJ, Blazer DG, Krishnan KR, Sibert TE: Profile of depressive symptoms in younger and older medical inpatients with major depression. J Am Geriatr Soc 1993; 41:1169–76
56. Kurlowicz LH, Streim JE: Measuring depression in hospitalized, medically ill, older adults. Arch Psychiatr Nurs 1998; 12:209–18
57. Linden M, Borchelt M, Barnow S, Geiselmann B: The impact of somatic morbidity on the Hamilton depression rating scale in the very old. Acta Psychiatrica Scandinavica 1995; 92:150–4

58. Lyness JM, Cox C, Curry J, Conwell Y, King DA, Caine ED: Older age and the underreporting of depressive symptoms. J Am Geriatr Soc 1995; 43:216–21

59. Nebes RD, Pollock BG, Houck PR, Butters MA, Mulsant BH, Zmuda MD, Reynolds CF, 3rd: Persistence of cognitive impairment in geriatric patients following antidepressant treatment: a randomized, double-blind clinical trial with nortriptyline and paroxetine. J Psychiatr Res 2003; 37:99–108

60. Yesavage JA: Geriatric Depression Scale. Psychopharmacol Bull 1988; 24:709–11

61. Yesavage JA, Brink TL, Rose TL, Lum O, Huang V, Adey M, Leirer VO: Development and validation of a geriatric depression screening scale: a preliminary report. J Psychiatric Res 1982; 17:37–49

62. Burns A, Lawlor B, Craig S: Rating scales in old age psychiatry. Br J Psychiatry 2002; 180:161–7

63. Bent-Hansen J, Lunde M, Klysner R, Andersen M, Tanghoj P, Solstad K, Bech P: The validity of the depression rating scales in discriminating between citalopram and placebo in depression recurrence in the maintenance therapy of elderly unipolar patients with major depression. Pharmacopsychiatry 2003; 36:313–6

64. Wohlreich MM, Mallinckrodt CH, Watkin JG, Hay DP: Duloxetine for the long-term treatment of major depressive disorder in patients aged 65 and older: an open-label study. BMC Geriatr 2004; 4:11

65. Roose SP, Sackeim HA, Krishnan KR, Pollock BG, Alexopoulos G, Lavretsky H, Katz IR, Hakkarainen H: Antidepressant pharmacotherapy in the treatment of depression in the very old: a randomized, placebo-controlled trial. Am J Psychiatry 2004; 161:2050–9

66. Sheikh JI, Cassidy EL, Doraiswamy PM, Salomon RM, Hornig M, Holland PJ, Mandel FS, Clary CM, Burt T: Efficacy, safety, and tolerability of sertraline in patients with late-life depression and comorbid medical illness. J Am Geriatr Soc 2004; 52:86–92

67. Poznanski E, Mokros HB, Grossman J, Freeman LN: Diagnostic criteria in childhood depression. Am J Psychiatry 1985; 142:1168–73

68. Poznanski EO, Cook SC, Carroll BJ: A depression rating scale for children. Pediatrics 1979; 64:442–50

69. Poznanski EO, Grossman JA, Buchsbaum Y, Banegas M, Freeman L, Gibbons R: Preliminary studies of the reliability and validity of the children's depression rating scale. J Am Acad Child Psychiatry 1984; 23:191–7

70. Emslie GJ, Rush AJ, Weinberg WA, Kowatch RA, Hughes CW, Carmody T, Rintelmann J: A double-blind, randomized, placebo-controlled trial of fluoxetine in children and adolescents with depression. Arch Gen Psychiatry 1997; 54:1031–7

71. March J, Silva S, Petrycki S, Curry J, Wells K, Fairbank J, Burns B, Domino M, McNulty S, Vitiello B, Severe J: Fluoxetine, cognitive-behavioral therapy, and their combination for adolescents with depression: treatment for adolescents with depression study (TADS) randomized controlled trial. JAMA 2004; 292:807–20

72. Kovacs M: The children's depression, inventory (CDI). Psychopharmacol Bull 1985; 21:995–8

73. Reynolds WM, Graves A: Reliability of children's reports of depressive symptomatology. J Abnorm Child Psychol 1989; 17:647–55

74. Smucker MR, Craighead WE, Craighead LW, Green BJ: Normative and reliability data for the children's depression inventory. J Abnorm Child Psychol 1986; 14:25–39

75. Reynolds WM, Anderson G, Bartell N: Measuring depression in children: a multimethod assessment investigation. J Abnorm Child Psychol 1985; 13:513–26

76. Steer RA, Kumar G, Beck JS, Beck AT: Evidence for the construct validities of the Beck Youth Inventories with child psychiatric outpatients. Psychol Rep 2001; 89:559–65

77. Brooks SJ, Krulewicz SP, Kutcher S: The Kutcher adolescent depression scale: assessment of its evaluative properties over the course of an 8-week pediatric pharmacotherapy trial. J Child Adolesc Psychopharmacol 2003; 13:337–49

78. Cheng AT: Case definition and culture: are people all the same? Br J Psychiatry 2001; 179:1–3
79. Marsella AJ: Thoughts on cross-cultural studies on the epidemiology of depression. Cult Med Psychiatry 1978; 2:343–57
80. Stompe T, Ortwein-Swoboda G, Chaudhry HR, Friedmann A, Wenzel T, Schanda H: Guilt and depression: a cross-cultural comparative study. Psychopathology 2001; 34:289–98
81. Radford MH, Nakane Y, Ohta Y, Mann L, Kalucy RS: Decision making in clinically depressed patients. A transcultural social psychological study. J Nerv Ment Dis 1991; 179:711–9
82. Sonawalla SB, Kelly KE, Neault NB, Mischoulon D, Farabaugh AH, Pava JA, Yeung A, Fava M: Predictors of suicidal ideation in a college population., in 154th Annual Meeting of the American Psychiatric Association. New Orleans, LA, 2001
83. Posternak MA, Zimmerman M: Elevated rates of psychosis among treatment-seeking Hispanic patients with major depression. J Nerv Ment Dis 2005; 193:66–9
84. Simon GE, VonKorff M, Piccinelli M, Fullerton C, Ormel J: An international study of the relation between somatic symptoms and depression. N Engl J Med 1999; 341:1329–35
85. Marmanidis H, Holme G, Hafner RJ: Depression and somatic symptoms: a cross-cultural study. Aust N Z J Psychiatry 1994; 28:274–8
86. Waza K, Graham AV, Zyzanski SJ, Inoue K: Comparison of symptoms in Japanese and American depressed primary care patients. Fam Pract 1999; 16:528–33
87. Parker G, Cheah YC, Roy K: Do the Chinese somatize depression? A cross-cultural study. Soc Psychiatry Psychiatr Epidemiol 2001; 36:287–93
88. Ulusahin A, Basoglu M, Paykel ES: A cross-cultural comparative study of depressive symptoms in British and Turkish clinical samples. Soc Psychiatry Psychiatric Epidemiol 1994; 29:31–9
89. Fugita SS, Crittenden KS: Towards culture- and population-specific norms for self-reported depressive symptomatology. Int J Soc Psychiatry 1990; 36:83–92
90. Lam CY, Pepper CM, Ryabchenko KA: Case identification of mood disorders in Asian American and Caucasian American college students. Psychiatr Q 2004; 75:361–73
91. Shumway M, Sentell T, Unick G, Bamberg W: Cognitive complexity of self-administered depression measures. J Affect Disord 2004; 83:191–8
92. Moritz S, Meier B, Hand I, Schick M, Jahn H: Dimensional structure of the Hamilton depression rating scale in patients with obsessive-compulsive disorder. Psychiatry Res 2004; 125:171–80
93. Zigmond AS, Snaith RP: The hospital anxiety and depression scale. Acta Psychiatr Scand 1983; 67:361–70

Hamilton Depression Rating Scale (HAMD-17)

Instructions: To rate the severity of depression in patients who are already diagnosed as depressed, administer this questionnaire. The higher the score, the more severe the depression.

For each item, circle the number next to the correct item (only one response per item).

1. **Depressed Mood** (sadness, hopeless, helpless, worthless)
   - 0 - Absent
   - 1 - These feeling states indicated only on questioning
   - 2 - These feeling states spontaneously reported verbally
   - 3 - Communicates feeling states non-verbally – i.e., through facial expression, posture, voice, and tendency to weep
   - 4 - Patient reports VIRTUALLY ONLY these feeling states in his spontaneous verbal and non-verbal communication

2. **Feelings of Guilt**
   - 0 - Absent.
   - 1 - Self reproach, feels he has let people down
   - 2 - Ideas of guilt or rumination over past errors or sinful deeds
   - 3 - Present illness is a punishment. Delusions of guilt
   - 4 - Hears accusatory or denunciatory voices and/or experiences threatening visual hallucinations

3. **Suicide**
   - 0 - Absent
   - 1 - Feels life is not worth living
   - 2 - Wishes he were dead or any thoughts of possible death to self
   - 3 - Suicidal ideas or gesture
   - 4 - Attempts at suicide (any serious attempt rates 4)

4. **Insomnia Early**
   - 0 - No difficulty falling asleep
   - 1 - Complains of occasional difficulty falling asleep – i.e., more than 1/2 hour
   - 2 - Complains of nightly difficulty falling asleep

5. **Insomnia Middle**
   - 0 - No difficulty
   - 1 - Patient complains of being restless and disturbed during the night
   - 2 - Waking during the night – any getting out of bed rates 2 (except for purposes of voiding)

6. **Insomnia Late**
   - 0 - No difficulty
   - 1 - Waking in early hours of the morning but goes back to sleep
   - 2 - Unable to fall asleep again if he gets out of bed

7. **Work and Activities**
   - 0 - No difficulty
   - 1 - Thoughts and feelings of incapacity, fatigue or weakness related to activities, work or hobbies
   - 2 - Loss of interest in activity, hobbies or work – either directly reported by patient, or indirect in listlessness, indecision and vacillation (feels he has to push self to work or activities)

3 - Decrease in actual time spent in activities or decrease in productivity
4 - Stopped working because of present illness

8. Retardation: Psychomotor (slowness of thought and speech; impaired ability to concentrate; decreased motor activity)
0 - Normal speech and thought
1 - Slight retardation at interview
2 - Obvious retardation at interview
3 - Interview difficult
4 - Complete stupor

9. Agitation
0 - None
1 - Fidgetiness
2 - Playing with hands, hair, etc.
3 - Moving about, can't sit still.
4 - Hand wringing, nail biting, hair-pulling, biting of lips.

10. Anxiety (psychological)
0 - No difficulty
1 - Subjective tension and irritability
2 - Worrying about minor matters
3 - Apprehensive attitude apparent in face or speech
4 - Fears expressed without questioning

11. Anxiety Somatic: Physiological concomitants of anxiety (i.e., effects of autonomic overactivity, "butterflies," indigestion, stomach cramps, belching, diarrhea, palpitations, hyperventilation, paresthesia, sweating, flushing, tremor, headache, urinary frequency). Avoid asking about possible medication side effects (i.e., dry mouth, constipation)
0 - Absent
1 - Mild
2 - Moderate
3 - Severe
4 - Incapacitating

12. Somatic Symptoms (gastrointestinal)
0 - None.
1 - Loss of appetite but eating without encouragement from others. Food intake about normal
2 - Difficulty eating without urging from others. Marked reduction of appetite and food intake.

13. Somatic Symptoms General
0 - None
1 - Heaviness in limbs, back or head. Backaches, headache or muscle aches. Loss of energy and fatigability.
2 - Any clear-cut symptom rates "2"

14. Genital Symptoms (symptoms such as loss of libido; impaired sexual performance; menstrual disturbances)
0 - Absent
1 - Mild
2 - Severe

15. Hypochondriasis

    0 -   Not present
    1 -   Self-absorption (bodily)
    2 -   Preoccupation with health
    3 -   Frequent complaints, requests for help, etc.
    4 -   Hypochondriacal delusions

16. Loss of Weight

    0 -   No weight loss
    1 -   Probable weight loss associated with present illness
    2 -   Definite (according to patient) weight loss
    3 -   Not assessed

17. Insight

    0 -   Acknowledges being depressed and ill
    1 -   Acknowledges illness but attributes cause to bad food, climate, overwork, virus, need for
          rest, etc.
    2 -   Denies being ill at all

Total Score (total of circled responses): _____

Montgomery Asberg Depression Rating Scale

1. Apparent Sadness

Representing despondency, gloom and despair (more than just ordinary transient low spirits) reflected in speech, facial expression, and posture. Rate by depth and inability to brighten up.

0 - No sadness.
2 - Looks dispirited but does brighten up without difficulty.
4 - Appears sad and unhappy most of the time.
6 - Looks miserable all the time. Extremely despondent.

2. Reported Sadness

Representing reports of depressed mood, regardless of whether it is reflected in appearance or not. Includes low spirits, despondency or the feeling of being beyond help and without hope.

0 - Occasional sadness in keeping with the circumstances.
2 - Sad or low but brightens up without difficulty.
4 - Pervasive feelings of sadness or gloominess. The mood is still influenced by external circumstances.
6 - Continuous or unvarying sadness, misery or despondency.

3. Inner Tension

Representing feelings of ill-defined discomfort, edginess, inner turmoil, mental tension mounting to either panic, dread or anguish. Rate according to intensity, frequency, duration and the extent of reassurance called for.

0 - Placid. Only fleeting inner tension.
2 - Occasional feelings of edginess and ill-defined discomfort.
4 - Continuous feelings of inner tension or intermittent panic which the patient can only master with some difficulty.
6 - Unrelenting dread or anguish. Overwhelming panic.

4. Reduced Sleep

Representing the experience of reduced duration or depth of sleep compared to the subject's own normal pattern when well.

0 - Sleeps as normal.
2 - Slight difficulty dropping off to sleep or slightly reduced, light or fitful sleep.
4 - Moderate stiffness and resistance.
6 - Sleep reduced or broken by at least 2 hours.

5. Reduced Appetite

Representing the feeling of a loss of appetite compared with when well. Rate by loss of desire for food or the need to force oneself to eat.

0 - Normal or increased appetite.
2 - Slightly reduced appetite.
4 - No appetite. Food is tasteless.
6 - Needs persuasion to eat at all.

6. Concentration Difficulties

Representing difficulties in collecting one's thoughts mounting to an incapacitating lack of concentration.

0 - No difficulties in concentrating.
2 - Occasional difficulties in collecting one's thoughts.

4 - Difficulties in concentrating and sustaining thought which reduced ability to read or hold a conversation.
6 - Unable to read or converse without great difficulty.

7. Lassitude

Representing difficulty in getting started or slowness in initiating and performing everyday activities.

0 - Hardly any difficulty in getting started. No sluggishness.
2 - Difficulties in starting activities.
4 - Difficulties in starting simple routine activities which are carried out with effort.
6 - Complete lassitude. Unable to do anything without help.

8. Inability to Feel

Representing the subjective experience of reduced interest in the surroundings or activities that normally give pleasure. The ability to react with adequate emotion to circumstances or people is reduced.

0 - Normal interest in the surroundings and in other people.
2 - Reduced ability to enjoy usual interests.
4 - Loss of interest in the surroundings. Loss of feelings for friends and acquaintances.
6 - The experience of being emotionally paralyzed, inability to feel anger, grief or pleasure and a complete or even painful failure to feel for close relatives and friends.

9. Pessimistic Thoughts

Representing thoughts of guilt, inferiority, self-reproach, sinfulness, remorse, and ruin.

0 - No pessimistic thoughts.
2 - Fluctuating ideas of failure, self-reproach or self-depreciation.
4 - Persistent self-accusations or definite but still rational ideas of guilt or sin. Increasingly pessimistic about the future.
6 - Delusions of ruin, remorse or irredeemable sin. Self-accusations which are absurd and unshakable.

10. Suicidal Thoughts

Representing the feeling that life is not worth living, that a natural death would be welcome, suicidal thoughts, and preparations for suicide. Suicide attempts should not in themselves influence the rating.

0 - Enjoys life or takes it as it comes.
2 - Weary of life. Only fleeting suicidal thoughts.
4 - Probably better off dead. Suicidal thoughts are common, and suicide is considered as a possible solution, but without specific plans or intentions.
6 - Explicit plans for suicide when there is an opportunity. Active preparations for suicide.

Total Score (total of circled responses): _____

QIDS-SR16

Instructions: Please circle one response to each item that best describes you for the past 7 days.

During the Past 7 Days. . .

---

1. Falling Asleep

0 - I never take longer than 30 min to fall asleep.
1 - I take at least 30 min to fall asleep, less than half the time.
2 - I take at least 30 min to fall asleep, more than half the time.
3 - I take more than 60 min to fall asleep, more than half the time.

2. Sleep During the Night

0 - I do not wake up at night.
1 - I have a restless, light sleep with a few brief awakenings each night.
2 - I wake up at least once a night, but I go back to sleep easily.
3 - I awaken more than once a night and stay awake for 20 min or more, more than half the time.

3. Waking Up Too Early

0 - Most of the time, I awaken no more than 30 min before I need to get up.
1 - More than half the time, I awaken more than 30 min before I need to get up.
2 - I almost always awaken at least 1 hour or so before I need to, but I go back to sleep eventually.
3 - I awaken at least 1 hour before I need to, and can't go back to sleep.

4. Sleeping Too Much

0 - I sleep no longer than 7–8 hours/night, without napping during the day.
1 - I sleep no longer than 10 hours in a 24-hour period including naps.
2 - I sleep no longer than 12 hours in a 24-hour period including naps.
3 - I sleep longer than 12 hours in a 24-hour period including naps.

5. Feeling Sad

0 - I do not feel sad.
1 - I feel sad less than half the time.
2 - I feel sad more than half the time.
3 - I feel sad nearly all of the time.

Please Complete Either 6 or 7 (Not Both)

---

6. Decreased Appetite

0 - There is no change in my usual appetite.
1 - I eat somewhat less often or lesser amounts of food than usual.
2 - I eat much less than usual and only with personal effort.
3 - I rarely eat within a 24-hour period, and only with extreme personal effort or when others persuade me to eat.

-Or-

7. Increased Appetite

0 - There is no change from my usual appetite.
1 - I feel a need to eat more frequently than usual.
2 - I regularly eat more often and/or greater amounts of food than usual.
3 - I feel driven to overeat both at mealtime and between meals.

Please Complete Either 8 or 9 (Not Both)

---

8. Decreased Weight (Within the Last 2 Weeks)

0 - I have not had a change in my weight.
1 - I feel as if I've had a slight weight loss.
2 - I have lost 2 pounds or more.
3 - I have lost 5 pounds or more.

-Or-

9. Increased Weight (Within the Last 2 Weeks)

0 - I have not had a change in my weight.
1 - I feel as if I've had a slight weight gain.
2 - I have gained 2 pounds or more.
3 - I have gained 5 pounds or more.

10. Concentration/Decision Making

0 - There is no change in my usual capacity to concentrate or make decisions.
1 - I occasionally feel indecisive or find that my attention wanders.
2 - Most of the time, I struggle to focus my attention or to make decisions.
3 - I cannot concentrate well enough to read or cannot make even minor decisions.

11. View of Myself

0 - I see myself as equally worthwhile and deserving as other people.
1 - I am more self-blaming than usual.
2 - I largely believe that I cause problems for others.
3 - I think almost constantly about major and minor defects in myself.

12. Thoughts of Death or Suicide

0 - I do not think of suicide or death.
1 - I feel that life is empty or wonder if it's worth living.
2 - I think of suicide or death several times a week for several minutes.
3 - I think of suicide or death several times a day in some detail, or I have made specific plans for suicide or have actually tried to take my life.

13. General Interest

0 - There is no change from usual in how interested I am in other people or activities.
1 - I notice that I am less interested in people or activities.
2 - I find I have interest in only one or two of my formerly pursued activities.
3 - I have virtually no interest in formerly pursued activities.

14. Energy Level

0   There is no change in my usual level of energy.
1 - I get tired more easily than usual.

2 - I have to make a big effort to start or finish my usual daily activities (for example, shopping, homework, cooking or going to work).

3 - I really cannot carry out most of my usual daily activities because I just don't have the energy.

15. Feeling Slowed Down

0 - I think, speak, and move at my usual rate of speed.

1 - I find that my thinking is slowed down or my voice sounds dull or flat.

2 - It takes me several seconds to respond to most questions and I'm sure my thinking is slowed.

3 - I am often unable to respond to questions without extreme effort.

16. Feeling Restless

0 - I do not feel restless.

1 - I'm often fidgety, wring my hands, or need to shift how I am sitting.

2 - I have impulses to move about and am quite restless.

3 - At times, I am unable to stay seated and need to pace around.

Total Score*: _____

*Total of circled items including *either* 6 or 7, but not both, and *either* 8 or 9 but not both

Zung Self-Rating Depression Scale

Instructions: Please read each statement and decide how much of the time the statement describes how you have been feeling during the past several days. Make a check mark (√) in the appropriate column.

	A little of the time	Some of the time	Good part of the time	Most of the time
1. I feel down-hearted and blue				
2. Morning is when I feel the best				
3. I have crying spells or feel like it				
4. I have trouble sleeping at night				
5. I eat as much as I used to				
6. I still enjoy sex				
7. I notice that I am losing weight				
8. I have trouble with constipation				
9. My heart beats faster than usual				
10. I get tired for no reason				
11. My mind is as clear as it used to be				
12. I find it easy to do the things I used to				
13. I am restless and can't keep still				
14. I feel hopeful about the future				
15. I am more irritable than usual				
16. I find it easy to make decisions				
17. I feel that I am useful and needed				
18. My life is pretty full				
19. I feel that others would be better off if I were dead				
20. I still enjoy the things I used to do				

Total Score*: _____
*refer to scoring key

Zung Self-Rating Depression Scale Scoring Key

*A total score is derived by summing the individual item scores (1–4) and ranges from 20 to 80. The items are scored: 1 = a little of the time, through 4 = most of the time, *except* for items 2, 5, 6, 11, 12, 14, 16, 17, 18, and 20 which are scored inversely (4 = a little of the time)

Chapter 3
Rating Scales for Anxiety Disorders

Luana Marques, Anne Chosak, Naomi M. Simon, Dieu-My Phan, Sabine Wilhelm, and Mark Pollack

Abstract Anxiety is defined by the Diagnostic and Statistical Manual of Mental Disorders (DSM-IV; American Psychiatric Association (Diagnostic and Statistical Manual of Mental Disorders, 2000)) as an "apprehensive anticipation of future danger or misfortune accompanied by a feeling of dysphoria or somatic symptoms of tension" (American Psychiatric Association (Diagnostic and Statistical Manual of Mental Disorders, 2000 p. 820)). The anxiety disorders in the DSM-IV include panic disorder with and without agoraphobia, generalized anxiety disorder, social phobia, specific phobia, posttraumatic stress disorder, and obsessive compulsive disorder. Measures for evaluating anxiety disorders can be useful in clinical practice and research as a tool for measuring change due to treatment, comparing disorder severity and symptom presentation across groups, motivating patients by systematically discussing the extent of their symptoms and impairment, and informing the clinician of symptom presentation and areas of impairment in each individual patient. This chapter is designed to aid clinicians and researchers in choosing empirically driven measures to guide their clinical and research endeavors for each of the aforementioned anxiety disorders. Whenever appropriate, measures are reprinted to facilitate this process.

Keywords Anxiety · GAD · OCD · Panic disorder · Social anxiety · Rating scales · Questionnaires · Assessment · Psychiatry

Anxiety is defined by the *Diagnostic and Statistical Manual of Mental Disorders* (DSM-IV; [1]) as an "apprehensive anticipation of future danger or misfortune accompanied by a feeling of dysphoria or somatic symptoms of tension" ([1], p. 820). The anxiety disorders in the DSM-IV are as follows: panic disorder with and without agoraphobia, generalized anxiety disorder, social phobia, specific phobia, posttraumatic stress disorder, and obsessive compulsive disorder. In addition to

S. Wilhelm (✉)
Department of Psychiatry, Body Dysmorphic Disorder Clinic, Massachusetts General Hospital and Harvard Medical School, Boston, MA 02114, USA
e-mail: wilhelm@psych.mgh.harvard.edu

L. Baer, M.A. Blais (eds.), *Handbook of Clinical Rating Scales and Assessment in Psychiatry and Mental Health*, Current Clinical Psychiatry, DOI 10.1007/978-1-59745-387-5_3,
© Humana Press, a part of Springer Science+Business Media, LLC 2010

being a core feature of anxiety disorders, which are fully described in the DSM-IV [1], anxiety itself is also associated with several other psychiatric conditions (e.g., hypochondriasis, in which the individual is preoccupied or anxious about having a serious medical condition despite contrary evidence from doctors). Thus, it is important for clinicians to conduct a comprehensive assessment that identifies and differentiates among anxiety disorders and other potential disorders that have anxiety as a core feature.

There are several reasons for clinicians to use rating scales in their clinical and research endeavors. Clinicians frequently use rating scales before treatment to aid in differential diagnosis (in tandem with a diagnostic interview), as well as to describe the disorder, to guide case formulation and treatment planning, and as a pre-treatment severity indicator. Rating scales that assess focus of apprehension can help with the tricky differential diagnoses characteristic of anxiety disorders. For example, symptoms such as panic attacks might be indicative of different disorders (i.e., out of the blue attacks in panic disorder versus worry-cued panic attacks associated with generalized anxiety disorder). Clinicians will often use self-report measures at various points during treatment to monitor treatment progress and to determine if a particular treatment component is helping. Finally, clinicians and clinical researchers will utilize these rating scales at post-treatment to evaluate whether the treatment was successful and, if so, to what extent.

A plethora of assessment measures have been empirically tested within the anxiety disorders. Clinicians will often begin their assessment with broad screening questions (e.g., "Have you ever experienced a traumatic event?") to determine if further assessment is warranted. In research clinics, often these screening questions are taken from structured and semi-structured diagnostic interviews. Following are the two semi-structured interviews often used by clinical researchers studying anxiety disorders: (1) The Anxiety Disorders Interview Schedule for DSM-IV (ADIS-IV; [2]) and (2) The Structured Clinical Interview for DSM-IV (SCID-IV; [3]). The ADIS-IV [2] is a semi-structured interview designed to assess the diagnostic criteria and severity of each anxiety disorder and other comorbid DSM-IV disorders. Similar information can be obtained by using the SCID-IV [3]. Both of these semi-structured interviews have good psychometric properties [4–7]. One of the shortcomings of these interviews is that they are time-consuming and often require additional training, which may be why they are primary measures in research trials but not in clinical practice. The MINI Plus International [8] was developed to offer a quicker semi-structured interview, but there are a number of versions and it is somewhat less comprehensive than the ADIS or the SCID. Fortunately, a wide range of briefer clinician-administered interviews/questionnaires and self-report measures are also empirically supported for the assessment of anxiety disorders. This chapter will focus primarily on easy-to-use and routinely administered measures in clinical practice. We will highlight the gold standard measure for each disorder and provide copies of these measures when possible. In addition, we will describe scoring keys and psychometric properties for each measure. Finally, we will summarize additional empirically supported measures that clinicians might want to also consider.

General Measure of Anxiety

Several disorders, in addition to the anxiety disorders as classified in the DSM-IV, include anxiety symptoms as an important feature. Clinicians may therefore administer general anxiety measures in conjunction with disorder-specific measures to get an overall sense of a patient's trait anxiety level.

Gold Standard Measures:

- Beck Anxiety Inventory
- Hamilton Rating Scale for Anxiety

Gold Standard Scale: Beck Anxiety Inventory

The Beck Anxiety Inventory (BAI; [9]) is the gold standard self-report measure of general anxiety symptoms. (The BAI is copyrighted by the Psycholological Corporation, and is not reproduced in this chapter). The BAI was designed to assess anxiety severity among adults and is intended to distinguish anxiety from comorbid conditions such as depressive symptoms. Because of this specificity, some researchers have suggested that the measure is overly focused on physical symptoms of anxiety [10].

Application of Scale

The BAI is a 21-item self-report measure of anxiety that was designed to assess anxiety severity in adults, while being able to discriminate from comorbid conditions such as depressive symptoms. It is often used as a weekly measure of anxiety symptoms.

Scoring Key

The BAI is a self-administered measure that takes between 5 and 10 min to complete [11], with scores ranging from 0 to 63. It is rated on a Likert scale from "not at all" to "severely."

Cut-Off Scores

Scores of 0–7 reflect minimal anxiety, 8–15 mild anxiety, 16–25 moderate anxiety, and scores above 26 represent severe anxiety [11].

Reliability and Validity

The BAI has received extensive empirical support, with excellent internal consistency within psychiatric samples ($\alpha = 0.92$; [9] and anxiety disorders samples αs 0.85–0.93; [11]). The original article suggested adequate 1-week test–retest reliability ($r = 0.75$; [9]). Subsequent research has also shown adequate 5-week test–retest reliability among individuals diagnosed with panic disorder and agoraphobia ($r = 0.83$; [12]). In addition, the BAI has demonstrated good convergent validity by significantly correlating with other measures of anxiety ($r = 0.48$) among clinical samples [9]. The BAI also has shown good discriminant validity with respect to measures of depression as compared to other anxiety-specific measures such as the State-Trait Anxiety Scale (STAI; [13]). In addition, results from newer research designed to examine whether the BAI was uniquely able to serve as an screening tool for different anxiety disorders (e.g., generalized anxiety disorder, specific or social phobia, panic disorder with or without agoraphobia, obsessive-compulsive disorder) reported that the BAI is able to better differentiate between individuals with panic disorder versus no panic in comparison to other anxiety disorders [14]. Thus, these investigators suggest that the BAI might be an appropriate screening measure to inquire whether individuals suffer from panic disorder.

Source and Alternative Forms

The manual and forms for the BAI are available from the Psychological Corporation, 555 Academic Court, San Antonio, TX 78204-2498, USA. Website: www.psychocorp.com. The Psychological Corporation has a computerized and a Spanish version of the BAI.

Gold Standard Scale: The Hamilton Rating Scale for Anxiety (HAM-A)

The HAM-A is described in detail below in the description of scales for assessing Generalized Anxiety Disorder, and is reproduced in the appendix to this chapter [57, 58].

Panic Disorder and Agoraphobia

Panic disorder without agoraphobia (PD) is a disorder characterized by recurrent, unexpected panic attacks, combined with a persistent concern about future panic attacks [1]. Agoraphobia refers to a fear or avoidance of situations where escape might be difficult or embarrassing, or of situations where help might not be easily accessible in the event of a panic attack. A few special considerations must be taken into account when discussing measures of these disorders. Accurate differential diagnosis is essential, as some medical and substance-induced disorders can mimic panic attacks (for a review see [15]). In addition, it is important to distinguish PD from other anxiety disorders. Comprehensive diagnostic interviews such as the ADIS-IV [2] and the SCID-IV [3] are optimal instruments to make these distinctions. To that end, clinicians have to be able to differentiate between cued (i.e., triggered) versus uncued (i.e., out-of-the blue) panic attacks, with the latter being necessary at some point in the course of illness for a diagnosis of PD. It is important to keep in mind that, as the PD progresses, it is not uncommon for uncued panic attacks to start being cued, so this should also be assessed.

Furthermore, clinicians might want to inquire about the focus of the apprehension during the panic attack. Individuals who suffer from PD are afraid of the experience of the panic attack itself, often associated with a concern that they might be having a heart attack or going crazy, whereas individuals who have panic attacks associated with other conditions tend to be concerned about the consequences associated with their fear (e.g., individuals with social anxiety disorder are afraid of negative evaluation). Finally, individuals with PD and panic disorder with agoraphobia (PDA) begin avoiding situations, activities, and even physical sensations they associate with panic attacks. Therefore, it is important that clinicians assess patients' interoceptive (sensation-focused) anxiety, panic-related cognitions, and agoraphobic avoidance.

Gold Standard Measure: Panic Disorder Severity Scale (PDSS)

The PDSS (reproduced in the appendix to this chapter) is a 7-item clinician-administered scale designed to measure the following dimensions of panic: frequency and distress during panic attacks, severity of anticipatory anxiety, fear and avoidance of agoraphobic situations, fear and avoidance of panic-related sensations, impairment in work and social functioning [16].

Application of Scale

The PDSS is a clinician-administered scale that takes between 10 and 15 min to administer. The PDSS is usually administered as an outcome measure, and may be given pre- and post-treatment.

Scoring Key

The total PDSS is rated on a five-point scale from 0 (none or not present) to 4 (extreme, pervasive, near-constant symptoms, disabling, and incapacitating), with symptoms being rated in the past month. Scores on each dimension range from 0 to 4. The total score is the average of the scores for each of the seven items.

Cut-Off Scores

Recent studies confirmed the reliability and validity of this measure and suggested that a cut-off score of 8 is appropriate to differentiate between patients with PD versus those without [17]. The PDSS has been shown to be sensitive to changes in medication [18, 19] and cognitive behavioral therapy trials [20].

Reliability and Validity

The reliability of the PDSS has been examined in a sample of patients with PD [21]. In this study, reliability for individual items ranged from 0.73 to 0.87 and yielded an intra-class correlation coefficient of 0.88, indicating high inter-rater reliability [21]. However, internal consistency was low in this study ($\alpha = 0.65$; [21]). Shear et al.

[21] also examined the factor structure of the PDSS, with results suggesting that a two-factor model provided the best fit. Specifically, items 1 and 2 (panic frequency and distress) loaded on the first factor, while the remaining items loaded on a different factor. These investigators suggested that the PDSS tends to be sensitive enough to monitor change in treatment.

Source and Alternative Forms

The PDSS is reprinted at the end of this chapter. A self-report version has also been empirically validated and shown to be a reliable, easy-to-complete measure that can be given to a patient prior to a visit to monitor treatment progress [22]. In addition, the PDSS has been translated into Turkish [23] and also has been examined in a Japanese sample [24].

Other Empirically Driven Scales for PD and PDA

Several other measures have been empirically validated to assess PD and PDA. Examples are as follows.

The Anxiety Sensitivity Index

The Anxiety Sensitivity Index (ASI; [25, 26]) is a widely used self-report measure that assesses individuals' tendency to be distressed in response to anxiety-related symptoms. It takes approximately 5 min to administer and has shown strong psychometric properties [25–28].

Agoraphobic Cognitions Questionnaire (ACQ) and the Body Sensation Questionnaire (BSQ)

In addition, the Agoraphobic Cognitions Questionnaire (ACQ; [29]) and the Body Sensation Questionnaire (BSQ; [29]) are two commonly used self-report measures. The ACQ and BSQ are easy and fast (between 5 and 10 min) to administer and have demonstrated acceptable reliability and validity [29, 30]. One of the advantages of these two measures is that they examine different facets of the panic response, with the ACQ focusing on specific cognitions that one might experience during a panic attack, and the BSQ focusing primarily on feared bodily sensations.

Social Anxiety Disorder

Social anxiety disorder (SAD) is a commonly occurring psychiatric disorder characterized by persistent, uncontrollable, and debilitating fear of social situations, where the individual often fears that he/she will act in ways that might be humiliating or embarrassing [1]. Exposures to social situations are associated with an increase in anxiety, which in turn accounts for why individuals with SAD often either avoid

social situations or endure them with high anxiety. Individuals may also have anticipatory anxiety about social situations, which in turn can become associated with
more avoidance. Individuals with SAD may have variable levels of avoidance of
social interactions (e.g., going on dates, meeting new people, etc.) and/or performance situations (e.g., public speaking, eating in public, etc.). It is important for the
clinician to keep in mind that an in-person assessment itself may represent an exposure to the patient's social evaluative concerns, and may be avoided by individuals
who have SAD. When assessing SAD, it is important to assess behavioral as well
as cognitive components, as these areas are core features of cognitive behavioral
models of SAD and are implicated in the maintenance of the disorder [31]. Patients
with SAD may be reluctant or unable to describe their symptoms or their changes
in detail, so use of a rating scale both for initial assessment and for monitoring of
outcomes in response to treatment over time is particularly helpful for this disorder.
Several of the most widely used measures for social phobia are reviewed below.

Gold Standard Measure: Liebowitz Social Anxiety Scale (LSAS)

The LSAS (reproduced in the appendix to this chapter) is a widely used clinician-
administered 24-item interview that assesses fear and avoidance of specific social
situations for people who suffer from social phobia [32].

Application of Scale

The LSAS is an interview measure that takes approximately 30 minutes to administer. It is often used as an outcome measure, administered pre- and post-treatment.

Scoring Key

The LSAS contains two subscales: (1) Fear of Social Interaction (11 items) and
(2) Performance (13 items). Fear is rated on a four-point scale from 0 (none) to 3
(severe), and avoidance is rated on a four-point scale ranging from 0 (never) to 3
(usually 67–100%) to rate symptom severity in the past week. Summing items for
each subscale creates the final scores, with the following indices available: (1) *Total
Fear* (sum of fear ratings on all 24 items), (2) *Fear of Social Situation* (sum of fear
ratings for items 5, 7, 10–12, 15, 18, 19, 22–24), (3) *Fear of Performance* (sum
of fear ratings for items 1–4, 6, 8, 9, 13, 14, 16, 17, 20, 21), (4) *Total Avoidance*
(sum of avoidance ratings for items 5, 7, 10–12, 15, 18, 19, 22–24), (5) *Avoidance
of Performance* (sum of avoidance ratings for items 1–4, 6, 8, 9, 13, 14, 16, 17, 20,
21), and (6) *Total Fear and Avoidance* (sum of total fear and total avoidance scores).

Cut-Off Scores

Researchers have examined cut-off scores that might aid clinicians in identifying
patients who meet criteria for SAD in clinical practice, with results suggesting that

a cut-off of 50 or 60 for its generalized subtype is appropriate [33], while remission has been defined for the generalized subtype as an LSAS score ≤ 30 [34]. The LSAS has also demonstrated significant clinical change in numerous controlled trials [35–38].

Reliability and Validity

The LSAS has demonstrated good reliability across studies, with Cronbach's alpha ranging from 0.81 to 0.92 for the fear subscales, from 0.83 to 0.92 for the avoidance subscales, and 0.96 for the total score [39]. In addition, several studies have examined the validity of the LSAS. For example, Heimberg et al. [35] reported that the LSAS was significantly correlated with clinician rating of social anxiety from a structured interview ($r = 0.52$), as well as several self-report measures ($r = 0.49$–0.73), documenting the convergent validity of the measure. In addition, consistent with the original citation, the fear and avoidance subscales were highly correlated, thus indicating that they might not be distinct constructs in clinical samples. The factor structure of the LSAS has also been examined, with a study suggesting that the measure has four distinct factors: (1) social interaction, (2) public speaking, (3) observation by others, and (4) eating and drinking in public [40].

Source and Alternative Forms

The LSAS is available at the end of the chapter. The LSAS has been translated and validated in French [41], Turkish [42], Hebrew [43], and Spanish [41]. In addition, a computer-administered form has been designed and successfully tested in a pharmaceutical trial [44]. There is also a self-report version of the LSAS, which has demonstrated adequate psychometric properties and can be given to the patient in the waiting room or at the start of a clinical appointment to aid in monitoring outcomes [45–47].

Other Empirically Based Scales for SAD

The Social Phobia and Anxiety Inventory (SPAI)

The SPAI is a 45-item self-report instrument that has been widely used to assess the cognitive, somatic, and behavioral dimensions of SAD [48]. This measure has demonstrated sound psychometric properties [49–51] and has been shown to reliably predict change in treatment outcome [52].

In addition, the Social Phobia Scale (SPS) and Social Interaction Anxiety Scale (SIAS [53]) are two other widely used self-report measures of social anxiety, with sound psychometric properties [53–55]. These measures are helpful as they evaluate central aspects of social anxiety in an easy, time-efficient way, each taking not more than 5 minutes to administer. The SPS measures social evaluations by others when the patient is engaged in activities such as eating and writing, while the

SIAS measures cognitive, behavioral, and affective reactions to interaction situations. Investigators have documented a mean score of 32.8 (SD = 14.9) on the SPS and 49.0 (SD = 15.6) on the SIAS for individuals diagnosed with SAD, and mean scores of 12.5 (SD=11.5; SPS) and 19.9 (SD = 14.2) for healthy controls (e.g., community sample) [54].

Generalized Anxiety Disorder

Generalized anxiety disorder (GAD) is characterized by chronic, excessive worry about several different aspects of life such as health, job, and day-to-day matters [1]. The core feature of GAD is excessive worry that is difficult to control [56]. When assessing GAD, it is helpful to examine several aspects of worry that have been implicated in the maintenance of GAD. For example, one might want to assess the frequency with which the worry occurs. Also, it is important to examine the individual's perception of control over the worry and possible positive beliefs associated with the function of the worry (e.g., If I worry about my mother's health, I will be more prepared to handle it when she gets sick). Patients with GAD might also attempt to control or suppress their worries by engaging in avoidance strategies.

Gold Standard Measure: The Hamilton Rating Scale for Anxiety (HAM-A)

The HAM-A (reproduced in the appendix to this chapter) is a clinician-administered, typically semi-structured interview designed to assess anxiety symptoms not specific to any disorder [57, 58]. A structured interview guide is available as well for the Hamilton Anxiety Rating Scale (SIGH-A) [59], which has demonstrated adequate reliability and validity. The HAM-A is most widely used as an outcome measure in therapeutic trials of GAD. It has 14 items, each measuring specific anxiety symptom clusters (e.g., tension, insomnia, respiratory) which are rated by the interviewer on a scale from 0 (not present) to 4 (very severe/incapacitating) [57].

Application of Scale

The HAM-A takes between 15 and 30 minutes to administer and is often used as an outcome measure in pharmacological and psychosocial outcome research, typically administered at pre- and post-treatment.

Scoring Key

A total score is obtained by summing the 14 items (higher scores indicating more anxiety). In addition to a total score, two subscales have been suggested: psychic subscale (sum of items 1–6 and 14) and somatic subscale (sum of items 7–13).

Cut-Off Scores

Total scores above 16 on the HAM-A are generally considered indicative of symptomatic GAD [58]. The HAM-A has been shown to be sensitive to change in medication trials [19, 60–65].

Reliability and Validity

Internal consistency for the HAM-A ranges from adequate (α ranging from 0.77 to 0.81; [66]) to excellent (α=0.92; [67]) depending on the study considered. The HAM-A has also demonstrated excellent 1-week test–retest reliability (α=0. 96; [68]). Inter-rater reliability of the original study was strong (α=0.89; [69]), but subsequent studies showed lower estimates (e.g., α=0.65; [66]).

Source and Alternative Forms

The HAM-A is included at the end of the chapter. A computer-administered version of the HAM-A has also been designed and has demonstrated a high correlation with the clinician-administered version [67].

Other Empirically Driven Scales for GAD

Several other measures have been empirically validated to assess GAD, and may be somewhat less cumbersome to use in clinical practice.

For example, the Penn State Worry Questionnaire (PSWQ; [70]) is a widely used self-report measure of intensity and excessiveness of worries that contains 16 items rated on a scale from 1 (not at all typical) to 5 (very typical) of the individual.

In addition, a newly empirically validated measure, the *GAD-7*, is a promising measure to quickly screen and assess GAD [71].

Finally, the BAI, described above can also be used as a measure of generalized anxiety symptoms.

Obsessive Compulsive Disorder

Obsessive compulsive disorder (OCD) is characterized by repetitive, intrusive impulses, thoughts, or images that trigger anxiety. "Obsessions" are defined as intrusive, recurrent, distressing, thoughts, images, or impulses that a person attempts to suppress or ignore [1]. "Compulsions" are repetitive behaviors or mental rituals that the individual performs in an attempt to minimize the anxiety generated by the obsessions [1]. Although individuals suffering with OCD might be able to postpone their compulsive rituals, they often cannot stop them.

In contrast to other anxiety disorders in which there is a great deal of symptom commonality, OCD symptoms tend to have a wide variability in clinical presentation. For example, patients might engage in ordering and arranging rituals, excessively wash their hands, seek reassurance, count, pray to neutralize religious obsessions, etc. When assessing OCD, the clinician should be mindful of the wide range in presentation.

Gold Standard Measure: Yale-Brown Obsessive Compulsive Scale (YBOCS)

There are two types of YBOCS forms described in the literature: the YBOCS *symptom checklist* interview and the YBOCS *symptom severity scale* (both are reproduced in the appendix to this chapter) [72, 73]. Clinicians should begin an OCD assessment by administering the YBOCS symptom checklist interview, which is a 64-item clinician-administered checklist that examines present and past obsessions and compulsions [72, 73]. Specifically, the checklist helps clinicians to identify 36 different types of obsessions and 23 types of compulsions, covering the following types of symptoms: harming, contamination/washing, sexual, hoarding/saving, religious, symmetry/exactness, somatic, and miscellaneous. In addition, some symptoms of OC spectrum conditions (e.g., trichotillomania, hypochondriasis) are also included. Next, clinicians will commonly use the 10-item clinician-administered semi-structured severity scale to assess the severity of obsessions and compulsions [72, 73]. This 10-item scale rates the severity of obsessions and compulsions on a five-point scale ranging from 0 (no symptoms) to 4 (extremely severe symptoms), with respect to time spent, interference, distress, resistance, and control with total scores ranging from 0 to 40.

Application of Scale

The time needed to administer the YBOCS symptom checklist depends on the number of symptoms endorsed by the patient. The checklist is usually administered at the beginning of the treatment or at times when the patient might report a shift in OCD symptoms. The YBOCS interview can take approximately 20 minutes to administer and is often used as an outcome measure in studies, administered pre- and post-treatment.

Scoring Key

There is no scoring for the YBOCS checklist. The YBOCS interview provides a total symptom severity scale that can be obtained by summing up all of the items in the scale. In addition, one can also get a separate score for the severity of obsessions (items 1–5) and compulsions (items 6–10) by summing these items respectively.

Cut-Off Scores

A YBOCS score equal to or greater than 16 is the cut-off score commonly used in therapeutic trials to identify clinically symptomatic levels of OCD (see [74]). In addition, scores from 0 to 7 are considered indicative of subclinical OCD symptoms, 8–15 mild, 16–23 moderate, 24–31 severe, and 32–40 extreme. The YBOCS has become the gold standard for most recent pharmacological and behavioral treatment trials because it can be used to measure severity regardless of the types of obsessions and compulsions the subject exhibits.

Reliability and Validity

Inter-rater reliability for the OCD severity score has been estimated at 0.95 [72, 73] and it has been shown to be sensitive to treatment effects [75].

Source and Alternative Forms

The YBOCS checklist and interview are reprinted at the end of the chapter. A self-report version of the YBOCS has been created and has shown good psychometric properties [76].

Other Empirically Driven Scales for OCD

Several other measures have been empirically validated to assess OCD. For example, the *Obsessive Beliefs Questionnaire* (OBQ; [77, 78]), which is a recently developed measure designed to examine dysfunctional beliefs held by patients with OCD, has received increased interest in the literature [79–83]. In addition, the *Obsessive Compulsive Inventory* (OCI; [84]) is another established measure within the OCD literature designed to measure the severity of specific OCD symptoms [85–88]. Finally, researchers have extended the YBOCS to measure the different dimensions of OCD, creating the dimensional YBOCS (DY-BOCS) [89]. The DY-BOCS consists of a symptom checklist divided into six different dimensions. The scale is completed by the patient, who endorses the symptom as present, (1) in the past week, (2) ever in the past, or (3) never present. In a second part of the DY-BOCS, a clinician rates the severity of each symptom and overall impairment on a scale from 0 (no symptoms) to 10 (symptoms are extremely troublesome). Patients are also asked the degree of avoidance related to each specific symptom on a scale from 0 (never) to 5 (extreme, very extensive avoidance). Psychometric analyses have indicated excellent internal consistencies (alphas $\geq$ 0.94). Furthermore, the convergent validity, as measured by the correlation between the DY-BOCS and the YBOCS total score, is very good.

Posttraumatic Stress Disorder (PTSD)

The DSM-IV defines trauma as "the experience, witnessing, or confronting of an event that involves actual or threatened death or serious injury, or other threat to one's physical integrity" (Criterion A.1; [1]). To be considered a traumatic event, the individual's reaction to the event must involve "intense fear, helplessness, or horror" (Criterion A.2). To be diagnosed with PTSD, an individual must have been exposed to a traumatic event that meets Criterion A, report trauma symptoms from three diagnostic clusters, and have symptoms that have persisted at a distressing level for at least 1 month. Thus, when assessing PTSD, one must consider the symptoms from the three different symptom clusters. In addition, given that some trauma survivors experience shame associated with the trauma, and that simply asking detailed questions about the trauma may trigger anxiety and emotional distress, clinicians are advised to be particularly sensitive when assessing these symptoms.

Gold Standard: Clinician-Administered PTSD Scale

One of the gold standard measures to assess and diagnose PTSD is the *Clinician-Administered PTSD Scale* (CAPS; [90]), which is a structured interview that assesses PTSD symptoms. PTSD symptoms are usually assessed in the preceding month, using five-point Likert scale to assess frequency and intensity (e.g., 0 indicates that the symptom does not occur or does not cause distress, 4 indicates that the symptom occurs nearly every day or causes extreme distress and discomfort). The total severity score for the CAPS (CAPS-total) is computed by summing the frequency and intensity ratings for each symptom (range 0–136). Additionally, PTSD symptom cluster scores can be computed by summing the frequency and intensity ratings for each cluster [90]. Although the CAPS is a well-established and reliable measure, it is also time-consuming to administer (approximately an hour). Thus, the CAPS is not typically used as a clinical measure.

Short PTSD Rating Interview (SPRINT)

Other measures such as the *Short PTSD Rating Interview* (SPRINT; [91]) are more commonly used in clinical settings. The SPRINT (reproduced in the appendix to this chapter) is a 10-item clinician-administered scale which includes questions assessing the core symptoms of PTSD, as well as related aspects of somatic malaise, stress vulnerability, and functional impairment [92]. The SPRINT also has two additional items, which are designed to measure global improvement (i.e., percentage change) and a severity rating.

Application of Scale

The SPRINT requires approximately 5–10 minutes to administer and it is often used as an outcome measure in pharmacological and psychosocial outcome research, administered at pre- and post-treatment [93–95].

Scoring Key

The SPRINT is rated on a five-point scale: not at all (0), a little bit (1), moderately (2), quite a lot (3), and very much (4), with a maximum score of 32. A total score is obtained by summing the first eight items, with higher scores indicating more post-trauma symptoms.

Cut-Off Score

The original scale development article for the SPRINT suggests that scores between 14 and 17 were associated with 96% diagnostic accuracy. However, scores between 11 and 13 performed better in diagnostic prediction among clinical samples [92]. In some studies, a 25% reduction in the SPRINT was considered to indicate response to a drug trial [95]. The SPRINT has been shown to be sensitive to treatment changes in several medication trials [93, 95].

Reliability and Validity

The SPRINT has demonstrated adequate psychometric properties [92] and has been shown to be empirically similar to the CAPS [96]. For example, it has demonstrated good test–retest reliability, with high intra-class correlations $r = 0.778$ and internal consistency (α range 0.77–0.88) [92].

Source and Alternative Forms

The SPRINT is reprinted at the end of the chapter.

Other Empirically Driven Scales for PTSD

Several other measures have been empirically validated to assess PTSD. For example, the self-rated Davidson Trauma Scale (DTI; [97]), the PTSD Symptom Scale (PDS; [98]), and the self-rated Connors-Davidson Resilience Scale (CD-RISC; [99]). The PDS is widely used in the literature because it provides information on diagnosis, symptom severity and characteristics, and impairment. Additionally, the PDS has good internal reliability and convergence with other measures of PTSD and can be used to measure change with treatment as well as a diagnostic screening instrument in high-risk populations.

References

1. American Psychiatric Association. *Diagnostic and Statistical Manual of Mental Disorders*. Fourth, Text Revision ed. 2000, Washington, DC: American Psychiatric Association.
2. Brown, T.A., P.A. Di Nardo, and D.H. Barlow, *Anxiety Disorders Interview Schedule for DSM-IV*. 1994, San Antonio, TX: The Psychological Corporation.

3. First, M.B., et al., *Structured Clinical Interview for DSM-IV Axis I Disorders-Patient Editions (SCID-I/P, Version 2.0)*. 1996, New York: Biometrics Research Department, New York State Psychiatric Institute.

4. Blanchard, E.B., et al., *The utility of the Anxiety Disorders Interview Schedule (ADIS) in the diagnosis of the Post-traumatic Stress Disorder (PTSD) in Vietnam veterans*. Behaviour Research and Therapy, 1986. **24**(5): pp. 577–580.

5. Bouman, T.K. and C. de Ruiter, *The validity of the Anxiety Disorders Interview Schedule-Revised (ADIS-R): A pilot study*. Gedragstherapie, 1991. **24**(2): pp. 77–88.

6. Grisham, J.R., T.A. Brown, and L.A. Campbell, *The Anxiety Disorders Interview Schedule for DSM-IV (ADIS-IV)*, in *Comprehensive handbook of psychological assessment, Vol 2: Personality assessment*. 2004, John Wiley & Sons, Inc: Hoboken, NJ. pp. 163–177.

7. First, M.B. and M. Gibbon, *The Structured Clinical Interview for DSM-IV Axis I Disorders (SCID-I) and the Structured Clinical Interview for DSM-IV Axis II Disorders (SCID-II)*, in *Comprehensive handbook of psychological assessment, Vol 2: Personality assessment*. 2004, John Wiley & Sons, Inc: Hoboken, NJ. pp. 134–143.

8. Sheehan, D.V., et al., *The Mini-International Neuropsychiatric Interview (M.I.N.I.): the development and validation of a structured diagnostic psychiatric interview for DSM-IV and ICD-10*. Journal of Clinical Psychiatry, 1998. **59 Suppl 20**: pp. 22–33; quiz 34–57.

9. Beck, A.T., et al., *An Inventory for Measuring Clinical Anxiety: Psychometric Properties*. Journal of Consulting & Clinical Psychology, 1988. **56**(6): pp. 893–897.

10. Cox, B.J., et al., *Does the Beck Anxiety Inventory measure anything beyond panic attack symptoms?* Behaviour Research & Therapy, 1996. **34**(11–12): pp. 949–54; discussion 955–61.

11. Beck, A.T. and R.A. Steer, *Beck Inventory Manual*. 1993, San Antonio, TX: Psychological Coorporation.

12. de Beurs, E., et al., *Convergent and divergent validity of the Beck Anxiety Inventory for patients with panic disorder and agoraphobia*. Depression & Anxiety, 1997. **6**(4): pp. 140–6.

13. Creamer, M., et al., *The Beck Anxiety Inventory in a non-clinical sample*. Behaviour Research & Therapy, 1995. **33**(4): pp. 477–85.

14. Leyfer, O.T., et al., *Examination of the utility of the Beck Anxiety Inventory and its factors as a screener for anxiety disorders*. Journal of Anxiety Disorders, 2006. **20**(4): pp. 444–58.

15. Dattilio, F.M. and J. Salas-Auvert, *Panic Disorder: Assessment and treatment through a wide-angle lens*. 2000, Phoenix, AZ: Zeig, Tucker & Co.

16. Shear, M.K., et al., *Panic Disorder Severity Scale (PDSS)*. 1992, Pittsburg, PA: Department of Psychiatry, University of Pittsburg School of Medicine.

17. Shear, M.K., et al., *Reliability and validity of the Panic Disorder Severity Scale: replication and extension*. Journal of Psychiatric Research, 2001. **35**(5): pp. 293–6.

18. Pollack, M.H., et al., *Sertraline in the treatment of panic disorder: a flexible-dose multicenter trial*. Archives of General Psychiatry, 1998. **55**(11): pp. 1010–6.

19. Simon, N.M., et al., *An open-label trial of risperidone augmentation for refractory anxiety disorders*. Journal of Clinical Psychiatry, 2006. **67**(3): pp. 381–5.

20. Otto, M.W., et al., *Group cognitive-behavior therapy for patients failing to respond to pharmacotherapy for panic disorder: a clinical case series*. Behaviour Research and Therapy, 1999. **37**(8): pp. 763–770.

21. Shear, M.K., et al., *Multicenter collaborative panic disorder severity scale*. American Journal of Psychiatry, 1997. **154**(11): pp. 1571–5.

22. Houck, P.R., et al., *Reliability of the self-report version of the panic disorder severity scale*. Depression & Anxiety, 2002. **15**(4): pp. 183–5.

23. Monkul, E.S., et al., *Panic Disorder Severity Scale: reliability and validity of the Turkish version*. Depression & Anxiety, 2004. **20**(1): pp. 8–16.

24. Yamamoto, I., et al., *Cross-cultural evaluation of the Panic Disorder Severity Scale in Japan*. Depression & Anxiety, 2004. **20**(1): pp. 17–22.

25. Reiss, S., et al., *Anxiety sensitivity, anxiety frequency and the predictions of fearfulness*. Behaviour Research and Therapy, 1986. **24**(1): pp. 1–8.

26. Peterson, R.A. and S. Reiss, *Anxiety Sensitivity Index. Revised test manual*. 1993, Worthington, OH: IDS Publishing Corporation.
27. Peterson, R.A. and R.L. Heilbronner, *The Anxiety Sensitivity Index: Construct validity and factor analytic structure*. Journal of Anxiety Disorders, 1987. **1**(2): pp. 117–121.
28. Zinbarg, R.E., et al., *Anxiety sensitivity, panic, and depressed mood: A reanalysis teasing apart the contributions of the two levels in the hierarchical structure of the Anxiety Sensitivity Index*. Journal of Abnormal Psychology, 2001. **110**(3): pp. 372–377.
29. Chambless, D.L., et al., *Assessment of fear of fear in agoraphobics: The Body Sensations Questionnaire and the Agoraphobic Cognitions Questionnaire*. Journal of Consulting & Clinical Psychology, 1984. **52**(6): pp. 1090–1097.
30. Khawaja, N.G., *Revisiting the Factor Structure of the Agoraphobic Cognitions Questionnaire and Body Sensations Questionnaire: A Confirmatory Factor Analysis Study*. Journal of Psychopathology & Behavioral Assessment, 2003. **25**(1): pp. 57–63.
31. Heimberg, R.G., *Cognitive assessment strategies and the measurement of outcome of treatment for social phobia*. Behaviour Research and Therapy, 1994. **32**(2): pp. 269–280.
32. Liebowitz, M.R. and M.R. Liebowitz, *Social phobia*. Modern Problems of Pharmacopsychiatry, 1987. **22**: pp. 141–73.
33. Mennin, D.S., et al., *Screening for social anxiety disorder in the clinical setting: using the Liebowitz Social Anxiety Scale*. Journal of Anxiety Disorders, 2002. **16**(6): pp. 661–73.
34. Liebowitz, M.R., et al., *A randomized controlled trial of venlafaxine extended release in generalized social anxiety disorder*. Journal of Clinical Psychiatry, 2005. **66**(2): pp. 238–47.
35. Heimberg, R.G., et al., *Psychometric properties of the Liebowitz Social Anxiety Scale*. Psychological Medicine, 1999. **29**(1): pp. 199–212.
36. Baldwin, D., et al., *Paroxetine in social phobia/social anxiety disorder: Randomized, double-blind, placebo-controlled study*. British Journal of Psychiatry, 1999. **175**(Aug 1999): pp. 120–126, Royal College of Psychiatrists.
37. Bouwer, C. and D.J. Stein, *Use of the selective serotonin reuptake inhibitor citalopram in the treatment of generalized social phobia*. Journal of Affective Disorders, 1998. **49**(1): pp. 79–82.
38. Lott, M., et al., *Brofaromine for social phobia: A multicenter, placebo-controlled, double-blind study*. Journal of Clinical Psychopharmacology, 1997. **17**(4): pp. 255–260.
39. Liebowitz, M.R., et al., *Pharmacotherapy of social phobia. A condition distinct from panic attacks*. Psychosomatics, 1987. **28**(6): pp. 305–8.
40. Safren, S.A., et al., *Factor structure of social fears: The Liebowitz Social Anxiety Scale*. Journal of Anxiety Disorders, 1999. **13**(3): pp. 253–70.
41. Yao, S.N., et al., *Social anxiety in patients with social phobia: validation of the Liebowitz social anxiety scale: the French version*. Encephale, 1999. **25**(5): pp. 429–35.
42. Soykan, C., et al., *Liebowitz social anxiety scale: the Turkish version*. Psychological Reports, 2003. **93**(3 Pt 2): pp. 1059–69.
43. Levin, J.B., et al., *Psychometric properties and three proposed subscales of a self-report version of the Liebowitz Social Anxiety Scale translated into Hebrew*. Depression & Anxiety, 2002. **16**(4): pp. 143–51.
44. Kobak, K.A., et al., *Computer-administered rating scales for social anxiety in a clinical drug trial. [see comment]*. Depression & Anxiety, 1998. **7**(3): pp. 97–104.
45. Baker, S.L., et al., *The liebowitz social anxiety scale as a self-report instrument: a preliminary psychometric analysis*. Behaviour Research & Therapy, 2002. **40**(6): pp. 701–15.
46. Cox, B.J., et al., *A comparison of social phobia outcome measures in cognitive-behavioral group therapy*. Behavior Modification, 1998. **22**(3): pp. 285–97.
47. Fresco, D.M., et al., *The Liebowitz social anxiety scale: a comparison of the psychometric properties of self-report and clinician-administered formats*. Psychological Medicine, 2001. **31**(6): pp. 1025–1035.
48. Turner, S.M., et al., *An empirically derived inventory to measure social fears and anxiety: The Social Phobia and Anxiety Inventory*. Psychological Assessment, 1989. **1**: pp. 35–40.

49. Peters, L. and L. Peters, *Discriminant validity of the Social Phobia and Anxiety Inventory (SPAI), the Social Phobia Scale (SPS) and the Social Interaction Anxiety Scale (SIAS).* Behaviour Research & Therapy, 2000. **38**(9): pp. 943–50.
50. Rodebaugh, T.L., et al., *Convergent, discriminant, and criterion-related validity of the Social Phobia and Anxiety Inventory.* Depression & Anxiety, 2000. **11**(1): pp. 10–4.
51. Beidel, D.C., et al., *The social phobia and anxiety inventory: concurrent validity with a clinic sample.* Behaviour Research & Therapy, 1989. **27**(5): pp. 573–6.
52. Beidel, D.C., et al., *Assessing reliable and clinically significant change in social phobia: validity of the social phobia and anxiety inventory.* Behaviour Research & Therapy, 1993. **31**(3): pp. 331–7.
53. Mattick, R.P. and J.C. Clarke, *Development and validation of measures of social phobia scrutiny fear and social interaction anxiety.* Behaviour Research & Therapy, 1998. **36**(4): pp. 455–70.
54. Heimberg, R.G., et al., *Assessment of anxiety in social interaction and being observed by others: The Social Interaction Anxiety Scale and the Social Phobia Scale.* Behavior Therapy, 1992. **23**(1): pp. 53–73.
55. Osman, A., et al., *The Social Phobia and Social Interaction Anxiety Scales: Evaluation of psychometric properties.* Journal of Psychopathology and Behavioral Assessment, 1998. **20**(3): pp. 249–264.
56. Borkovec, T., *The nature, functions, and origins of worry*, in *Worrying: Perspectives on theory, assessment and treatment.* 1994, John Wiley & Sons: Oxford, England. pp. 5–33.
57. Hamilton, M., *Diagnosis and rating of anxiety.* British Journal of Psychiatry, 1969. Special Publication No 3.: pp. 76–79.
58. Hamilton, M., *The assessment of anxiety states by rating.* British Journal of Medical Psychology, 1959. **32**: pp. 50–55.
59. Shear, M.K., et al., *Reliability and validity of a structured interview guide for the Hamilton Anxiety Rating Scale (SIGH-A).* Depression & Anxiety, 2001. **13**(4): pp. 166–78.
60. Kim, T.S., et al., *Comparison of venlafaxine extended release versus paroxetine for treatment of patients with generalized anxiety disorder.* Psychiatry & Clinical Neurosciences, 2006. **60**(3): pp. 347–51.
61. Brawman-Mintzer, O., et al., *Adjunctive risperidone in generalized anxiety disorder: a double-blind, placebo-controlled study. [see comment].* Journal of Clinical Psychiatry, 2005. **66**(10): pp. 1321–5.
62. Nimatoudis, I., et al., *Remission rates with venlafaxine extended release in Greek outpatients with generalized anxiety disorder. A double-blind, randomized, placebo controlled study.* International Clinical Psychopharmacology, 2004. **19**(6): pp. 331–6.
63. Perugi, G., et al., *Open-label evaluation of venlafaxine sustained release in outpatients with generalized anxiety disorder with comorbid major depression or dysthymia: effectiveness, tolerability and predictors of response.* Neuropsychobiology, 2002. **46**(3): pp. 145–9.
64. Montgomery, S.A., et al., *Characterization of the longitudinal course of improvement in generalized anxiety disorder during long-term treatment with venlafaxine XR.* Journal of Psychiatric Research, 2002. **36**(4): pp. 209–17.
65. Meoni, P., et al., *Pattern of symptom improvement following treatment with venlafaxine XR in patients with generalized anxiety disorder.* Journal of Clinical Psychiatry, 2001. **62**(11): pp. 888–93.
66. Moras, K., P.A. di Nardo, and D.H. Barlow, *Distinguishing anxiety and depression: Reexamination of the reconstructed Hamilton scales.* Psychological Assessment, 1992. **4**(2): pp. 224–227.
67. Kobak, K.A., W.M. Reynolds, and J.H. Greist, *Development and validation of a computer-administered version of the Hamilton Rating Scale.* Psychological Assessment, 1993. **5**(4): pp. 487–492.
68. Maier, W., et al., *The Hamilton anxiety scale: reliability, validity and sensitivity to change in anxiety and depressive disorders.* Journal of Affective Disorders, 1988. **14**(1): pp. 61–8.

69. Bruss, G.S., et al., *Hamilton anxiety rating scale interview guide: joint interview and test-retest methods for interrater reliability.* Psychiatry Research, 1994. **53**(2): pp. 191–202.

70. Meyer, T., et al., *Development and validation of the Penn State worry questionnaire.* Behaviour Research and Therapy, 1990. **28**(6): pp. 487–495.

71. Spitzer, R.L., et al., *A brief measure for assessing generalized anxiety disorder: the GAD-7.* Archives of Internal Medicine, 2006. **166**(10): pp. 1092–7.

72. Goodman, W.K., et al., *The Yale-brown obsessive compulsive scale. II. Validity.* Archives of General Psychiatry, 1989. **46**(11): pp. 1012–6.

73. Goodman, W.K., et al., *The Yale-Brown Obsessive Compulsive Scale: I. Development, use, and reliability.* Archives of General Psychiatry, 1989. **46**(11): pp. 1006–1011.

74. Tolin, D.F., J.S. Abramowitz, and G.J. Diefenbach, *Defining Response in Clinical Trials for Obsessive-Compulsive Disorder: A Signal Detection Analysis of the Yale-Brown Obsessive Compulsive Scale.* Journal of Clinical Psychiatry, 2005. **66**(12): pp. 1549–1557.

75. DeVeaugh-Geiss, J., P. Landau, and R. Katz, *Preliminary results from a multicenter trial of clomipramine in obsessive-compulsive disorder.* Psychopharmacological Bulletin, 1989. **25**: pp. 36–40.

76. Steketee, G., et al., *The Yale-Brown Obsessive Compulsive Scale: interview versus self-report.* Behaviour Research & Therapy, 1996. **34**(8): pp. 675–84.

77. Steketee, G., et al., *Psychometric validation of the Obsessive Beliefs Questionnaire and the Interpretation of Intrusions Inventory: Part I.* Behaviour Research and Therapy, 2003. **41**(8): pp. 863–878.

78. Steketee, G. and R. Frost, *Development and initial validation of the Obsessive Beliefs Questionnaire and the Interpretation of Intrusions Inventory.* Behaviour Research and Therapy, 2001. **39**(8): pp. 987–1006.

79. Aardema, F., K.P. O'Connor, and P.M. Emmelkamp, *Inferential Confusion and Obsessive Beliefs in Obsessive-Compulsive Disorder.* Cognitive Behaviour Therapy, 2006. **35**(3): pp. 138–147.

80. Julien, D., et al., *The specificity of belief domains in obsessive-compulsive symptom subtypes.* Personality and Individual Differences, 2006. **41**(7): pp. 1205–1216.

81. Taylor, S., D. McKay, and J.S. Abramowitz, *Hierarchical structure of dysfunctional beliefs in obsessive-compulsive disorder.* Cognitive Behaviour Therapy, 2005. **34**(4): pp. 216–228.

82. Taylor, S., J.S. Abramowitz, and D. McKay, *Are There Interactions Among Dysfunctional Beliefs in Obsessive Compulsive Disorder?* Cognitive Behaviour Therapy, 2005. **34**(2): pp. 89–98.

83. Woods, C.M., D.F. Tolin, and J.S. Abramowitz, *Dimensionality of the Obsessive Beliefs Questionnaire (OBQ).* Journal of Psychopathology and Behavioral Assessment, 2004. **26**(2): pp. 113–125.

84. Foa, E.B., et al., *The validation of a new obsessive-compulsive disorder scale: the obsessive-compulsive inventory.* Psychological Assessment, 1998. **10**(3): pp. 206–214.

85. Simonds, L.M., S.J. Thorpe, and S.A. Elliott, *The Obsessive Compulsive Inventory: psychometric properties in a nonclinical student sample.* Behavioural and Cognitive Psychotherapy, 2000. **28**(2): pp. 153–159.

86. Wu, K.D. and D. Watson, *Further investigation of the obsessive-compulsive inventory: Psychometric analysis in two non-clinical samples.* Journal of Anxiety Disorders, 2003. **17**(3): pp. 305–319.

87. Abramowitz, J.S., D.F. Tolin, and G.J. Diefenbach, *Measuring Change in OCD: Sensitivity of the Obsessive- Compulsive Inventory-Revised.* Journal of Psychopathology and Behavioral Assessment, 2005. **27**(4): pp. 317–324.

88. Abramowitz, J.S. and B.J. Deacon, *Psychometric properties and construct validity of the Obsessive-Compulsive Inventory-Revised: Replication and extension with a clinical sample.* Journal of Anxiety Disorders, 2006. **20**(8): pp. 1016–1035.

89. Rosario-Campos, M.C., et al., *The Dimensional Yale-Brown Obsessive-Compulsive Scale (DY-BOCS): an instrument for assessing obsessive-compulsive symptom dimensions.* Molecular Psychiatry, 2006. **11**(5): pp. 495–504.
90. Blake, D.D., et al., *The development of a Clinician-Administered PTSD Scale.* Journal of Traumatic Stress, 1995. **8**(1): pp. 75–90.
91. Connor, K.M., et al., *SPRINT: a brief global assessment of post-traumatic stress disorder.* International Clinical Psychopharmacology, 2001. **16**(5): pp. 279–84.
92. Connor, K.M. and J. Davidson, *SPRINT: A brief global assessment of post-traumatic stress disorder.* International Clinical Psychopharmacology, 2001. **16**(5): pp. 279–284.
93. Davidson, J.R., et al., *Mirtazapine vs. placebo in posttraumatic stress disorder: A pilot trial.* Biological Psychiatry, 2003. **53**(2): pp. 188–191.
94. Bahk, W.-M., et al., *Effects of mirtazapine in patients with post-traumatic stress disorder in Korea: A pilot study.* Human Psychopharmacology: Clinical and Experimental, 2002. **17**(7): pp. 341–344.
95. Kim, W., et al., *The effectiveness of mirtazapine in the treatment of post-traumatic stress disorder: a 24-week continuation therapy.* Psychiatry and Clinical Neurosciences, 2005. **59**(6): pp. 743–747.
96. Vaishnavi, S., et al., *A comparison of the SPRINT and CAPS assessment scales for posttraumatic stress disorder.* Depression & Anxiety, 2006. **23**(7): pp. 437–40.
97. Davidson, J.R., H.M. Tharwani, and K.M. Connor, *Davidson Trauma Scale (DTS): normative scores in the general population and effect sizes in placebo-controlled SSRI trials.* Depression & Anxiety, 2002. **15**(2): pp. 75–8.
98. Foa, E.B., et al., *The validation of a self-report measure of posttraumatic stress disorder: The Posttraumatic Diagnostic Scale.* Psychological Assessment, 1997. **9**(4): pp. 445–451.
99. Connor, K.M., et al., *Development of a new resilience scale: the Connor-Davidson Resilience Scale (CD-RISC).* Depression & Anxiety, 2003. **18**(2): pp. 76–82.

Panic Disorder Severity Scale

General Instructions for Raters

The goal is to obtain a measure of overall severity of DSM-IV symptoms of panic disorder, with or without agoraphobia. Ratings are generally made for the past month, to allow for a stable estimation of panic frequency and severity. Users may choose a different time frame, but time frame should be consistent for all items.

Each item is rated from 0 to 4, where 0 = none or not present; 1 = mild, occasional symptoms, slight interference; 2 = moderate, frequent symptoms, some interference with functioning, but still manageable; 3 = severe, preoccupying symptoms, substantial interference in functioning, and 4 = extreme, pervasive near constant symptoms, disabling/incapacitating.

A suggested script is provided as a guide to questioning, but is not essential. Probes should be used freely to clarify ratings. As an overall caution, please note that this not an observer administered self-rating scale. The patient is not asked to rate a symptom as "mild, moderate or severe." Rather the symptom is explored and rated by the interviewer. However, to clarify a boundary between two severity levels, it is appropriate to utilize the descriptors above. For example, the interviewer might ask the patient whether it is more accurate to describe a given symptom as occurring "frequently, with definite interference but still manageable," or if it is "preoccupying, with substantial interference." Similarly, it may be appropriate to ask whether a symptom is "preoccupying, with substantial interference," or "pervasive, near constant, and incapacitating."

In rating items 6 and 7, the interviewer should be alert to inconsistencies. For example, sometimes a subject will describe a symptom from items 1 to 5 as causing substantial impairment in functioning, but then will report that overall panic disorders symptoms cause only mild or moderate work and social impairment. This should be pointed out and clarified.

There are some types of anxiety, common in panic disorder patients, but not rated by this instrument. Anticipatory anxiety about situations feared for reasons other than panic (e.g., related to a specific phobia or social phobia) is not considered panic-related anticipatory anxiety and is not rated by this instrument. Similarly, generalized anxiety is not rated by this instrument. The concerns of someone experiencing generalized anxiety are focused on the probability of adverse events in the future. Such worries often include serious health problems in oneself or a loved one, financial ruin, job loss, or other possible calamitous outcomes of daily life problems.

1. Panic Attack Frequency, Including Limited Symptom Episodes

Begin by explaining to the patient that we define a *Panic Attack* as a feeling of fear or apprehension that begins suddenly and builds rapidly in intensity, usually reaching a peak in less than 10 min. This feeling is associated with uncomfortable physical sensations like racing or pounding heart, shortness of breath, choking, dizziness, sweating, trembling. Often there are distressing, catastrophic thoughts such as fear of losing control, having heart attack or dying. A **Limited Symptom Episode (LSE)** is similar to a full panic attack, but has fewer than 4 symptoms. Given these definitions, please tell me

Q: In the past month, how many full panic attacks did you experience, the kind with 4 or more symptoms? How about limited symptom episodes, the kind with less than 4 symptoms? On average, did you have more than one limited symptom episode/day? (*Calculate weekly frequencies by dividing the total number of full panic attacks over the rating interval by the number of weeks in the rating interval.*)

0 = No panic or limited symptom episodes.
1 = Mild, less than an average of one full panic a week, and no more than 1 limited symptom episode/day.
2 = Moderate, one or two full panic attacks a week, and/or multiple limited symptom episode/day.
3 = Severe, more than 2 full attacks/week, but not more than 1/day on average.
4 = Extreme, full panic attacks occur more than once a day, more days than not.

2. Distress During Panic Attacks, Include Limited Symptom Episodes

Q: Over the past month, when you had panic or limited symptom attacks, how much distress did they cause you? I am asking you now about the distress you felt during the attack itself.

(This item rates the average degree of distress and discomfort the patient experienced during panic attacks experienced over the rating interval. Limited symptom episodes should be rated only if they caused more distress than full panic. Be sure to distinguish between distress DURING panic and anticipatory fear that an attack will occur.)

Possible further probes: How upset or fearful did you feel during the attacks? Were you able to continue doing what you were doing when panic occurred? Did you lose your concentration? If you had to stop what you were doing, were you able to stay in the situation where the attack occurred or did you have leave?

0 = No panic attacks or limited symptoms episodes, or no distress during episodes.
1 = Mild distress but able to continue activity with little or no interference.
2 = Moderate distress, but still manageable, able to continue activity and/or maintain concentration, but does so with difficulty.
3 = Severe, marked distress and interference, loses concentration, loses concentration and/or must stop activity, but able to remain in the room or situation.
4 = Extreme, severe and disabling distress, must stop activity, will leave the room or situation if possible, otherwise remains, unable to concentrate, with extreme distress.

3. Severity of Anticipatory Anxiety (panic-related fear, apprehension or worry)

Q: Over the past month, on average, how much did you worry, feel fearful or apprehensive about when your next panic would occur or about what panic attacks might mean about your physical or mental health? I am asking about times you were not actually having a panic attack.

(Anticipatory anxiety can be related to the meaning of the attacks rather than having an attack, so there can be considerable anxiety about having an attack even if the distress during the attack was low. Remember that sometimes a patient does not worry about when the next attack will occur, but instead worries about the meaning of the attacks for his or her physical or mental health.)

Possible further probes: How intense was your anxiety? How often did you have these worries or fears? Did the anxiety get to the point where it interfered with your life? IF SO, How much did it interfere?

0 = No concern about panic.
1 = Mild, there is occasional fear, worry or apprehension about panic.
2 = Moderate, often worried, fearful or apprehensive, but has periods without anxiety. There is a noticeable modification of lifestyle, but anxiety is still manageable and overall functioning is not impaired.

3 = Severe, preoccupied with fear, worry or apprehension about panic, substantial interference with concentration and/or ability to function effectively.

4 = Extreme, near constant and disabling anxiety, unable to carry out important task because of fear, worry or apprehension about panic.

4. Agoraphobic Fear/Avoidance

Q: Over the past month, were there places where you felt afraid, or that you avoided, because you thought if you had a panic attack, it could be difficult to get help or to easily leave?

Possible further probes: Situations like using public transportation, driving in a car, being in a tunnel or a bridge, going to the movies, to a mall or supermarket, or being in other crowded places? Anywhere else? Were you afraid of being at home alone or completely alone in other places? How often did you experience fear of these situations? How intense was the fear? Did you avoid any of those situations? Did having a trusted companion with you make a difference? Were there things you would do with a companion that you would not do alone? How much did the fear and/or avoidance affect your life? Did you need to change your lifestyle to accommodate your fears?

0 = None, no fear or avoidance.

1 = Mild, occasional fear and/or avoidance, but will usually confront or endure the situation. There is little or no modification of lifestyle.

2 = Moderate, noticeable fear and/or avoidance, but still manageable, avoids feared situations but can confront with a companion. There is some modification of lifestyle, but overall functioning is not impaired.

3 = Severe, extensive avoidance; substantial modification of lifestyle is required to accommodate phobia, making it difficult to manage usual activities.

4 = Extreme pervasive disabling fear and/or avoidance. Extensive modification in lifestyle is required such that important tasks are not performed.

5. Panic-Related Sensation Fear/Avoidance

Q: Sometimes people with panic disorder experience physical sensations that may be reminiscent of panic and cause them to feel frightened or uncomfortable. Over the past month, did you avoid doing anything because you thought it would cause this kind of uncomfortable physical sensation?

Possible further probes: For example, things that made your heart beat rapidly, such as strenuous exercise or walking? Playing sports? Working in the garden? What about exciting sports events, frightening movies or having an argument? Sexual activity or orgasm? Did you fear or avoid sensations on your skin such as heat or tingling? Sensations of feeling dizzy or out of breath? Did you avoid any food, drink or other substance because it might bring on physical sensations, such as coffee or alcohol or medications like cold medication? How much did the avoidance situations or activities like these affect your life? Did you need to change your lifestyle to accommodate your fears?

0 = No fear or avoidance of situations or activities that provoke distressing physical sensations.

1 = Mild, occasional fear and/or avoidance, but usually will confront or endure with little distress activities and situations which provoke physical sensations. There is little modification of lifestyle.

2 = Moderate, noticeable avoidance, but still manageable, there is definite, but limited modification of lifestyle, such that overall functioning not impaired.

3 = Severe, extensive avoidance, causes substantial modification of lifestyle or interference in functioning.

4 = Extreme pervasive and disabling avoidance. Extensive modification in lifestyle is required such that important tasks or activities are not performed.

6. **Impairment/Interference in Work Functioning Due to Panic Disorder**

(*Note to raters: This item focuses on work. If the person is not working, ask about school, and if not in school full time, ask about household responsibilities.*)

Q: Over the past month, considering all the symptoms, the panic attacks, limited symptom episodes, anticipatory anxiety and phobic symptoms, how much did your panic disorder interfere with your ability to do your job (or your schoolwork or carry out responsibilities at home)?

Possible further probes: Did the symptoms affect the quality of your work? Were you able to get things done as quickly and effectively as usual? Did you notice things you were not doing because of your anxiety, or things you couldn't do as well? Did you take shortcuts or request assistance to get things done? Did you or anyone else notice a change in your performance? Was there a formal performance review or warning about work performance? Any comments from coworkers or from family members about your work?

0 = No impairment from panic disorder symptoms.

1 = Mild, slight interference, feels job is harder to do but performance is still good.

2 = Moderate, symptoms cause regular, definite interference but still manageable. Job performance has suffered but others would say work is still adequate.

3 = Severe, causes substantial impairment in occupational performance, such that others have noticed, may be missing work or unable to perform at all on some days.

4 = Extreme, incapacitating symptoms, unable to work (or go to school or carry out household responsibilities).

7. **Impairment/Interference in Social Functioning Due to Panic Disorder**

Q: Over the past month, considering all the panic disorder symptoms together, how much did they interfere with your social life?

Possible further probes: Did you spend less time with family or other relatives than you used to? Did you spend less time with friends? Did you turn down opportunities to social-ize because of panic disorder? Did you have restrictions about where or how long you would socialize because of panic disorder? Did the panic disorder symptoms affect your relationships with family members or friends?

0 = No impairment.

1 = Mild, slight interference, feels quality of social behavior is somewhat impaired but social functioning is still adequate.

2 = Moderate, definite, interference with social life but still manageable. There is some decrease in frequency of social activities and/or quality of interpersonal interactions but still able to engage in most usual social activities.

3 = Severe, cause substantial impairment in social performance. There is marked decrease in social activities, and/or marked difficulty interacting with others; can still force self to interact with others, but does not enjoy or function well in most social or interpersonal situations.

4 = Extreme, disabling symptoms, rarely goes out or interacts with others, may have ended a relationship because of panic disorder.

Total Score (sum of items 1–7):_____

Liebowitz Social Anxiety Scale

Instructions: The clinician should rate each item with 0 (none), 1 (mild), 2 (moderate) or 3 (severe) based upon the patient's actual experience of the past week. Each item should be given only one score for fear and one score for avoidance. If the patient did not enter the feared situation in the past week, rate the item according to what would have been the patient's level of fear if the feared situation was encountered and would the patient have avoided it.

Fear or Anxiety Scoring Key:	Avoidance Scoring Key:
0 = None	0 = Never (0% of the time)
1 = Mild	1 = Occasionally (1–33% of the time)
2 = Moderate	2 = Often (33–67% of the time)
3 = Severe	3 = Usually (67–100% of the time)

	Fear or Anxiety	Avoidance
1. Telephoning in public (P)		
2. Participating in small groups (P)		
3. Eating in public places (P)		
4. Drinking with others in public places (P)		
5. Talking to people in authority (S)		
6. Acting, performing or giving a talk in front of audience (P)		
7. Going to party (S)		
8. Working while being observed (P)		
9. Writing while being observed (P)		
10. Calling someone you don't know very well (S)		
11. Talking with people you don't know very well (S)		
12. Meeting strangers (S)		
13. Urinating in a public bathroom (P)		
14. Entering a room when others are already seated (P)		
15. Being the center of attention (P)		
16. Speaking up at a meeting (P)		
17. Taking a test (P)		
18. Expressing a disagreement or disapproval to people you don't know very well (S)		
19. Looking at people you don't know very well in the eyes (S)		
20. Giving a report to a group (P)		
21. Trying to pick up someone (P)		
22. Returning goods to a store (S)		
23. Giving a party (S)		
24. Resisting a high pressure salesperson (S)		

Performance (P) Anxiety subscore: [Add all (P) scores]: _____   Avoidance (Ps) _____

Social (S) Anxiety subscore: [Add all (S) scores]: _____   Avoidance (Ss) _____

Total Anxiety (P + S):   _____
Total Avoidance (P + S): _____

Hamilton Anxiety Rating Scale (HAM-A)

> **Scoring Key: 0 = none; 1 = mild; 2 = moderate; 3 = severe; 4 = very severe, grossly disabling**

1. Anxious Mood	Worries, anticipation of the worst apprehension (fearful anticipation) irritability	0 1 2 3 4
2. Tension	Feelings of tension, fatigability, inability to relax, startle response, moved to tears easily, trembling, feelings of restlessness	0 1 2 3 4
3. Fears	Of dark, strangers, being left alone, large animals, traffic, crowds	0 1 2 3 4
4. Insomnia	Difficulty in falling asleep, broken sleep, unsatisfying sleep and fatigue on waking, dreams, nightmares, night terrors	0 1 2 3 4
5. Intellectual (Cognitive)	Difficulty in concentration, poor memory	0 1 2 3 4
6. Depressed Mood	Loss of interest, lack of pleasure in hobbies, depression, early waking, diurnal swing	0 1 2 3 4
7. General Somatic (Muscular)	Muscular pains and aches, muscular stiffness, muscular twitching, clonic jerks, grinding of teeth, unsteady voice	0 1 2 3 4
8. General Somatic (Sensory)	Tinnitus, blurring of vision, hot and cold flushes, feelings of weakness, pricking sensations	0 1 2 3 4
9. Cardiovascular Symptoms	Tachycardia, palpitations, pain in chest, throbbing of vessels, fainting feelings, missing beat	0 1 2 3 4
10. Respiratory Symptoms	Pressure or constriction in chest, choking feelings, sighing, dyspnea	0 1 2 3 4
11. Gastrointestinal Symptoms	Difficulty in swallowing, wind, dyspepsia, pain before and after meals, burning sensations, fullness, waterbrash, nausea, vomiting, sinking feelings, "working" in the abdomen, borborygmi, looseness of bowels, loss of weight, constipation	0 1 2 3 4
12. Genito-Urinary	Frequency of micturition, urgency of micturition, amenorrhea, menorrhagia, development of frigidity, premature ejaculation, loss of erection, impotence	0 1 2 3 4
13. Autonomic Symptoms	Dry mouth, flushing, pallor, tendency to sweat, giddiness, tension headache, raising of hair	0 1 2 3 4

Total Score (sum of circled responses): _____

Y-BOCS Symptom Checklist

Instructions: Check all that apply, but clearly mark the principal symptoms with a "P." (Rater must ascertain whether reported behaviors are bona fide symptoms of OCD, and not symptoms of another disorder such as simple phobia or hypochondriasis. Items marked "∗" may or may not be OCD phenomena.)_____

————————————————*Obsessions*————————————————

Current	Past	
		Aggressive Obsessions
_____	_____	Fear might harm self
_____	_____	Fear might harm others
_____	_____	Violent or horrific images
_____	_____	Fear of blurting out obscenities or insults
_____	_____	Fear of doing something else embarrassing∗
_____	_____	Fear will act on unwanted impulses (e.g., to stab friend)
_____	_____	Fear will steal things
_____	_____	Fear will harm others because not careful enough (e.g., hit/run MVA)
_____	_____	Fear will be responsible for something else terrible happening (e.g., fire, burglary)
_____	_____	Other

Current	Past	
		Contamination Obsessions
_____	_____	Concerns or disgust with bodily waste or secretions (e.g., urine, feces, saliva)
_____	_____	Concern with dirt or germs
_____	_____	Excessive concerns with environmental contaminants (e.g., asbetios, radiations, toxic waste)
_____	_____	Excessively concerned with animals or insects
_____	_____	Bothered by sticky substances or residues
_____	_____	Concerned will get ill because of contamination
_____	_____	Concerned will get others ill because of contamination
_____	_____	Concerned will get others ill because of spreading contamination (aggressive)
_____	_____	No concern with consequences of contamination other than how it might feel
_____	_____	Other

Current	Past	
		Sexual Obsessions
_____	_____	Forbidden or perverse sexual thoughts or images
_____	_____	Content involves children or incest
_____	_____	Content involveshomosexuality∗
_____	_____	Sexual behavior towards others (aggressive)∗
		Other

_____   _____   Hoarding/Saving Obsessions
                      (distinguish from hobbies and concern with objects
                      of monetary or sentimental value)

                      Religious Obsessions (scrupulosity)
_____   _____   Concerned with sacrilege and blasphemy
_____   _____   Excess concern with right/wrong, morality
_____   _____   Other _____

                      Obsession with Need for Symmetry or Exactness
_____   _____   Accompanied by magical thinking (e.g., concerned that mother
                      will have accident unless things are in the right place)
_____   _____   Not accompanied by magical thinking

                      Miscellaneous Obsessions
_____   _____   Need to know or remember
_____   _____   Fear of saying certain things
_____   _____   Fear of not saying just the right thing
_____   _____   Fear of losing things
_____   _____   Intrusive (non-violent) images
_____   _____   Intrusive nonsense sounds, words, or music
_____   _____   Bothered by certain sounds/noises*
_____   _____   Lucky/unlucky numbers
_____   _____   Colors with special significance
_____   _____   Superstitious fears
_____   _____   Other _____

                      Somatic Obsessions
_____   _____   Concern with illness or disease*
_____   _____   Excessive concern with body part or aspect of appearance
                      (e.g. dysmorphophobia)*
_____   _____   Other _____

—————————————————Compulsions—————————————

Current	Past	
		Cleaning/Washing Compulsions
_____	_____	Excessive or ritualized hand-washing
_____	_____	Excessive or ritualized showering, bathing, tooth-brushing, grooming, or toilet routines
_____	_____	Involves cleaning of household items or other inanimate objects excessively
_____	_____	Other measures to prevent or remove contact with contaminants
_____	_____	Other _____

Current	Past	
		Cleaning/Washing Compulsions
_____	_____	Checking locks, stove, appliances, etc.
_____	_____	Checking that did not/will not harm others
_____	_____	Checking that did not/will not harm self
_____	_____	Checking that nothing terrible did/will happen
_____	_____	Checking that did not make mistake
_____	_____	Checking tied to somatic obsessions
_____	_____	Other

Current	Past	
		Repeating Rituals
_____	_____	Re-reading or re-writing
_____	_____	Need to repeat routine activities (e.g., in/out doors, up/down from chair)
_____	_____	Other

Current	Past	
		Counting Compulsions
_____	_____	
		Ordering/Arranging Compulsions
_____	_____	

Current	Past	
		Hoarding/Collecting Compulsions
		[distinguish from hobbies and concern with objects of monetary or sentimental value (e.g., carefully reads junkmail, piles up newspapers, sorts through garbage, collects useless objects)]
_____	_____	

		Miscellaneous Compulsions
_____	_____	Mental rituals (other than checking/counting)
_____	_____	Excessive list-making
_____	_____	Need to tell, ask, or confess
_____	_____	Need to touch, tap, or rub*
_____	_____	Rituals involving blinking or staring*
_____	_____	Measures (not checking) to prevent: Harm to self ___; harm to others ___; terrible consequences ____
_____	_____	Ritualized eating behaviors*
_____	_____	Superstitious behaviors
_____	_____	Trichotillomania*
_____	_____	Other self-damaging or self-mutilating behaviors*
_____	_____	Other

Target Symptom List
Obsessions

1._____

2._____

3._____

Compulsions

1._____

2._____

3._____

Avoidance

1._____

2._____

3._____

Yale-Brown Obsessive Compulsive Scale (Y-BOCS)

> **Instructions:** "I am now going to ask several questions about your obsessive thoughts." [Make specific reference to the patient's target obsessions from the YBOCS checklist.]

1. **Time Occupied by Obsessive Thoughts**: "How much of your time is occupied by obsessive thoughts?"
   - 0 - None.
   - 1 - Mild, less than 1 hr/day or occasional intrusions.
   - 2 - Moderate, 1–3 hrs/day or frequent intrusions.
   - 3 - Severe, greater than 3 and up to 8 hrs/day or very frequently.
   - 4 - Extreme, greater than 8 hrs/day or near constant intrusion.

2. **Interference Due to Obsessive Thoughts**: "How much do your obsessive thoughts interfere with your social or work (or role) functioning? Is there anything that you don't do because of them?"
   - 0 - None.
   - 1 - Mild, slight interference with social or occupational activities, but overall performance not impaired.
   - 2 - Moderate, definite interference with social or occupational performance, but still manageable.
   - 3 - Severe, causes substantial impairment in social or occupational performance.
   - 4 - Extreme, incapacitating.

3. **Distress Associated with Obsessive Thoughts:** "How much distress do your obsessive thoughts cause you?"
   - 0 - None.
   - 1 - Mild, not too disturbing.
   - 2 - Moderate, disturbing, but still manageable.
   - 3 - Severe, very disturbing.
   - 4 - Extreme, near constant and disabling distress.

4. **Resistance Against Obsessions:** "How much of an effort do you make to resist the obsessive thoughts? How often do you try to disregard or turn your attention away from these thoughts as they enter your mind?"
   - 0 - Makes an effort to always resist, or symptoms so minimal doesn't need to actively resist.
   - 1 - Tries to resist most of the time.
   - 2 - Makes some effort to resist.
   - 3 - Yields to all obsessions without attempting to control them, but does so with some reluctance.
   - 4 - Completely and willingly yields to all obsessions.

5. **Degree of Control over Obsessive Thoughts:** "How much control do you have over your obsessive thoughts? How successful are you in stopping or diverting your obsessive thoughts? Can you dismiss them?"
   - 0 - Complete control.
   - 1 - Much control, usually able to stop or divert obsessions with some effort and concentration.
   - 2 - Moderate control, sometimes able to stop or divert obsessions.

3 - Little control, rarely successful in stopping or dismissing obsessions, can only divert attention with difficulty.

4 - No control, experienced as completely involuntary, rarely able to even momentarily.

> "The next several questions are about your compulsive behaviors." [Make specific reference to the patient's target compulsions from YBOCS Checklist.]

6. **Time Spent Performing Compulsive Behaviors:** "How much time do you spend performing compulsive behaviors?"

0 - None.

1 - Mild (spends less than 1 hr/day performing compulsions) or occasional performance of compulsive behaviors.

2 - Moderate (spends from 1 to 3 hrs/day performing compulsions) or frequent performance of compulsive behaviors.

3 - Severe (spends more than 3 and up to 8 hrs/day performing compulsions) or very frequent performance of compulsive behaviors.

4 - Extreme (spends more than 8 hrs/day performing compulsions) or near constant performance of compulsive behaviors (too numerous to count).

7. **Interference Due to Compulsive Behaviors:** "How much do your compulsive behaviors interfere with your social or work (or role) functioning? Is there anything that you don't do because of your compulsions?"

0 - None.

1 - Mild, slight interference with social or occupational activities, but overall performance not impaired.

2 - Moderate, definite interference with social or occupational performance, but still manageable.

3 - Severe, causes substantial impairment in social or occupational performance.

4 - Extreme, incapacitating.

8. **Distress Associated with Compulsive Behavior:** "How much of an effort do you make to resist the compulsion(s)? [Pause] How anxious would you become?"

0 - None.

1 - Mild only slightly anxious if compulsions prevented, or only slight anxiety during performance of compulsions.

2 - Moderate, reports that anxiety would mount but remain manageable if compulsions prevented, or that anxiety increases but remains manageable during the performance of compulsions.

3 - Severe, prominent and very disturbing increase in anxiety if compulsions interrupted, or prominent and very disturbing increase in anxiety during performance of compulsions.

4 - Extreme, incapacitating anxiety from any intervention aimed at modifying activity, or incapacitating anxiety develops during performance of compulsions.

9. **Resistance Against Compulsions:** "How much of an effort do you make to resist the compulsions?"

0 - Makes an effort to always resist, or symptoms so minimal doesn't need to actively resist

1 - Tries to resist most of the time

2 - Makes some effort to resist

3 - Yields to all compulsions without attempting to control them, but does so with some reluctance

4 - Completely and willingly yields to all compulsions

10. **Degree of Control over Compulsive Behavior:** "How strong is the drive to perform the compulsive behavior? [Pause] How much control do you have over the compulsions?"

   0 -   Complete control.
   1 -   Much control, experiences pressure to perform the behavior but usually able to exercise voluntary control over it.
   2 -   Moderate control, strong pressure to perform behavior, can control it only with difficulty.
   3 -   Little control, very strong drive to perform behavior, must be carried to completion, can only delay with difficulty.
   4 -   No control, drive to perform behavior experiences as completely involuntary, rarely able to even momentarily delay activity.

   Total Score (total of circled responses): _____

YBOCS Detailed Scoring Instructions

1. Time Occupied by Obsessive Thoughts

   Q: How much of your time is occupied by obsessive thoughts? [When obsessions occur as brief, intermittent intrusions, it may be difficult to assess time occupied by them in terms of total hours. In such cases, estimate time by determining how frequently they occur. Consider both the number of times the intrusions occur and how many hours of the day are affected. Ask:] How frequently do the obsessive thoughts occur? [Be sure to exclude ruminations and preoccupations which, unlike obsessions, are ego-syntonic and rational (but exaggerated).]

1b. Obsession-Free Interval (not included in total score)

   Q: On the average, what is the longest number of consecutive waking hours per day that you are completely free of obsessive thoughts? [If necessary, ask:] What is the longest block of time in which obsessive thoughts are absent?

   0 = No symptoms.
   1 = Long symptom-free interval, more than 8 consecutive hours/day symptom free.
   2 = Moderately long symptom-free interval, more than 3 and up to 8 consecutive hours/day symptom free.
   3 = Short symptom-free interval, from 1 to 3 consecutive hours/day symptom free.
   4 = Extremely short symptom-free interval, less than 1 consecutive hour/day symptom free.

2. Interference Due to Obsessive Thoughts

   Q: How much do your obsessive thoughts interfere with your social or work (or role) functioning? Is there anything that you don't do because of them? [If currently not working determine how much performance would be affected if patient were employed.]

3. Distress Associated with Obsessive Thoughts

   Q: How much distress do your obsessive thoughts cause you? [In most cases, distress is equated with anxiety; however, patients may report that their obsessions are "disturbing" but deny anxiety." Only rate anxiety that seems triggered by obsessions, not generalized anxiety or anxiety associated with other conditions]

4. Resistance Against Obsessions

   Q: How much of an effort do you make to resist the obsessive thoughts? How often do you try to disregard or turn your attention away from these thoughts as they enter your mind? [Only rate effort made to resist, not success or failure in actually controlling the obsessions. How much the patient resists the obsessions may or may not correlate with his/her ability to control them. Note that this item does not directly measure the severity of the intrusive thoughts; rather it rates a manifestation of health, i.e., the effort that patient makes to counteract the obsessions by means other than avoidance or the performance of compulsions. Thus, the more the patient tries to resist, the less impaired is this aspect of his/her functioning. There are "active" and "passive" forms of resistance. Patients in behavioral therapy may be encouraged to counteract their obsessive symptoms by not struggling against them (e.g., "just let the thoughts come"; passive opposition) or by intentionally bringing on the disturbing thoughts. For the purpose of this item, consider use of these behavioral techniques as forms of resistance. If the obsessions are minimal, the patient may not feel the need to resist them. In such cases, a rating of "0" should be given.]

5. Degree of Control over Obsessive Thoughts

   Q: How much control do you have over your obsessive thoughts? How successful are you in stopping or diverting your obsessive thoughts? Can you dismiss them? [In contrast to the proceeding item on resistance, the ability of the patient to control his obsessions is more closely related to the severity of the intrusive thoughts.]

6. Time Spent Performing Compulsive Behaviors

Q: How much time do you spend performing compulsive behaviors? [When rituals involving activities of daily living are chiefly present, ask:] How much longer than most people does it take to complete routine activities because of your rituals? [When compulsions occur as brief, intermittent behaviors, it may be difficult to assess time spent performing them in terms of total hours. In such cases, estimate time by determining how frequently they are performed. Consider the number of times compulsions are performed and how many hours of the day are affected. Count separate occurrences of compulsive behaviors, not number of repetitions; e.g., a patient who goes into the bathroom 20 different times a day to wash his hands 5 times very quickly, performs compulsions 20 times a day, not 5 or 5 x 20 = 100 Ask:] How frequently do you perform compulsions? [In most cases, compulsions are observable behaviors (e.g., hand washing), but some compulsions are covert (e.g., silent checking).]

6b. Compulsion-Free Interval (not included in total score)

Q: On average, what is the longest number of consecutive waking hours per day that you are completely free of compulsive behavior? [If necessary, ask:] What is the longest block of time in which compulsions are absent?

0 = No symptoms.
1 = Long symptom-free interval, more than 8 consecutive hours/day symptom free.
2 = Moderately long symptom-free interval, more than 3 and up to 8 consecutive hours/day symptom free.
3 = Short symptom-free interval, from 1 to 3 consecutive hours/day symptom free.
4 = Extremely short symptom-free interval, less than 1 consecutive hour/day symptom free.

7. Interference Due to Compulsive Behaviors

Q: How much do your compulsive behaviors interfere with your social or work (or role) functioning? Is there anything that you don't do because of your compulsions? [If currently not working determine how much performance would be affected if patient were employed.]

8. Distress Associated with Compulsive Behavior

Q: How much of an effort do you make to resist the compulsion(s)? [Pause] How anxious would you become? [Rate degree of distress patients would experience if performance of the compulsions were suddenly interrupted without reassurance offered. In most, but not all cases, performing compulsions reduces anxiety. If, in the judgment of the interviewer, anxiety is actually reduced by preventing compulsions in the manner described above, then ask:] How anxious do you get while performing compulsions until you are satisfied they are completed?

9. Resistance Against Compulsions

Q: How much of an effort do you make to resist the compulsions? [Only rate effort made to resist, not success or failure in actually controlling the compulsions. How much the patient resists the compulsions may or may not correlate with his ability to control them. Note that this item does not directly measure the severity of the compulsions; rather it rates a manifestation of health, i.e., the effort that patient makes to counteract the compulsions. Thus, the more the patient tries to resist, the less impaired is this aspect of his functioning. If the compulsions are minimal, the patient may not feel the need to resist them. In such cases, a rating of "0" should be given.]

10. Degree of Control over Compulsive Behavior

Q: How strong is the drive to perform the compulsive behavior? [Pause] How much control do you have over the compulsions? [In contrast to the proceeding item on resistance, the ability of the patient to control his compulsions is more closely related to the severity of the compulsions.]

Short PTSD Rating Scale

Identify the relevant trauma:

In the past week……	Not at all 0	A little bit 1	Moderately 2	Quite a lot 3	Very much 4
1 How much have you been bothered by unwanted memories, nightmares or reminders of the event?	☐	☐	☐	☐	☐
2 How much effort have you made to avoid thinking or talking about the event, or doing things which remind you of what happened?	☐	☐	☐	☐	☐
3 To what extent have you lost enjoyment for things, kept your distance from people, or found it difficult to experience feelings?	☐	☐	☐	☐	☐
4 How much have you been bothered by poor sleep, poor concentration, jumpiness, irritability or feeling watchful around you?	☐	☐	☐	☐	☐
5 How much have you been bothered by pain, aches, or tiredness?					
6 How much would you get upset when stressful events or setbacks happen to you?	☐	☐	☐	☐	☐
7 How much have the above symptoms interfered with your ability to work or carry out daily activities?	☐	☐	☐	☐	☐
8 How much have the above symptoms interfered with your relationships with family or friends?	☐	☐	☐	☐	☐

Total _____

9   How much better do you feel since beginning treatment? (as a percentage)

0   50   100

No change   As well as I could be

	Worse 5	No change 4	Minimally 3	Much 2	Very much 1
10 How much have the above symptoms improved since starting treatment?	☐	☐	☐	☐	☐

Total Score: _____

Total Score: _____

Chapter 4
Rating Scales for Bipolar Disorder

Roy H. Perlis

Abstract Patients with bipolar disorder may experience both manic and depressive symptoms which fluctuate over time, so appropriate monitoring includes assessment of both sets of symptoms. As these symptoms may persist even in the absence of a DSM-IV-defined mood episode, tools for monitoring must be sensitive to milder or subthreshold symptoms. In addition, as patients commonly experience concomitant axis I disorders, particularly anxiety disorders, symptom monitoring should address these symptoms as well.

Keywords Bipolar disorder · Mania · Depression · Mood · Rating scales · Questionnaires · Assessment · Psychiatry

Patients with bipolar disorder experience mood episodes, typically recurrent, which may be depressive, hypomanic, manic, or mixed. The evaluation of the bipolar patient therefore entails assessment of both manic/hypomanic and depressive symptoms. When evaluating the bipolar patient, three aspects of the evolving understanding of bipolar disorder bear consideration: (1) Patients may experience depressive symptoms during apparent manic episodes (and vice versa), so assessment of *both* kinds of mood states is important at every visit. (2) Many bipolar patients experience significant residual symptoms (particularly depressive symptoms) between episodes, so assessment should be sensitive to these "subthreshold" symptoms as well as full-blown manic or depressive episodes. (3) While not considered central to the diagnosis of bipolar disorder, a majority of patients experience symptoms of anxiety and/or substance use disorders. Therefore, it is crucial that these symptoms also be identified and monitored (for further discussion of assessing anxiety see Chapter 3, and for substance use disorders see Chapter 5).

R.H. Perlis (✉)
Department of Psychiatry, Bipolar Disorder Program, Massachusetts General Hospital and Harvard Medical School, Boston, MA 02114, USA
e-mail: rperlis@partners.org

L. Baer, M.A. Blais (eds.), *Handbook of Clinical Rating Scales and Assessment in Psychiatry and Mental Health*, Current Clinical Psychiatry, DOI 10.1007/978-1-59745-387-5_4, © Humana Press, a part of Springer Science+Business Media, LLC 2010

Assessment of Depressive Symptoms in Bipolar Disorder

Whether depressive symptoms differ between individuals with bipolar disorder and major depressive disorder remains a much-debated topic [1]. While not all studies find this association, some have suggested that atypical depressive symptoms, particularly hypersomnia and hyperphagia, may be more commonly seen in bipolar depression. Thus, the fact that some depression scales do not assess reverse neurovegetative signs can be a limitation for monitoring patients who have these symptoms.

Regardless of which measure is utilized, systematic assessment of suicidal thoughts and behaviors at every clinical visit is key to the management of bipolar disorder, because patients have a significantly elevated lifetime suicide risk. All of the depression measures described below include similar questions relating to suicidality, though none are sufficient to fully characterize these symptoms when clinically indicated.

Gold Standard Scale: The Hamilton Depression Rating Scale 31-Item Version (HDRS-31)

The HDRS is a 17-item scale requiring 15–20 min to perform (see Chapter 2 for detailed description of HDRS) [2]. One of the most widely used depression rating scales, it was originally developed to assess depressive symptom severity among inpatients. Interestingly, the intent of its developer was that two interviewers would perform ratings at the same time, though this is rarely if ever the case. The original HDRS includes 17 items, each scored 0–2 or 0–4. Multiple structured interviews have been developed to enhance the HDRS' reliability (Williams 1988), for example: http://www.ids-qids.org/translations/english/SIGHD-IDSCEnglish-USA.pdf. As noted above, one limitation of the 17-item HDRS pertinent to its use with bipolar patient is the lack of questions assessing reverse neurovegetative symptoms such as hypersomnia and hyperphagia (a limitation remedied in the longer 28- and 31-item versions). We typically rely on patient self-report measures for depression, such as the IDS-SR or QIDS-SR [3] (see below), and do not routinely utilize the HDRS in clinical practice. However, a reasonable practice would be quarterly assessment of mood state using a clinician-rated measure such as the HDRS-31 (reproduced in the appendix to this chapter).

Other Scales Available

The Montgomery Asberg Depression Rating Scale

MADRS [4] is a 10-item scale requiring 15 min or less to perform; it was designed in part to be sensitive to change during medication treatment (see Chapter 2 for detailed description of MADRS). Each of 10 items is scored on a 0–6 scale, with anchors every two points; a structured interview can be used but is not required. Like the HDRS, the MADRS does not specifically capture hypersomnia and hyperphagia.

Multiple recent bipolar depression trials relied on the MADRS in part because the scale gives less weight to sleep items. Regardless of which measure is utilized, systematic assessment of suicidal thoughts and behaviors at every clinical visit is also key to the management of bipolar disorder, because patients have a significantly elevated lifetime suicide risk.

The Inventory of Depressive Symptomatology

The Inventory of Depressive Symptomatology [5] was developed to measure depressive symptoms, but with broader coverage than other depression scales, particularly for depressive subtypes such as atypical depression (see Chapter 2 for full description of the IDS and QIDS) [2]. The IDS contains 30 items, most but not all of which are scored 0–3. The maximum score on the IDS is an 84, because some items are not included in the score. Of note, the IDS addresses the role of atypical neurovegetative symptoms by scoring only the maximum sleep and appetite symptom. Many of us utilize a short self-report form of the IDS, the QIDS-SR, in routine practice, completed by patients in the waiting room at each visit.

While newer than the HAM-D or MADRS, the IDS is used increasingly in clinical trials, and the self-report version was used as a primary outcome measure in the multicenter STAR*D study [6]. Two aspects of the IDS make it particularly useful in a clinical context. First, a self-report form has been developed and shown to be valid. Second, a shorter (16-item) form was developed [3], including only those items from the 30-item form which appeared to be most important in capturing change.

Assessment of Manic or Mixed symptoms in Bipolar Disorder

Gold Standard Rating Scale: The Young Mania Rating Scale

Most, though not all, recent randomized controlled trials utilize the Young Mania Rating Scale [7] (reproduced in the appendix to this chapter). This 11-item scale was developed to monitor manic symptoms on inpatient units; most items are scored 0–4, while items assessing behavior, thought content, speech, and irritability are scored 0–8, yielding a total score between 0 and 60. Because some items assess symptoms that may be present to a modest degree among euthymic patients (increase in energy or libido, for example), a "normal" score is not necessarily 0. Strengths include clear anchor points, ease of use, and the availability of a structured interview (Sachs GS, unpublished). The YMRS requires around 15–20 min to administer. In addition, it has good coverage of the major domains of manic symptomatology, and includes one question examining psychosis. Importantly, the interviewer is expected to incorporate observation as well as patient's responses in arriving at a score.

The major limitation of the YMRS is that, while it is sensitive to change in clinical trials, it may not be particularly sensitive to milder (hypomanic) symptoms. Indeed, self-report measures such as the Internal State Scale [8] (reproduced in the appendix to this chapter) may be more sensitive to these symptoms than the YMRS [9].

Assessment of Psychosis in Bipolar Disorder

Rating scales for psychosis per se are not routinely used in outpatient practice. At minimum, clinical trials which include psychotic bipolar patients often utilize the items in the Young Mania Rating Scale and depression rating scales which relate to delusions and hallucination. For more extensive assessment of psychotic symptoms, the Brief Psychiatric Rating Scale (BPRS) can be useful, though this is rarely necessary in clinical practice. For further details of the assessment of psychotic symptoms, see Chapter 10.

Integrated Symptom Assessment in Bipolar Disorder

As an alternative or supplement to the use of rating scales, the multicenter Systematic Treatment Enhancement Program for Bipolar Disorder (STEP-BD) study utilized the Clinical Monitoring Form [10] (reproduced in the appendix to this chapter). This clinician-rated form inquires about percent of time with depressive and manic/hypomanic symptoms in the past 10 days or 2 weeks, as well as each of the DSM-IV criteria for mood episode. The mood criteria are scored on a 0–2 scale, with "1" considered threshold or syndromal. (Some items, such as sleep, are scored on a –2 to +2 range, with negative indicating decrease and positive indicating increase.) Clinicians are encouraged to utilize fractions where appropriate. Anchor points at each $\frac{1}{2}$-point have been developed. The CMF also includes space for recording medications, adverse effects, and common associated symptoms such as anxiety or panic.

Utilizing the CMF is akin to performing the (current) mood module of the SCID at each visit, though without the structured interview. The CMF may also be used to derive ratings for depression and mania/hypomania which correlate with rating scales such as the HAM-D and YMRS. A strength of this assessment is that it explicitly captures subsyndromal or subthreshold symptoms (e.g., by rating a "1/2") and ensures that DSM criteria for current mood state are assessed at each visit. A patient-rated "waiting room" form also exists (also reproduced in the appendix to this chapter) which may aid the clinician in completing the CMF. Limitations include a lack of data about sensitivity to change and relatively little study of the CMF's psychometric properties.

References

1. Perlis RH, Ostacher MJ, Patel JK, Marangell LB, Zhang H, Wisniewski SR, Ketter TA, Miklowitz DJ, Otto MW, Gyulai L, Reilly-Harrington NA, Nierenberg AA, Sachs GS, Thase ME: Predictors of recurrence in bipolar disorder: primary outcomes from the systematic treatment enhancement program for bipolar disorder (STEP-BD). Am J Psychiatry 2006; 163(2):217–24
2. Hamilton M: A rating scale for depression. J Neurol Neurosurg Psychiatry 1960; 23:56–62
3. Rush AJ, Trivedi MH, Ibrahim HM, Carmody TJ, Arnow B, Klein DN, Markowitz JC, Ninan PT, Kornstein S, Manber R, Thase ME, Kocsis JH, Keller MB: The 16-item quick inventory of depressive symptomatology (QIDS), clinician rating (QIDS-C), and self-report (QIDS-SR): a psychometric evaluation in patients with chronic major depression. Biol Psychiatry 2003; 54(5):573–83
4. Montgomery SA, Asberg M: A new depression scale designed to be sensitive to change. Br J Psychiatry 1979; 134:382–9
5. Rush AJ, Gullion CM, Basco MR, Jarrett RB, Trivedi MH: The inventory of depressive symptomatology (IDS): psychometric properties. Psychol Med 1996; 26(3):477–86
6. Rush AJ, Trivedi MH, Wisniewski SR, Nierenberg AA, Stewart JW, Warden D, Niederehe G, Thase ME, Lavori PW, Lebowitz BD, McGrath PJ, Rosenbaum JF, Sackeim HA, Kupfer DJ, Luther J, Fava M: Acute and longer-term outcomes in depressed outpatients requiring one or several treatment steps: a STAR*D report. Am J Psychiatry 2006; 163:1905–17.
7. Young RC, Biggs JT, Ziegler VE, Meyer DA: A rating scale for mania: reliability, validity and sensitivity. Br J Psychiatry 1978; 133:429–35
8. Mark S. Bauer, MD; Paul Crits-Christoph, PhD; William A. Ball, MD, PhD; Edward Dewees; Thomas McAllister, MD; Peter Alahi; John Cacciola, PhD; Peter C. Whybrow, MD: Independent Assessment of Manic and Depressive Symptoms by Self-rating: Scale Characteristics and Implications for the Study of Mania. Arch Gen Psychiatry. 1991; 48(9):807–812
9. Cooke RG, Kruger S, Shugar G: Comparative evaluation of two self-report mania rating scales. Biological Psychiatry 1996; 40(4):279–283
10. Sachs GS, Guille C, McMurrich SL: A clinical monitoring form for mood disorders. Bipolar Disord 2002; 4(5):323–7

Hamilton Depression Rating Scale 31-Item Version (HDRS-31)

Instructions: To rate the severity of depression in patients who are already diagnosed as depressed, administer this questionnaire. The higher the score, the more severe the depression.

For each item, circle the number next to the correct item. (Only one response per item.)

1. **Depressed Mood** (sadness, hopeless, helpless, worthless)
   - 0 - Absent
   - 1 - These feeling states indicated only on questioning
   - 2 - These feeling states spontaneously reported verbally
   - 3 - Communicates feeling states non-verbally – i.e., through facial expression, posture, voice, and tendency to weep
   - 4 - Patient reports VIRTUALLY ONLY these feeling states in his spontaneous verbal and non-verbal communication

2. **Feelings of Guilt**
   - 0 - Absent
   - 1 - Self reproach, feels he has let people down
   - 2 - Ideas of guilt or rumination over past errors or sinful deeds
   - 3 - Present illness is a punishment. Delusions of guilt
   - 4 - Hears accusatory or denunciatory voices and/or experiences threatening visual hallucinations

3. **Suicide**
   - 0 - Absent
   - 1 - Feels life is not worth living
   - 2 - Wishes he were dead or any thoughts of possible death to self
   - 3 - Suicidal ideas or gesture
   - 4 - Attempts at suicide (any serious attempt rates 4)

4. **Insomnia Early**
   - 0 - No difficulty falling asleep
   - 1 - Complains of occasional difficulty falling asleep – i.e., more than 1/2 hour
   - 2 - Complains of nightly difficulty falling asleep

5. **Insomnia Middle**
   - 0 - No difficulty
   - 1 - Patient complains of being restless and disturbed during the night
   - 2 - Waking during the night – any getting out of bed rates 2 (except for purposes of voiding)

6. **Insomnia Late**
   - 0 - No difficulty
   - 1 - Waking in early hours of the morning but goes back to sleep
   - 2 - Unable to fall asleep again if he gets out of bed

7. **Work and Activities**
   - 0 - No difficulty
   - 1 - Thoughts and feelings of incapacity, fatigue or weakness related to activities, work or hobbies
   - 2 - Loss of interest in activity, hobbies or work – either directly reported by patient, or indirect in listlessness, indecision and vacillation (feels he has to push self to work or activities)
   - 3 - Decrease in actual time spent in activities or decrease in productivity
   - 4 - Stopped working because of present illness

8. Retardation: Psychomotor (slowness of thought and speech; impaired ability to concentrate; decreased motor activity)

   0 - Normal speech and thought
   1 - Slight retardation at interview
   2 - Obvious retardation at interview
   3 - Interview difficult
   4 - Complete stupor

9. Agitation

   0 - None
   1 - Fidgetiness
   2 - Playing with hands, hair, etc.
   3 - Moving about, can't sit still
   4 - Hand wringing, nail biting, hair-pulling, biting of lips

10. Anxiety (psychological)

   0 - No difficulty
   1 - Subjective tension and irritability
   2 - Worrying about minor matters
   3 - Apprehensive attitude apparent in face or speech
   4 - Fears expressed without questioning

11. Anxiety Somatic: Physiological concomitants of anxiety (i.e., effects of autonomic overactivity, "butterflies," indigestion, stomach cramps, belching, diarrhea, palpitations, hyperventilation, paresthesia, sweating, flushing, tremor, headache, urinary frequency). Avoid asking about possible medication side effects (i.e., dry mouth, constipation)

   0 - Absent
   1 - Mild
   2 - Moderate
   3 - Severe
   4 - Incapacitating

12. Somatic Symptoms (gastrointestinal)

   0 - None
   1 - Loss of appetite but eating without encouragement from others. Food intake about normal
   2 - Difficulty eating without urging from others. Marked reduction of appetite and food intake

13. Somatic Symptoms General

   0 - None
   1 - Heaviness in limbs, back, or head. Backaches, headache, or muscle aches. Loss of energy and fatigability
   2 - Any clear-cut symptom rates "2"

14. Genital Symptoms (symptoms such as loss of libido, impaired sexual performance, menstrual disturbances)

   0 - Absent
   1 - Mild
   2 - Severe

15. Hypochondriasis

   0 - Not present
   1 - Self-absorption (bodily)
   2 - Preoccupation with health

3 - Frequent complaints, requests for help, etc.
4 - Hypochondriacal delusions

16. Loss of Weight
0 - No weight loss
1 - Probable weight loss associated with present illness
2 - Definite (according to patient) weight loss
3 - Not assessed

17. Insight
0 - Acknowledges being depressed and ill
1 - Acknowledges illness but attributes cause to bad food, climate, overwork, virus, need for rest, etc.
2 - Denies being ill at all

18. Diurnal Variation

A. Note whether symptoms are worse in morning or evening. If NO diurnal variation, mark none:
_____ no variation OR not currently depressed
_____ worse in A.M.
_____ worse in P.M.
B. When present, mark the severity of the variation:
0 - none
1 - mild
2 - severe

19. Depersonalization and Derealization (such as feelings of unreality and nihilistic ideas)
0 - Absent
1 - Mild
2 - Moderate
3 - Severe
4 - Incapacitating

20. Paranoid Symptoms
0 - None
1 - Suspicious
2 - Ideas of reference
3 - Delusions of reference and persecution

21. Obsessional and Compulsive Symptoms
0 - Absent
1 - Mild
2 - Severe

22. Hypersomnia – Early Bedtime
0 - No
1 - Mild, infrequent – less than 60 min
2 - Obvious/definite – more than 60 min earlier most nights

23. Hypersomnia – Oversleeping (sleeping more than usual)
0 - No
1 - Mild, infrequent – less than an hour
2 - Obvious/definite – oversleeps more than an hour, most days

24. Hypersomnia – Napping
   0 - Absent
   1 - Mild, infrequent – naps less than 30 min, or reports excessive daytime sleepiness
   2 - Obvious/definite – naps more than 30 min most days

25. Increased Appetite (change in appetite marked by increased food intake, or excessive cravings)
   0 - Absent
   1 - Minimal – light increase in appetite; food cravings
   2 - Definite – marked increase in food intake, or cravings

26. Weight Gain
   0 - Absent
   1 - Doubtful/minimal – less than one pound
   2 - Obvious, one pound or more weight gain

27. Psychic Retardation (slowness of speech and thought process: describes inhibition of will or feeling as if thought processes are paralyzed. Rate on basis of both observation and self-report but separate from actual motoric retardation)
   0 - Absent
   1 - Mild – slight slowing of speech, thought process
   2 - Moderate – delay in answering questions, describes volitional inhibition
   3 - Severe – slowness of speech and thought process sufficient to markedly prolong the interview
   4 - Extreme – nearly mute, minimally responsive

28. Motoric Retardation
   0 - Absent
   1 - Mild – slight flattening of affect, fixity of expression
   2 - Moderate – monotonous voice and decrease in spontaneous movements
   3 - Severe – obvious slowness of movement, gait; blunted affect
   4 - Extreme – stuporous; marked motoric retardation observed in gait and posture

29. Helplessness
   0 - Not present
   1 - Subjective feelings elicited only by inquiry
   2 - Patient volunteers helpless feelings
   3 - Requires urging, guidance, and reassurance to accomplish ward chores
   4 - Requires physical assistance for dress, grooming, eating, or personal hygiene

30. Hopelessness
   0 - Not present
   1 - Intermittently doubts that "things will improve" but can be reassured
   2 - Consistently feels "hopeless" but accepts reassurances
   3 - Expresses feelings of discouragement, despair, pessimism about future, which cannot be dispelled
   4 - Spontaneously and inappropriately perseverates, "I'll never get well" or its equivalent

31. Worthlessness
   0 - Not present
   1 - Indicates feelings of worthlessness (loss of self-esteem) only on questioning
   2 - Spontaneously indicates feelings of worthlessness
   3 - Different from (2) above by degree; patient volunteers that he/she is "no good," "inferior"
   4 - Delusional notions of worthlessness

   Total Score (total of circled responses): _____

Young Mania Rating Scale

Instructions: The purpose of each item is to rate the severity of that abnormality in the patient. When several keys are given for a particular grade of severity, the presence of only one is required to qualify for that rating.

The keys provided are guides. One can ignore the keys if that is necessary to indicate severity, although this should be the exception rather than the rule.

Scoring between the points given (whole or half points) is possible and encouraged after experience with the scale is acquired. This is particularly useful when severity of a particular item in a patient does not follow the progression indicated by the keys.

1. Elevated Mood

0 - Absent
1 - Mildly or possibly increased on questioning
2 - Definite subjective elevation; optimistic, self-confident; cheerful; appropriate to content
3 - Elevated; inappropriate to content; humorous
4 - Euphoric; inappropriate laughter; singing

2. Increased Motor Activity-Energy

0 - Absent
1 - Subjectively increased
2 - Animated; gestures increased
3 - Excessive energy; hyperactive at times; restless (can be calmed)
4 - Motor excitement; continuous hyperactivity (cannot be calmed)

3. Sexual Interest

0 - Normal; not increased
1 - Mildly or possibly increased
2 - Definite subjective increase on questioning
3 - Spontaneous sexual content; elaborates on sexual matters; hypersexual by self-report
4 - Overt sexual acts (toward patients, staff, or interviewer)

4. Sleep

0 - Reports no decrease in sleep
1 - Sleeping less than normal amount by up to one hour
2 - Sleeping less than normal by more than one hour
3 - Reports decreased need for sleep
4 - Denies need for sleep

5. Irritability

0 - Absent
2 - Subjectively increased
4 - Irritable at times during interview; recent episodes of anger or annoyance on ward
6 - Frequently irritable during interview; short, curt throughout
8 - Hostile, uncooperative; interview impossible

6. Speech (rate and amount)

0 - No increase
2 - Feels talkative
4 - Increased rate or amount at times, verbose at times
6 - Push; consistently increased rate and amount; difficult to interpret
8 - Pressured; uninterruptible, continuous speech

7. Language-Thought Disorder

- 0 - Absent
- 1 - Circumstantial
- 2 - Distractible, loses goal of thought; changes topics frequently; racing thoughts
- 3 - Flight of ideas; tangentiality; difficult to follow; rhyming, echolalia
- 4 - Incoherent; communication impossible

8. Content

- 0 - Normal
- 2 - Questionable plans, new interests
- 4 - Special project(s); hyper-religious
- 6 - Grandiose or paranoid ideas; ideas of reference

9. Disruptive-Aggressive Behavior

- 0 - Absent, cooperative
- 2 - Sarcastic; loud at times, guarded
- 4 - Demanding; threats on ward
- 6 - Threatens interviewer; shouting; interview difficult
- 8 - Assaultive; destructive; interview impossible

10. Appearance

- 0 - Appropriate dress and grooming
- 1 - Minimally unkempt
- 2 - Poorly groomed; moderately disheveled; overdressed
- 3 - Disheveled; partly clothed; garish make-up
- 4 - Completely unkempt; decorated; bizarre garb

11. Insight

- 0 - Present; admits illness; agrees with need for treatment
- 1 - Possibly ill
- 2 - Admits behavior change, but denies illness
- 3 - Admits possible change in behavior, but denies illness
- 4 - Denies any behavior change

Total Score (total of circled responses): _____

Internal State Scale (ISS)

Instructions: For each of the following statements, please mark an "X" at the point on the line that best describes the way you have felt *over the past 24 hours*. While there may have been some change during that time, try to give a single summary rating for each item.

	Not at all, rarely	Very much so, much of the time
1. Today my mood is changeable	0 ——————————————— 100	
2. Today I feel irritable	0 ——————————————— 100	
3. Today I feel like a capable person	0 ——————————————— 100	
4. Today I feel like people are out to get me	0 ——————————————— 100	
5. Today I actually feel great inside	0 ——————————————— 100	
6. Today I feel impulsive	0 ——————————————— 100	
7. Today I feel depressed	0 ——————————————— 100	
8. Today my thoughts are going fast	0 ——————————————— 100	
9. Today it seems like nothing will ever work out for me	0 ——————————————— 100	
10. Today I feel overactive	0 ——————————————— 100	
11. Today I feel as if the world is against me	0 ——————————————— 100	
13. Today I feel restless	0 ——————————————— 100	
14. Today I feel argumentative	0 ——————————————— 100	
15. Today I feel energized	0 ——————————————— 100	

Total Score: _____

Clinical Monitoring Form

Clinical Monitoring Form

Dept. of Psychiatry Clinical Monitoring: Treatment and Symptoms   E   V   Quarterly:____   Date __ / __ / __

Name:_____   ID# __ __ __-__ __-__ __ __ __ __   Others:_____   Physician:____CPT code:____   Visit Type:_____

Over the past 10 days, how many days have you been/had . . .

DSM Criteria Satisfied

	% days	Severity (0–4)	DSM Criteria	No	Probable	Definite
. . . depressed most of day:	____%	__	Depressed most of the day nearly every day for ≥ 2wk	__	__	__
. . . less interest in most activities or found you couldn't enjoy even pleasurable activities through most of the day:	____%	__	Decreased interest or diminished pleasure in most activities most of the day nearly every day for ≥ 2wks	__	__	__
. . . any period of abnormal mood elevation	____%	__	Mood Elevation (high, euphoric, expansive) to a significant degree over a 4 – 7 day period	__	__	__
. . . any period of abnormal initability	____%	__	Irritability to a significant degree over a 4 – 7 day period	__	__	__
. . . any abnormal anxiety	____%					

Rate Associated Symptoms for PAST WEEK

Much more +2 ____ 0 ____ –2 Much less
0 = usual/none

MDE	Depressed mood	Sleep	Interest	Guilt/SE	Energy	Conc/Distr	Appetite	PMR/PMA	SI
requires ≥ 5 (including depressed mood and/or interest	__	__	__ or __	__	__ or __	__	__ or __	__
Sleeps ____ - ____ hours	__ EBT __ DFA __ MCA __ EMA	__ DGOOB	__ Naps __ anhedonia		__ LNWL __ Passive __ Active

Elevation	Self Esteem	Need for sleep	Talking	FOI/Racing thoughts	Distractible	Goal directed activity/PMA	High Risk Behavior
Mania/hypomania requires ≥ 3 unless only irritable, then ≥ 4 moderate sxs are required (do not count elevation of irritability) towards dx of hypomania of mania	__	__	__	__	__	__ or	__

Y   N   New major stressor, if yes _____

____ c/d caffeine   ____ ppd nicotine   Onset of menses ____ / ____ / ____   early   late   NA

Y   N   Alcohol abuse ____ ____   Y   N   Headaches   Y   N   Binge/ Purge   Y   N   Additional Psych tx: OP   ER   Hosp

Y   N   Substance abuse ____ ____   Y   N   Migraines   Y   N   Panic attacks   Y   N   Additional Gen Med tx: OP   ER   Hosp

Y   N   Significant Medical illness, if yes _____   - Weight _____

Current Treatments						**Adverse Effects**	
Mood Stabilizers	Dose Mg 24 hr total	Mg Missed Past 7 days		Dose Mg 24 hr total	Mg Missed past 7 days	Severity 0-4	
						Tremor	__
						Dry Mouth	__
Anxiolytics/Hypnotics						Sedation	__
						Constipation	__
						Diarrhea	__
Antidepressants						Headache	__
						Poor Memory	__
						Sexual Dysfunction	__
Antipsychotics						Increased Appetite	__
				PRN	x	Other	__
				PRN	x	_____	__
						_____	__
						_____	__
						EPS _____	__

Psychosocial Interventions ____/mo ECT ____/mo Other _____ ____/mo
Y   N   Significant Noncompliance, if yes _____

Selected Mental Status   Severity 0–4
PI ___   IOR ___   OC ___
Hallucinations ___   Delusions ___

Last Labs   Date __ / __ / __
Li = ___   VPA = ___
Creat = ___   TSH = ___

Current Clinical Status (check one)
__ Depression   __ Continued Sx
__ Hypomania   __ Recovering
__ Mania   __ Recovered
__ Mixed*   __ Roughening
If new episode, estimate omest date: /   /
Other Dx:
CGI __   GAF __ __   GAF __ __
(1–7) week (1–90)   month (1–90)

Comments:

Path ___ ___ ___   **Phase: A C M T**
Path ___ ___ ___   **Phase: A C M T**

Plan:

RTC _____   Version 2.00   8/20/2001   Physician's Signature _____

Clinical Self-Report Form

Clinical Self report form

Name: _____   ID# _____   Clinician: _____   Date: _ _ / _ _ / _ _ _ _

During the last week: Check

Has there been a period of time when you were feeling down or depressed most of the day, nearly everyday?		☐ Yes ☐ No
If Yes, Did it last as long as two weeks?		☐ Yes ☐ No
What about being a lot less interested in most things or unable to enjoy things you usually enjoy?		☐ Yes ☐ No
If Yes, Did it last as long as 2 weeks?		☐ Yes ☐ No
Has there been a period of time when your were feeling so good or so hyper people thought you were not your normal self or you were so hyper you got in trouble?		☐ Yes ☐ No
If Yes, Was it more than just feeling good?		☐ Yes ☐ No
Did anyone say you were manic?		☐ Yes ☐ No
What about a period of time when you were so irritable that you would shout at people or start fights of arguments?		☐ Yes ☐ No
Have you experienced a major stress that you feel has caused your mood to change?		☐ Yes ☐ No

If yes (describe) _____

Have you experienced a other medical problems?   ☐ Yes ☐ No

If yes (describe) _____

Used additional psychiatric care/treatment ☐ Yes ☐ No Other medical treatment ☐ Yes ☐ No   Onset of last menses _ _ / _ _ / _ _

Over the past 10 days how many days have you been/had. . .

. . . depressed most of the day _____ /10 Days   . . . unable to experience pleasure most of the day _____ /10 Days

. . . any period of abnormal mood elevation _____ /10 Days   . . . any period of abnormal irritability _____ /10 Days

. . . any period of abnormal anxiety _____ /10 Days   . . . at least 20 minutes of exercise _____ /10 Days

During the past week . . .

What is the least you have slept in any one day _ _ hrs   What is the most you have slept any one day _ _ hrs

Have you had: Panic Attacks ___   Binge/Purge ___   Headaches ___   Weight _ _ _

Indicate your use of : Caffeine ___ cups/day   Nicotine ___ peaks/day   Alcohol ___ drinks/week Drugs _ _ _

For each item rate this week
compared to your usual (when well)

← ← ← ← ←Decreased ←Well→ Increased → → → → →

	Constant and Severe	Nearly Every Day	Often	Rarely and/or mild	Well	Rarely and/or mild	Often	Nearly Every Day	Constant and Severe
Sleep	O	O	O	O	O	☐ Normal	O	O	O	O
Ability to enjoy pleasant things/usual interests	O	O	O	O	O	☐ Normal	O	O	O	O
Self confidence/Sself Esteem	O	O	O	O	O	☐ Normal	O	O	O	O
Energy	O	O	O	O	O	☐ Normal	O	O	O	O
Ability to Concentrate	O	O	O	O	O	☐ Normal	O	O	O	O
Distractibility						☐ None	O	O	O	O
Appetite	O	O	O	O	O	☐ Normal	O	O	O	O
Physical restlessness/agitation						☐ None	O	O	O	O
Rare of speech or thoughts	O	O	O	O	O	☐ Normal	O	O	O	O
Feel life isn't worth living of suicidal thoughts						☐ None	O	O	O	O
Talking	O	O	O	O	O	☐ Normal	O	O	O	O
Racing thoughts						☐ None	O	O	O	O
Making plans or or getting new projects started	O	O	O	O	O	☐ Normal	O	O	O	O
Behaviors others regards as excessive, foolish or risky						☐ None	O	O	O	O

Please complete for all medications used since your last visit

Medication	Total daily done	Mg missed this week	Comments/adverse effects ☐ Check if no adverse effects
	_ _ _ Mg	_ _ _ Mg	
	_ _ _ Mg	_ _ _ Mg	
	_ _ _ Mg	_ _ _ Mg	
	_ _ _ Mg	_ _ _ Mg	
	_ _ _ Mg	_ _ _ Mg	
	_ _ _ Mg	_ _ _ Mg	
	_ _ _ Mg	_ _ _ Mg	
	_ _ _ Mg	_ _ _ Mg	
	_ _ _ Mg	_ _ _ Mg	

Chapter 5
Rating Scales for Alcohol and Nicotine Addictions

Julie Yeterian, Gladys Pachas, Eden Evins, and John Kelly

Abstract Alcohol and tobacco are among the leading causes of preventable deaths and are frequently used in combination. Because of the exceptional morbidity and mortality associated with the use of these substances, it is important to maximize opportunities for the detection of maladaptive use and subsequent intervention whenever a healthcare point of contact is made. This chapter provides a brief description of the health impact of these substances, as well as concise descriptions of helpful alcohol- and tobacco-related screening and assessment tools. The tools that are highlighted were chosen because of their excellent psychometric properties, but also for their high clinical utility and free availability for ease of use in a busy practice setting.

Keywords Addiction · Alcoholism · Nicotine · Smoking · Rating scales · Questionnaires · Assessment

Alcohol and tobacco are among the leading causes of preventable deaths in the United States [1] and are frequently used in combination. Because of the exceptional morbidity and mortality associated with the use of these substances, it is important to maximize opportunities for the detection of maladaptive use and subsequent intervention whenever a healthcare point of contact is made. Consequently, following a brief description of the health impact of these substances, we provide succinct descriptions of helpful alcohol- and tobacco-related screening and assessment tools. Our goal is not to provide a comprehensive overview of all available assessment measures. Rather, the tools we highlight are chosen because they are easy to use and score and have utility for the busy clinician in everyday clinical practice. We also provide copies of the measures. We begin first with alcohol and then focus on tobacco use.

J. Kelly (✉)

Department of Psychiatry, Massachusetts General Hospital and Harvard Medical School, Boston, MA 02114, USA

e-mail: jkelly11@partners.org

L. Baer, M.A. Blais (eds.), *Handbook of Clinical Rating Scales and Assessment in Psychiatry and Mental Health*, Current Clinical Psychiatry, DOI 10.1007/978-1-59745-387-5_5, © Humana Press, a part of Springer Science+Business Media, LLC 2010

Alcohol-Related Problems

Alcohol misuse is one of the leading causes of preventable morbidity and mortality in the United States. It is estimated that approximately 30% of US adults consume alcohol at harmful or hazardous levels. Of these, about 25% meet current criteria for an alcohol use disorder, such as the DSM-IV criteria for alcohol abuse or alcohol dependence [2].

Individuals who consume alcohol to excess have elevated risk for physical, mental, and social problems, such as motor vehicle and other accidents, violence and vandalism, unwanted sexual experiences, liver and cardiovascular diseases, cancers, fetal alcohol spectrum disorders, depression, panic attacks, and suicide [3]. It is estimated that alcohol causes about 20–30% of esophageal cancer, liver cancer, cirrhosis of the liver, homicide, epileptic seizures, and motor vehicle accidents worldwide [4]. Excessive or risky alcohol consumption is the third leading cause of death in the United States, accounting for approximately 85,000 mortalities each year [1]. The economic burden attributed to alcohol-related problems in the United States approaches $200 billion annually [5].

Despite its public health impact, risky alcohol consumption often goes undetected, and if detected, rarely receives the types of clinical attention considered to be "best practice" [6]. Many health-care providers may be reluctant to ask about alcohol use because they feel uncomfortable themselves, have little confidence in their ability to deal with alcohol-related issues, or believe that patients will become defensive when asked about their alcohol consumption. However, contrary to many clinicians' expectations, patients are often likely to be receptive and ready to make salutary changes in their alcohol use when approached in a respectful way in a medical setting. Furthermore, even brief interventions can make a difference in reducing harmful drinking [7]. Some drinkers who are alcohol dependent will accept referral to a specialty addiction program, and for others who will not accept a referral, an ongoing, empathic focus on their alcohol use can still be helpful [8].

Consequently, health-care providers are in a prime position to address and to make a difference in patients' drinking behavior. It is possible to screen effectively and efficiently for the presence of alcohol-related problems or alcohol use disorders using very brief, validated measures. Early detection and discussion of harmful or hazardous alcohol use can be an important first step that can ultimately make a substantial difference in the lives of patients and their families. As mentioned above, this chapter is intended to describe some helpful screening and assessment measures that have utility as clinical tools for the busy clinician. Within six assessment domains, we present valid and reliable measures that are designed to be quick and easy to administer and score. These measures cover screening for alcohol misuse, quantity and frequency of alcohol use and harmful use, severity of dependence, alcohol withdrawal symptoms, consequences or problems arising from alcohol use, and assessment of relapse risk.

These assessment domains and their associated measures are summarized in Table 5.1. This table contains the name of the recommended scale, the method and

Table 5.1 Measures for the assessment of alcohol-related problems

Name of scale	Method and timing of administration	Scoring key; how to interpret results	Cutoff scores for mild, moderate, and severe symptoms	Reliability	Validity
Alcohol Use Disorders Identification Test (AUDIT)	Self-report or interview 2 min	Total score (range=0–40) is the sum of individual question scores (ranges=0–4). Higher scores indicate increased likelihood of hazardous and harmful drinking, as well as dependence.	• 8–15=moderate alcohol problems • 16–19=high level of alcohol problems • >19=severe problems; possible dependence • Examination of subscales allows for more detailed evaluation	High internal consistency High test-retest reliability (r=0.86)	Thoroughly validated across populations, settings, and cultures in a large number of studies Convergent validity with the MAST (r=0.88) and the CAGE (r=0.78)
Leeds Dependence Questionnaire (LDQ)	Self-report or interview 2–5 min	Total score (range=0–30) is the sum of individual question scores (ranges=0–3). Higher scores indicate more severe dependence.	• <15=mild alcohol dependence • 16–23=moderate alcohol dependence • 24–30=severe alcohol dependence	High internal consistency (a=0.90) High test-retest reliability (r=0.95) over 2–5 days	Concurrent validity: Correlated with SADQ (r=0.69, p<0.0001) Convergent validity: Correlated with clinical ratings (r=0.60, p<0.01)
Clinical Institute Withdrawal Assessment for Alcohol-Revised (CIWA-Ar)	Interview and observation 2–5 min	Total score (range=0–67) is the sum of individual items (ranges=0–7, 0–4). Higher scores indicate more severe withdrawal.	• <15=mild withdrawal • 16–20=moderate withdrawal • >20=severe withdrawal • Pharmacological treatment indicated for those with a score of 10 or greater	High inter-rater reliability (r>0.9)	Frequently used in clinical trials of pharmacological treatments for alcohol withdrawal; sensitive to change

Table 5.1 (continued)

Name of scale	Method and timing of administration	Scoring key; how to interpret results	Cutoff scores for mild, moderate, and severe symptoms	Reliability	Validity
Short Index of Problems (SIP)	Self-report or interview 2 min	Total score (range=0–45) is the sum of individual question scores (ranges=0–3). Higher scores indicate more drinking-related consequences.	• Normative data and percentile scores available from Project MATCH data • Roughly, 0–14=very low level of consequences • 14–19=low level of consequences • 20–25=medium level of consequences • 26–32=high level of consequences • 33–45=very high level of consequences • These cutoffs vary slightly by gender	High internal consistency (a=0.81–0.95) High test-retest reliability (r=0.74–0.94)	High convergent validity with full DrInC (r=0.97) Correlated with DSM-IV criteria for alc dependence (r=0.36, p<0.001) and urges to drink (r=0.17, p=0.04)
Advanced Warning of Relapse (AWARE)	Self-report or interview 5 min	Total score (range=28–196) is the sum of individual question scores (ranges=1–7), with items 8, 14, 20, 24, and 26 reverse-scored. Higher scores represent greater relapse risk.	• Can use AWARE score and drinking status to assess risk for relapse over next 2 months • Predicted Relapse$_{x+2mo}$ = −0.031 + 0.465 Relapse$_x$ + 0.00337 AWARE	High internal consistency (a=0.91) High test-retest reliability (r=0.80)	Convergent validity: Correlated with Inventory of Drinking Situations (r=0.36, p<0.001) Highly correlated with measures of psychological distress (e.g., BDI)

approximate time needed for administration, the scoring key, how to interpret results and cutoff scores, and other psychometric properties of the measure. We begin first with efficient detection of harmful alcohol use.

Screening for Alcohol Misuse

Gold Standard Rating Scale: The Alcohol Use Disorders Identification Test (AUDIT)

Given the regrettable impact that a failure to detect and intervene with alcohol problems can have, routine screening for alcohol misuse should be standard in all clinical settings. There are a variety of brief and effective screening measures that can yield high rates of detection of these pervasive and debilitating disorders. Due to their speed of administration and empirical support for their utility, the National Institute on Alcohol Abuse and Alcoholism (NIAAA) has recommended either the use of a single alcohol screening question (SASQ) or administration of the Alcohol Use Disorders Identification Test (AUDIT) questionnaire as standard screening procedures for the detection of alcohol-related problems.

The AUDIT [9] (reproduced in the appendix to this chapter) contains 10 face-valid questions that screen for alcohol misuse in the past year across three dimensions: hazardous drinking (which increases the risk for future alcohol-related problems; items 1–3), harmful drinking (which has already caused physical, mental, or social problems; items 7–10), and alcohol dependence (a syndrome characterized by symptoms such as tolerance, withdrawal, and reduced control; items 4–6). The AUDIT can be administered as a self-report measure or an interview, and it takes about 2–5 min to complete.

Scoring

The total score (range = 0–40) is the sum of scores on individual questions (ranges = 0–4). Higher scores indicate greater likelihood of hazardous and harmful drinking, as well as dependence. In general, scores from 8 to 15 represent moderate alcohol problems and indicate the need for advice on reducing hazardous drinking, scores from 16 to 19 imply a high level of alcohol problems and implicate the need for brief counseling and further monitoring, and scores of 20 or more represent severe problems and are cause for a more thorough evaluation of the presence of alcohol dependence. Examination of the three subscale dimensions mentioned above can provide more specific insight into particular problems. Scores greater than or equal to 1 on questions 2 or 3 of the AUDIT indicate the presence of hazardous drinking; scores greater than or equal to 1 on questions 4, 5, or 6 indicate that alcohol dependence is present or developing; and scores greater than or equal to 1 on questions 7, 8, 9, or 10 indicate that alcohol-related problems are present or have been experienced in the past year. The AUDIT is easy to administer and is considered appropriate for use in a variety of settings, including primary care and psychiatric settings. The measure has been found to be both sensitive and specific in the detection of alcohol use disorders [10–12] and its reliability and validity have been established across many different countries and population subgroups [10]. It is a useful tool for identifying people who would benefit from reducing their drinking, even if they are not alcohol-dependent.

Other Measures

While the AUDIT is the preferred screening measure for alcohol misuse, there are several other commonly used alternatives. As mentioned, clinicians might choose to use the SASQ, where the patient is simply asked whether he has consumed five or more standard drinks at any one time during the last year (four or more drinks for a woman). A positive response may indicate an alcohol-related problem and requires a more detailed assessment [13]. When used by itself, the SASQ allows for greater sensitivity in the detection of alcohol problems at the expense of specificity.

A more traditional alternative screening interview is captured by the "CAGE" acronym, which stands for: "C" – Have you ever felt you should *C*ut down on your drinking?, "A" – Have people *A*nnoyed you by criticizing your drinking?, "G" – Have you ever felt bad or *G*uilty about your drinking?, and "E" – Have you ever had a drink first thing in the morning to steady your nerves or to get rid of a hangover (*E*ye opener)? Having two or more "yes" responses on the CAGE questionnaire indicates a possible alcohol-related problem or disorder. However, compared to the SASQ and the AUDIT, the CAGE lacks sensitivity to detect hazardous and harmful drinking. The Michigan Alcoholism Screening Test (MAST) is another self-report measure with good psychometric properties, but at 22 questions, it is longer than the AUDIT.

Given the subjective nature of self-report and the perceived social undesirability for some patients in disclosing heavy drinking, additional objective clinical screening procedures such as laboratory assay tests may be used to further assess chronic drinking problems (e.g., hand or tongue tremor, apparent blood vessels on face, and elevated liver enzymes, such as GGT, CDT, AST, ALT).

An additional resource for clinicians that thoroughly covers the topic of screening for alcohol misuse is the NIAAA manual *Helping Patients Who Drink Too Much* [13], which is a useful and practical guide to implementing alcohol screening and intervention procedures into clinical practice. This guide recommends screening with the AUDIT or the SASQ and provides useful algorithms to facilitate further assessment for alcohol use disorders (e.g., with DSM-IV criteria) for those with positive screens. It also provides guidelines for brief interventions for those who demonstrate at-risk drinking, abuse, or dependence. The guide is available for free and can be downloaded at: http://pubs.niaaa.nih.gov/publications/Practitioner/CliniciansGuide2005/guide.pdf.

Assessing Frequency and Quantity of Alcohol Use

For patients who screen positive on the AUDIT (total score ≥ 8) or SASQ (one or more heavy drinking days), it is useful to obtain an estimate of the frequency and quantity of their alcohol use in order to get a more detailed assessment of recent use and to monitor changes in use. To obtain such an estimate, we recommend using five simple questions about the frequency and quantity of alcohol use in the past 30 days (reproduced in the appendix to this chapter).

An alternative method of assessing the quantity and frequency of use is to use a timeline follow-back (TLFB [14]) method, where patients are given a calendar of a recent time period (e.g., past month) and are asked to provide their best estimate of items such as the days on which they drank, the total number of drinking days in the period, and how much they drank on average or on each occasion. The TLFB method is more time-consuming than using the questions listed above, but it is likely to be more accurate. Another alternative to the quantity–frequency questions is to ask patients to keep a daily diary of their use over a period of a couple of weeks. This prospective method is more accurate than questions that require retrospective recall, but is more time-consuming for the patient and is thereby limited by the amount of time that can be covered (e.g., 2 weeks rather than the past 2 months).

Assessing Severity of Dependence

Gold Standard Scale: The Leeds Dependence Questionnaire (LDQ)

Clinicians treating patients who show signs of alcohol dependence on the AUDIT (score ≥ 1 on questions 4–6) or who meet DSM-IV criteria for dependence (e.g., tolerance, withdrawal, unsuccessful attempts to cut down or stop, continued drinking despite physical or psychological problems) may find it helpful to assess patients' severity of dependence to plan the course of treatment, determine treatment goals, and assess treatment outcomes. The Leeds Dependence Questionnaire (LDQ [15]; reproduced in the appendix to this chapter), a 10-item, self-administered measure, is designed to assess severity of dependence upon alcohol and other substances. Participants are asked to think about their drinking and/or other drug use during the past few weeks when completing the measure. The LDQ examines the psychological characteristics of dependence, and as such, does not explicitly address the physical presence or absence of tolerance and withdrawal. Instead, to examine these features, the measure uses questions relating to maximizing the drug effect (question 5), the perceived importance of obtaining an effect (question 8), and maintaining a constant drug state (question 9), which can be considered responses to tolerance and withdrawal. Each of the 10 questions on the LDQ addresses a different psychological feature of dependence, similar to those in ICD-10 [16], which together yield a single, internally consistent measure of dependence. The measure is not substance-specific, and has been used to assess the degree of dependence in patients who use a variety of other substances, such as opiates [17].

Scoring

The LDQ is scored by adding the response scores for individual questions, which range from 0 to 3, to yield a total score that ranges from 0 to 30. Higher scores indicate more severe dependence. Heather et al. [17] provide normative data for the scale based on 821 patients at two addiction treatment centers with alcohol as their primary problem substance. A score of less than 15 on the LDQ indicates mild dependence, while a score of 16–23 indicates moderate dependence, and a score of 24–30 is indicative of severe dependence. However, the utility of the scale appears to be limited by a ceiling effect, and no suggested cutoff score is given to indicate the absence of dependence. The scale has high internal consistency ($\alpha = 0.90$) and high test–retest reliability over 2–5 days ($r = 0.95$). The scale also demonstrates high concurrent validity with a measure of psychobiological dependence, the Severity of Alcohol Dependence Questionnaire (SADQ [18]; $r = 0.69$, $p < 0.0001$) and high convergent validity with clinical ratings of substance misuse/dependence and psychosocial functioning ($r = 0.60$, $p < 0.01$) [15].

Other Measures

The SADQ [18] can also be used to assess patients' severity of dependence. It is a 20-item questionnaire that assesses the degree of alcohol dependence with regard to five dimensions: physical withdrawal, affective withdrawal, relief drinking, frequency of alcohol consumption, and withdrawal onset speed. Unlike the LDQ, the SADQ focuses on psychobiological, rather than purely psychological, symptoms. On this measure, respondents are asked to recall how they would feel after a typical heavy drinking period within the past 6 months. The measure is designed for use with adult problem drinkers, and is widely used in inpatient, outpatient, and community treatment centers. The total SADQ score (range 0–60) is the sum of individual question scores (ranges 0–3), with higher scores indicating a greater degree of dependence. Scores of 15 or below indicate mild dependence, while scores of 16–30 indicate moderate dependence, and scores greater than 30 indicate severe dependence. Detoxification is recommended for those who score greater than 16.

Assessing Alcohol Withdrawal Symptoms

Gold Standard Scale: The Revised Clinical Institute Withdrawal Assessment for Alcohol (CIWA-Ar)

The syndrome of alcohol withdrawal can range from mild discomfort that requires no medication to organ failure and death. Uncomplicated withdrawal is surprisingly common and is frequently missed [20]. Although more than 90% of individuals who experience alcohol withdrawal need nothing more than supportive treatment, those hospitalized with co-morbid medical conditions have a higher rate of complications [19]. The most common features of uncomplicated alcohol withdrawal emerge within hours, and resolve after 3–5 days. Early features of uncomplicated withdrawal symptoms include loss of appetite, irritability, and tremor.

Systematic assessment of the severity of alcohol withdrawal symptoms is important for providing ongoing guidance on the appropriate level of care needed to prevent serious medical complications during withdrawal. The revised CIWA-Ar [20] (reproduced in the appendix to this chapter) is a short, semi-structured, clinician-administered interview and observation that is used to assess and quantify the severity of alcohol withdrawal symptoms at the present time, and thereby inform the need for and response to treatment on an ongoing basis (e.g., hour by hour). The CIWA-Ar follows from the earlier 15-item CIWA-A [21] and includes the 10 items from that measure that contribute most to the total score.

Scoring

The scale is based on DSM-III-R criteria for alcohol withdrawal syndrome and assesses 10 symptom categories: sweating; tremor; agitation; nausea and/or vomiting; anxiety; tactile, auditory, and visual disturbances; headache; and orientation. The first three symptoms listed are assessed through observation of the patient and the latter seven are assessed by asking the patient semi-structured questions about each symptom. Symptoms are rated on scales of 0–7, with the exception of orientation, which is rated on a scale of 0–4, and the total score (range 0–67) is the sum of the individual symptom scores, where higher scores indicate more severe withdrawal. A score below 15 is considered to be mild withdrawal, while between 16 and 20 is moderate withdrawal, and a score greater than 20 is severe withdrawal. A score of 10 or greater on the CIWA-Ar indicates the need for pharmacological treatment (e.g., with benzodiazepines [20, 22]).

The CIWA-Ar has been shown to have high inter-rater reliability for the total score and for individual item scores ($r > 0.9$ [20]). In clinical trials of pharmacological treatments for alcohol withdrawal, the assessment is often used as a measure of change in alcohol withdrawal symptoms over time, to compare the efficacy of different medications in reducing alcohol withdrawal symptoms, and as a guide to the dosing and timing of pharmacological interventions (e.g., [23–25]). As such, the measure is clearly sensitive to change over time, and possesses great clinical utility as a guide to the need for and necessary level of pharmacological treatment during alcohol withdrawal.

Other Measures

There is a newer version of the CIWA-Ar, the CIWA-AD [26], which may have several advantages over the older version. First, it is likely to be less subjective, as it condenses the three perceptual disturbance questions from the CIWA-Ar into a single question and includes an objective measure of pulse rate, thereby lessening the influence of subjective responses on the total score [22]. The CIWA-AD is also more consistent with DSM-IV criteria for alcohol withdrawal syndrome, in that it contains an assessment of pulse rate and does not include an assessment of orientation/sensory clouding. Still, the CIWA-AD and CIWA-Ar share six identical items (sweating, tremor, agitation, nausea or vomiting, anxiety, and headache), and scores on the two measures are highly correlated [22]. Scores on the eight-item CIWA-AD range from 0 to 56. Sellers et al. [26] present an alternative scoring method for the CIWA-AD, where a score greater than 2 for a particular symptom is considered positive, and the number of positive symptoms indicates the severity of withdrawal, such that one positive symptom is very mild, two positive symptoms are mild, three moderate, and four severe. While the CIWA-AD may have some advantages over the CIWA-Ar, its psychometric properties have not been established. However, like the CIWA-Ar, the CIWA-AD is likely to be an efficient and reliable assessment tool that can prevent serious life-threatening problems and help determine the necessary level of care.

Assessing Alcohol-Related Consequences

Gold Standard Scales: The Short Index of Problems (SIP)

For a more detailed assessment of whether or how alcohol use is affecting a patient's functioning in terms of physical and mental health, social and family life, and/or occupational roles, clinicians may wish to employ measures of alcohol-related consequences. The Short Index of Problems (SIP [27]) (reproduced in the appendix to this chapter), an abbreviated version of the Drinker Inventory of Consequences (DrInC [27]), is designed to assess alcohol-related consequences across five dimensions – physical, intrapersonal, social, interpersonal, and impulse control – independently of the intensity of use and the presence of dependence. It can be used to assess the incidence of consequences throughout the lifetime and the incidence, frequency, and intensity of consequences within a shorter time period, such as the past 3 months. The 15-item SIP was derived from the original 50-item DrInC by selecting the three items from each of the five DrInC subscales that were most strongly related to the overall subscale score. Even though it is not as comprehensive in content as the DrInC, scores on the SIP are very highly correlated with scores on the DrInC ($r = 0.97$) and the SIP significantly predicts scores on the DrInC at a later time-point ($R^2 = 0.51$, $p < 0.001$; [28]). Therefore, the SIP appears to be just as useful as the DrInC, especially when time is limited, and takes just 2 min to complete by self-report or interview.

Scoring

The SIP is scored by summing the scores for individual responses, which range from 0 to 3, to yield a total score that ranges from 0 to 45, with higher scores representing a higher level of alcohol-related consequences. Miller et al. [27] give normative data and percentile values for scores on the measure. Normative data vary slightly by gender, but roughly speaking, a score from 0 to 14 represents a very low level of consequences, 15–19 low level of consequences, 20–25 medium, 26–32 high, and 33–45 very high. Individual subscale scores can also be examined. The SIP possesses good psychometric properties for both the lifetime and past 3-month versions. Internal consistency ranges from 0.81 for the lifetime version [27] to 0.95 for the 3-month [28]. Test–retest reliability is also high ($r = 0.74$–0.94). There is high convergent validity between the SIP and the full DrInC ($r = 0.97$), as mentioned above, and between the SIP and the partial DrInC with SIP items removed ($r = 0.87$; [29]). Baseline (i.e., pretreatment) SIP scores in a sample of heavy drinkers were correlated with the number of DSM-IV alcohol dependence criteria met ($r = 0.36, p < 0.001$) and urges to drink ($r = 0.17, p = 0.04$), but were unrelated to the quantity and frequency of heavy drinking [29].

Other Measures

While the SIP is appropriate for use with adult and college student populations [30], clinicians working with adolescents might use an alternative measure, the Rutgers Alcohol Problem Index (RAPI [31]), to gauge the level of alcohol-related consequences in these younger patients. In addition to assessing symptoms of problem drinking such as tolerance, withdrawal, and attempts to cut down, the RAPI examines negative consequences of drinking that are more specific to a younger population (e.g., drinking interferes with getting homework done, causes absence from school). With 23 items, the RAPI takes about 5 min to complete as a self-report or interview. The timeframe of assessment is the past 3 years, but can be adjusted to reflect a shorter period of time (e.g., past 6 months). The total score (range = 0–69) is the sum of individual item scores (ranges = 0–3), with higher scores indicating more negative consequences of drinking. In a clinical sample of youth aged 14–18, mean scores on the RAPI ranged from 21 to 25, while non-clinical sample (ages 15 and 18) means ranged from 4 to 8, depending on age and sex. The RAPI has high internal consistency ($\alpha = 0.92$) and has convergent validity with other measures of alcohol use and dependence (e.g., Alcohol Dependence Scale, Adolescent Involvement Scale, DSM-III-R; $r > 0.70$).

Assessing Relapse Risk

Gold Standard Scale: Assessment of Warning Signs of Relapse scale (AWARE [32])

The revised, 28-item version of the Assessment of Warning-signs of Relapse scale (AWARE [32] (reproduced in the appendix to this chapter)) provides a way for clinicians to assess the degree of risk for relapse among patients receiving treatment for alcohol dependence based on their score on the measure and their recent drinking status. The measure is based on Gorski's [33] 37-step theoretical model of progression to relapse and post-acute withdrawal syndrome. As such, the scale originally contained 37 items, but Miller and Harris [32] reduced it to the 28 items that loaded most strongly onto a single primary factor. The scale can be administered in approximately 5 min as a self-report or interview.

Scoring

The AWARE is scored by adding individual item scores (ranges = 1–7), with items 8, 14, 20, 24, and 26 reverse scored, to obtain a total score that ranges from 28 to 196 (see appendix to this chapter). In general, higher scores represent a greater risk for relapse. However, clinicians can use the AWARE score and the patient's drinking status over the past 2 months (i.e., relapse to drinking vs. abstinence) to more specifically predict the probability of relapse over the next 2 months for that patient, as detailed in Table 5.2.

Table 5.2 Probablility of relapse during the next 2 months based on AWARE score

AWARE score	If *already* drinking in the prior 2 months (%)	If *abstinent* during the prior 2 months (%)
28–55	37	11
56–69	62	21
70–83	72	24
84–97	82	25
98–111	86	28
112–125	77	37
126–168	90	43
169–196	>95	53

Clinicians may also use the following equation to predict relapse at Time $x + 2$ *months* with AWARE (the total raw score at *Time x*) and relapse at *Time x* as predictors:

$$\text{Predicted Relapse}_{x+2 \text{ months}} = -0.031 + 0.465 \, \text{Relapse}_x + 0.00337 \, \text{AWARE}$$

The AWARE has high internal consistency ($\alpha = 0.91$) and appears to be reliable over time ($r = 0.80$) [32]. The scale has predictive validity, in that it can predict slips and relapses over the next 2 months even after controlling for drinking status at the time of administration, which is itself a strong predictor of future drinking. The AWARE also demonstrates convergent validity with another relapse risk assessment, the Inventory of Drinking Situations ($r = 0.36$, $p < 0.001$), but appears to be more strongly correlated with measures of psychological and emotional distress, such as the Beck Depression Inventory (BDI; $r = 0.69$), Beck Anxiety Inventory (BAI; $r = 0.62$), and Spielberger Anger Expression Inventory trait scale ($r = 0.53$). In addition, the AWARE is strongly negatively associated with purpose in life (PIL; $r = -0.74$) and strongly positively associated with a desire for greater meaning in life ($r = 0.53$). As such, Miller and Harris [32] concluded that the AWARE is actually measuring a generalized demoralization and decreased purpose in life, along with negative emotional states such as depression, anxiety, and anger, and note that many of the items on the scale have face validity for this concept. The AWARE does not appear to be related to measures of alcohol cravings or urges, motivation for change, or coping style.

Nicotine-Related Problems

Smoking is the leading cause of preventable mortality in developed countries, and there are reportedly 1.3 billion smokers worldwide. It is estimated that 2.1 million people died from tobacco-related illnesses in the year 2000 in the developed world [34]. Unless current smoking trends are reversed, it is estimated that the death toll will rise to 10 million per year by the year 2020.

In 2005, an estimated 71.5 million Americans aged 12 or older were current (past month) users of a tobacco product, representing 29.4% of the population in that age range. In addition, 60.5 million persons (24.9% of the population) were current cigarette smokers; 13.6 million (5.6%) smoked cigars; 7.7 million (3.2%) used smokeless tobacco; and 2.2 million (0.9%) smoked tobacco in pipes [35].

Most smokers are dependent on nicotine, and smokeless tobacco use can also lead to nicotine dependence [36]. Nicotine dependence is the most common form of chemical dependence in the United States [37]. Seventy percent of smokers report that they would like to quit smoking, and pharmacologic and behavioral interventions have been shown to be effective for smoking cessation. However, their effectiveness decreases over time as former smokers relapse to smoking. Relapse is associated with craving, negative affect and depressed mood, and with stimuli associated with drug use [38–43]. Tobacco dependence is a chronic condition that often requires repeated interventions.

After quitting, many smokers experience symptoms of nicotine withdrawal. These include anxiety, restlessness, anger, irritability, sadness, difficulty concentrating, increase in appetite, weight gain, difficulty sleeping, and craving for tobacco [44, 45]. Withdrawal symptoms begin within a few hours and peak 24–48 hours after smoking cessation. Most symptoms last an average of 4 weeks [44]. Cessation of smoking can cause slowing on EEG, decreases in cortisol and catecholamine levels [46], sleep EEG changes, and a decline in metabolic rate. The mean heart rate decline is about eight beats per minute, and the mean weight gain is 3–5 kg [47]. As with all withdrawal syndromes, the severity varies among individuals.

Cessation of smoking can produce clinically significant changes in the blood levels of several medications [48]. This effect appears to be due, not to nicotine, but rather to the effects of benzopyrenes and related compounds on the P450 system. Withdrawal symptoms can also mimic, disguise, or aggravate the symptoms of other psychiatric disorders or side effects of medications. Also, although uncommon, cessation appears to be able to precipitate a relapse of major depression, bipolar disorder, and alcohol/drug problems [49].

Here we present several measures that are useful in the assessment of nicotine use and smoking history, current smoking status, and the degree of nicotine dependence. These measures, which are summarized in Table 5.3, are brief and easy to use in regular clinical practice.

Table 5.3 Measures for the assessment of nicotine-related problems

Name of scale	Method and timing of administration	Scoring key: how to interpret results	Cutoff scores	Reliability	Validity
Fagerström test for nicotine dependence (FTND)	Self-report	• Higher scores indicate more severe dependence. • 0–2 = very low • 3–4 = low • 5 = Moderate • 6–7 = high • 8–10 = very high	• Categorical variables: ranges=0–3 • Dichotomous variables: range=0–2 • Total score (range=0–10) is the sum of individual items	• The most widely used • Provides a robust quantitative measure of nicotine dependence	Internal Consistency $\alpha = 0.68$ [a]
Wisconsin smoking withdrawal scale	Self-report	Contains 7 factors • Urge to smoke: items 9, 11, 20, 26 • Irritability: 13, 15, 18 • Depression: 7*,12,19,24* • Increased appetite: 1*,14,16,21,28 • Difficulty concentrating: 4*,23,27 • Insomnia: 2*,5,17*,22*,25 • Anxiety: 3,6,8,10* * reverse scoring	• Consists of 28 items that are rated on a 5-point Likert scale: Strongly disagree–strongly agree) ranges 0–4	• Sensitive to smoking withdrawal, is predictive of smoking cessation outcomes, and yields data that conform to a 7-factor structure. [b]	Internal Consistency prequit α coefficients ranged from 0.81 to 0.89 (over last 24 hrs) and prequit coefficients alpha ranged from 0.70 to 0.88 (over last week). Post-quit α coefficients for the whole scale range from 0.90 to 0.91 and the factors ranged from 0.75 to 0.93 [b].

Table 5.3 (continued)

Name of scale	Method and timing of administration	Scoring key: how to interpret results	Cutoff scores	Reliability	Validity
Tiffany QSU brief form	Self-report	• Factor 1 (items 1, 3, 6, 7, 10) represents a desire and intention to smoke with smoking perceived as rewarding • Factor 2 (items 2, 4, 5, 8, 9) represents an anticipation of relief from negative affect with an urgent desire to smoke • Higher scores indicate more severe craving.	• Consists of 10 items that are rated on a 5-point Likert scale (very little–very much) ranges 0–5 • Total score (range=10–50) is the sum of individual items.	• QSU-Brief demonstrated high reliability as a measure of global craving in both the Initial and Follow-up Sessions [c]	High internal consistency across settings with smokers at differing stages of drug use, providing convenient and reliable assessment of desire to smoke. (Initial and Follow-up Sessions α =0.89 and 0.87, respectively) [c]

[a] A comparison of the content-, construct- and predictive validity of the cigarette dependence scale and the Fagerstrom test for nicotine dependence [64]
[b] Development and validation of the Wisconsin smoking withdrawal scale [60].
[c] Evaluation of the brief questionnaire of smoking urges (QSU-brief) in laboratory and clinical settings [56]

Assessing Nicotine Use

Smoking History Information

When evaluating an individual's cigarette smoking behavior, it is useful to begin by obtaining a general overview of their smoking history and degree of nicotine dependence. These topics can be assessed with the following items:

– Age of onset of tobacco use
– Number of cigarettes smoked (packs/years)
– Number of prior quit attempts
– Reasons for treatment failure or relapse (determine whether patients have failed previous attempts to quit with adequate trials of medications; i.e., bupropion and/or nicotine replacement therapy)
– Time from waking up to first cigarette of the day (to assess degree of dependence)

Assessing Smoking Status and Outcomes

An individual's current smoking status can be assessed through self-report (i.e., reported number of cigarettes smoked in the past 24 hours) or with objective measures of the level of saliva cotinine (the primary nicotine metabolite) and/or expired carbon monoxide (CO). Seven-day point prevalence smoking abstinence can be defined as a self-report of smoking no cigarettes for the past 7 days, which is then confirmed by a saliva cotinine level that is less than 10 ng/ml and/or expired air CO less than 8 ppm. That is, individuals are considered to be smokers when their cotinine value exceeds 10 ng/ml or when their expired CO level exceeds 8 ppm.

Cotinine has a half-life of about 12 hours, and cotinine concentration is considered to reflect the degree of nicotine administration over the past 2–3 days [50]. Saliva cotinine levels can be assessed with a saliva collection kit that is then analyzed using Accutest® Nicalert™ Strip Test Kits, a semi-quantitative method for measuring cotinine levels. This test provides a reading 10 min after performing the test. It may also be assessed by using a braided dental roll, which is chewed gently for 30 seconds and then placed into a polypropylene sample vial. The sensitivity and accuracy of saliva cotinine measurements are comparable at 90 and 98%, respectively [51]. As mentioned, the cutoff value for saliva cotinine is 10 ng/ml [52]. Levels higher than this are interpreted as consistent with recent active smoking, whereas lower levels are consistent with sustained abstinence or passive smoking.

Carbon monoxide (CO) is a product of combustion and as such is a component of cigarette smoke. Measurements of end-expiratory levels of CO and blood carboxyhemoglobin have been used to verify smoking abstinence with comparable sensitivity [53]. End-expiratory CO levels greater than 8–9 ppm are considered an accurate measure of current cigarette use, whereas levels less than 8 ppm indicate abstinence. It is important to note that there is a marked diurnal variability of CO in the body and that levels can be influenced by even low-level exposure to atmospheric pollutants. In addition, physical exercise as well as lactose intolerance in subsets of the population can yield variations in CO levels. Furthermore, CO measurements cannot reliably differentiate light smokers from non-smokers [54]. Despite these limitations, CO measurements are useful, as their results are immediately available. However, a standardized time of testing, generally late in the day (1600 h), is considered optimal. Levels of CO can be measured in end-expiratory air following a 15 seconds breath hold using a Bedfont Smokerlyzer III [55].

Assessing of Nicotine Craving, Withdrawal, and Dependence

Nicotine Craving

There are a number of questionnaires that clinicians may wish to employ in order to assess nicotine craving and withdrawal symptoms. For instance, The Tiffany QSU Brief Form [56] (reproduced in the appendix to this chapter) is a self-rating scale that evaluates the **intensity of nicotine craving** and urges to smoke. Participants rate the extent to which each item applies to them at the present time on a scale of 1 (*very little*) to 5 (*very much*). The 10-item scale is divided into two factors. Factor 1 (items 1, 3, 6, 7, 10) assesses craving associated with anticipation of pleasure from smoking, while factor 2 (items 2, 4, 5, 8, 9) measures craving associated with anticipation of relief from negative affect secondary to nicotine abstinence. The total score (range=10–50) is the sum of individual items where higher scores indicate more severe craving. Tiffany QSU-Brief has demonstrated high reliability as a measure of global craving in both initial and follow-up sessions [56]. High internal consistency across settings with smokers at differing stages of drug use, providing convenient and reliable assessment of desire to smoke. (Initial and Follow-up Sessions α =0.89 and 0.87, respectively) [56].

In addition, clinicians might also administer the Smoking Self-Efficacy Questionnaire (SSEQ) [57], which is a 17-item self-report scale that assesses an individual's belief in their ability to resist the urge to smoke. The SSEQ has been shown to predict smoking behavior at 3 and 6 months following smoking cessation.

Nicotine Withdrawal

To assess **withdrawal symptoms** from nicotine, clinicians may choose to use the Wisconsin Smoking Withdrawal Scale [60], a self-rated 28-item scale that measures current symptoms of nicotine and smoking withdrawal on a Likert scale ranging from 0 (*strongly disagree*) to 4 (*strongly AQ4 agree*). The Scale contains 7 factors:

- Urge to smoke: items 9,11,20, 26
- Irritability: 13,15,18
- Depression: 7*,12,19,24*
- Increased appetite: 1*,14,16,21,28
- Difficulty concentrating: 4*,23,27

- Insomnia: 2*,5,17*,22*,25
- Anxiety: 3,6,8,10*

*reverse scoring

The WSWS is sensitive to smoking withdrawal, is predictive of smoking cessation outcomes, and yields data that conform to a 7-factor structure [60]. Internal consistency prequit α coefficients that ranged from 0.81 to 0.89 (over last 24 hrs) and prequit coefficients alpha ranged from 0.70 to 0.88 (over last week). Post-quit α coefficients for the whole scale range from 0.90 to 0.91 and the factors ranged from 0.75 to 0.93 [60]. Also the Tobacco Withdrawal Questionnaire (TWQ [59]), which is a 15-item self-rating scale that evaluates the degree of withdrawal discomfort and includes the DSM-IV criteria for tobacco withdrawal syndrome.

Nicotine Dependence

The Fagerström Test for Nicotine Dependence (FTND [61] (reproduced in the appendix to this chapter)) is a brief six-item scale that provides a robust quantitative measure of nicotine dependence [62]. The scale includes two categorical variables and four dichotomous variables, and is useful in predicting the severity of nicotine craving and withdrawal. The categorical variables, smoking rate and length of time between waking and the first cigarette, are scored from 0 to 3, with lower scores indicating fewer cigarettes smoked per day and a longer length of time between waking and the first cigarette of the day. The dichotomous variables include smoking even when ill, difficulty refraining from smoking in places where it is forbidden, smoking more heavily in the morning, and reporting that the first cigarette of the day would be the most difficult to give up, and are scored as yes (1) or no (0). Scoring for the FTND is as follows: 0–2 is very low, 3–4 low, 5 moderate, 6–7 high, and 8–10 very high. An FTND score of six or greater is considered indicative of high nicotine dependence, while a score of less than six is considered indicative of low/moderate nicotine dependence. Internal Consistency α = 0.68 [61].

The Heaviness of Smoking Index (HSI) is a two-item self-rating scale that performs as well as the FTND and correlates with biochemical indices of nicotine intake.

The two items are

1. "How soon after you wake do you smoke your first cigarette?"
2. "How many cigarettes do you smoke a day?"

The HSI is used to assess an individual's degree of dependence on a scale from 0 to 6. Individuals who smoke at least 10 cigarettes per day or smoke within 60 min of waking up are considered to be moderately dependent upon nicotine. Individuals who smoke at least 20 cigarettes per day or smoke within 30 min of waking are considered to be highly dependent.

References

1. Mokdad AH, Marks JS, Stroup DF, Gerberding JL. Actual causes of death in the united states, 2000. JAMA 2004;291(10):1238–1245.
2. National Institue on Alcohol Abuse and Alcoholism. Unpublished data from the 2001–2002 national epidemiologic survey on alcohol and related conditions (nesarc), a nationwide survey of 43,093 U.S. Adults aged 18 or older. In; 2004.
3. National Institute on Alcohol Abuse and Alcoholism. 10th special report to the us congress on alcohol and health: Highlights from current research from the secretary of health and human services; 2000.
4. World Health Organization. Global status report on alcohol. Geneva, Switzerland; 2002.
5. Harwood H. Updating estimates of the economic cost of alcohol abuse in the united states: Estimates, update methods, and data: National Institute on Alcohol Abuse and Alcoholism; 2000.
6. McGlynn E, Asch S, Adams J, et al. The quality of health care delivered to adults in the united states. N Engl J Med 2003;348(26):2635–2645.
7. Fleming M, Mundt M, French M, Manwell L, Staauffacher E, Barry K. Brief physician advice for problem drinkers: Long-term efficacy and cost-benefit analysis. Alcohol Clin Exp Res 2002;26(1):36–43.
8. Anton R, O'Malley S, Ciraulo D, et al. Combined pharmacotherapies and behavioral interventions for alcohol dependence: The combine study: A randomized controlled trial. JAMA 2006;295:2003–2017.
9. Babor TF, Higgins-Biddle JC, Saunders JB, Monteiro MG. The alcohol use disorders identification test: Guidelines for use in primary care. 2nd ed. Geneva, Switzerland: World Health Organization; 2001.
10. Allen JP, Litten RZ, Fertig JB, Babor TF. A review of research on the alcohol use disorders identification test (AUDIT). Alcohol Clin Exp Res 1997;21(4):613–619.
11. Cherpitel CJ. Analysis of cut points for screening instruments for alcohol problems in the emergency room. J Stud Alcohol 1995;56:695–700.
12. Conigrave KM, Hall WD, Saunders JB. The AUDIT questionnaire: Choosing a cut-off score. Addiction 1995;90:1349–1356.
13. National Institue on Alcohol Abuse and Alcoholism. Helping patients who drink too much. Rockville, MD: NIAAA Publications; 2005.
14. Sobell LC, Sobell MB. Timeline follow-back: A technique for assessing self-reported alcohol consumption. In: Litten JR, Allen J, eds. Measuring alchol consumption. Totowa, NJ: Humana, 1992:41–72.
15. Raistrick D, Bradshaw J, Tober G, Weiner J, Allison J, Healey C. Development of the leeds dependence questionnaire (ldq): A questionnaire to measure alcohol and opiate dependence in the context of a treatment evaluation package. Addiction 1994;89:563–572.
16. World Health Organization. International classification of diseases, 10th revision. Geneva, Switzerland: World Health Organization.; 1994.
17. Heather N, Raistrick D, Tober G, Godfrey C, Parrott S. Leeds dependence questionnaire: New data from a large sample of clinic attenders. Addiction Res Theory 2001;9(3):253–269.
18. Stockwell T, Murphy D, Hodgson R. The severity of alcohol dependence questionnaire: Its use, reliability and validity. Br J Addiction 1983;78(2):145–155.
19. Castenada R, Cushman P. Alcohol withdrawal: A review of clinical management. J Clin Psychiatry 1989;50:278–284.
20. Sullivan JT, Sykora K, Schneiderman J, Naranjo CA, Sellers EM. Assessment of alcohol withdrawal: The revised clinical institute withdrawal assessment for alcohol scale (CIWA-Ar). Br J Addiction 1989;84:1353–1357.
21. Shaw JM, Kolesar GS, Sellers EM, Kaplan HL, Sandor P. Development of optimal treatment tactics for alcohol withdrawal. I. Assessment and effectiveness of supportive care. J Clin Psychopharmacol 1981;1:382–389.

22. Reoux JP, Oreskovich MR. A comparison of two versions of the clinical institute withdrawal assessment for alcohol: The CIWA-Ar and CIWA-Ad. Am J Addict 2006;15:83–93.
23. Favre J, Allain H, Aubin H, et al. Double-blind study of cyamemazine and diazepam in the alcohol withdrawal syndrome. Human Psychopharmacol: Clin Exp 2005;20(7):511–519.
24. Myrick H, Taylor B, LaRowe S, et al. A retrospective chart review comparing tiagabine and benzodiazepines for the treatment of alcohol withdrawal. J Psychoactive Drugs 2005;37(4):409–414.
25. Weaver M, Hoffman H, Johnson R, Mauck K. Alcohol withdrawal pharmacotherapy for inpatients with medical comorbidity. J Addict Dis 2006;25(2):17–24.
26. Sellers EM, Sullivan JT, Somer G, Sykora K. Characterization of DSM-III-r criteria for uncomplicated alcohol withdrawal provides an empirical basis for DSM-IV. Arch Gen Psychiatry 1991;48(5):442–447.
27. Miller WR, Tonigan JS, Longabaugh R. The drinker inventory of consequences (DrInc): An instrument for assessing adverse consequences of alcohol abuse. In: US Department of Health and Human Services PHS, National Institutes of Health, National Institute on Alcohol Abuse and Alcoholism, ed. Project MATCH Monograph Series. Rockville, MD; 1995.
28. Kenna G, Longabaugh R, Gogineni A, et al. Can the short index of problems (SIP) be improved? Validity and reliability of the three-month sip in an emergency department sample. J Stud Alcohol 2005;66:433–437.
29. Feinn R, Tennen H, Kranzler H. Psychometric properties of the short index of problems as a measure of recent alcohol-related problems. Alcohol Clin Exp Res 2003;27(9):1436–1441.
30. Tucker J, Vuchinich R, Murphy J. Substance use disorders. In: Antony M, Barlow D, eds. Handbook of assessment and treatment planning for psychological disorders. New York, NY: The Guilford Press, 2002.
31. White H, Labouvie E. Toward the assessment of adolescent problem drinking. J Stud Alcohol 1989;50:30–37.
32. Miller WR, Harris R. A simple scale of Gorski's warning signs for relapse. J Stud Alcohol 2000;61:759–765.
33. Gorski T, Miller M. Counseling for relapse prevention. Independence, MO: Herald House, Independence Press; 1982.
34. MacKay J, Eriksen M. The tobacco atlas. Geneva, Switzerland: World Health Organization; 2002.
35. Substance Abuse and Mental Health Services Administration. National survey on drug use and health. Rockville, MD: Department of Health and Human Services.; 2005.
36. Tobacco use among adults – United States, 2005. In: Morbidity and Mortality Weekly Report; 2006:1145–1148.
37. National Center for Health Statistics. Health, United States, 2004 with chart book on trends in the health of Americans. Hyattsville, MD; 2004.
38. Hall SM, Humfleet GL, Reus VI, Munoz RF, Hartz DT, Maude-Griffin R. Psychological intervention and antidepressant treatment in smoking cessation. Arch Gen Psychiatry 2002;59(10):930–936.
39. Hays JT, Hurt RD, Rigotti NA, et al. Sustained-release bupropion for pharmacologic relapse prevention after smoking cessation. A randomized, controlled trial. Ann Intern Med 2001;135(6):423–433.
40. Hurt RD, Sachs DP, Glover ED, et al. A comparison of sustained-release bupropion and placebo for smoking cessation. N Engl J Med 1997;337(17):195–1202.
41. Kenford SL, Smith SS, Wetter DW, Jorenby DE, Fiore MC, Baker TB. Predicting relapse back to smoking: contrasting affective and physical models of dependence. J Consult Clin Psychol 2002;70(1):216–227.
42. Swan GE, Ward MM, Jack LM. Abstinence effects as predictors of 28-day relapse in smokers. Addict Behav 1996;21(4):481–490.
43. Jorenby DE, Leischow SJ, Nides MA, et al. A controlled trial of sustained-release bupropion, a nicotine patch, or both for smoking cessation. N Engl J Med 1999;340(9):685–691.

44. Hughes JR, Higgins ST, Bickel WK. Nicotine withdrawal versus other drug withdrawal syndromes: Similarities and dissimilarities. Addiction 1994;89(11):1461–1470.
45. Patten CA, Martin JE. Measuring tobacco withdrawal. A review of self report questionnaires. J Substance Abuse 1996;8(1):93–113.
46. Benowitz NL, Fitzgerald GA, Wilson M, Zhang Q. Nicotine effects on eicosanoid formation and hemostatic function: Comparison of transdermal nicotine and cigarette smoking. J Am Coll Cardiol 1993;22(4):1159–1167.
47. Williamson DF, Madans J, Anda RF, Kleinman JC, Giovino GA, Byers T. Smoking cessation and severity of weight gain in a national cohort. N Engl J Med 1991;324(11):739–745.
48. Skogh E, Bengtsson F, Nordin C. Could discontinuing smoking be hazardous for patients administered clozapine medication? A case report. Ther Drug Monit 1999;21(5):580–582.
49. Covey LS, Glassman AH, Stetner F. Major depression following smoking cessation. Am J Psychiatry 1997;154(2):263–265.
50. Benowitz NL, Jacob P, 3rd. Nicotine and cotinine elimination pharmacokinetics in smokers and nonsmokers. Clin Pharmacol Ther 1993;53(3):316–323.
51. Machacek DA, Jiang NS. Quantification of cotinine in plasma and saliva by liquid chromatography. Clin Chem 1986;32(6):979–982.
52. Cummings SR, Richard RJ. Optimum cutoff points for biochemical validation of smoking status. Am J Public Health 1988;1988(78):574–575.
53. Galvin KT, Kerin MJ, Williams G, Gorst KL, Morgan RH, Kester RC. Comparison of three methods for measuring cigarette smoking in patients with vascular disease. Cardiovasc Surg 1994;2(1):48–51.
54. Gilbert DD. Chemical analyses as validators in smoking cessation programs. J Behav Med 1993;16(3):295–308.
55. Irving JM, Clark EC, Crombie IK, Smith WC. Evaluation of a portable measure of expired-air carbon monoxide. Prev Med 1988;17(1):109–115.
56. Cox LS, Tiffany ST, Christen AG. Evaluation of the brief questionnaire of smoking urges (QSU-brief) in laboratory and clinical settings. Nicotine Tob Res 2001;3(1):7–16.
57. Colletti G, Supnick JA, Payne TJ. The smoking self-efficacy questionnaire (SSEQ): Preliminary scale development and validation. Behav Assess 1985;7:249–260.
58. Schneider NG, Jarvik ME. Time course of smoking withdrawal symptoms as a function of nicotine replacement. Psychopharmacology (Berl) 1984;82(1–2):143–144.
59. Hughes JR, Hatsukami D. Signs and symptoms of tobacco withdrawal. Arch Gen Psychiatry 1986;43(3):289–294.
60. Welsch SK, Smith SS, Wetter DW, Jorenby DE, Fiore MC, Baker TB. Development and validation of the Wisconsin smoking withdrawal scale. Exp Clin Psychopharmacol 1999;7(4):354–361.
61. Heatherton TF, Kozlowski LT, Frecker RC, Fagerstrom KO. The Fagerstrom test for nicotine dependence: A revision of the Fagerstrom tolerance questionnaire. Br J Addict 1991;86(9):1119–1127.
62. Chabrol H, Niezborala M, Chastan E, Montastruc JL, Mullet E. A study of the psychometric properties of the Fagerstrom test for nicotine dependence. Addict Behav 2003;28(8):1441–1445.
63. Etter JF, Le Houezec J, Perneger TV. A self-administered questionnaire to measure dependence on cigarettes: the cigarette dependence scale. Neuropsychopharmacology 2003;28(2):359–370.
64. Ether JF. A comparison of the content-, construct- and predictive validity of the cigarette dependence scale and the Fagerstrom test for nicotine dependence, Drug Alcohol Depend. 2005 Mar 7;77(3):259–268.

The Alcohol Use Disorders Identification Test:
Interview Version

Read questions as written. Record answers carefully. Begin the AUDIT by saying "Now I am going to ask you some questions about your use of alcoholic beverages during this past year." Explain what is meant by "alcoholic beverages" by using local examples of beer, wine, vodka, etc. Code answers in terms of "standard drinks."

1. How often do you have a drink containing alcohol?

    (0) Never [Skip to Qs 9–10]
    (1) Monthly or less
    (2) 2–4 times a month
    (3) 2–3 times a week
    (4) 4 or more times a week

2. How many drinks containing alcohol do you have on a typical day when you are drinking?

    (0) 1 or 2
    (1) 3 or 4
    (2) 5 or 6
    (3) 7, 8, or 9
    (4) 10 or more

3. How often do you have six or more drinks on one occasion?

    (0) Never
    (1) Less than monthly
    (2) Monthly
    (3) Weekly
    (4) Daily or almost daily

Skip to Questions 9 and 10 if Total Score
for Questions 2 and 3 = 0

4. How often during the last year have you found that you were not able to stop drinking once you had started?

    (0) Never
    (1) Less than monthly
    (2) Monthly
    (3) Weekly
    (4) Daily or almost daily

5. How often during the last year have you failed to do what was normally expected from you because of drinking?

    (0) Never
    (1) Less than monthly
    (2) Monthly
    (3) Weekly
    (4) Daily or almost daily

6. How often during the last year have you needed a first drink in the morning to get yourself going after a heavy drinking session?

    (0) Never
    (1) Less than monthly

   (2) Monthly
   (3) Weekly
   (4) Daily or almost daily

7. How often during the last year have you had a feeling of guilt or remorse after drinking?

   (0) Never
   (1) Less than monthly
   (2) Monthly
   (3) Weekly
   (4) Daily or almost daily

8. How often during the last year have you been unable to remember what happened the night before because you had been drinking?

   (0) Never
   (1) Less than monthly
   (2) Monthly
   (3) Weekly
   (4) Daily or almost daily

9. Have you or someone else been injured as a result of your drinking?

   (0) No
   (2) Yes, but not in the last year
   (4) Yes, during the last year

10. Has a relative or friend or a doctor or another health worker been concerned about your drinking or suggested you cut down?

   (0) No
   (2) Yes, but not in the last year
   (4) Yes, during the last year

Assessment of the Frequency and Quantity of Alcohol Use in the Past 30 Days

During the past **30 days**…	
1. On how many days did you have at least one drink containing alcohol?	_____ days
2. On the days that you drank alcohol, on how many days did you have five or more drinks (for men; four or more drinks for women)?	_____ days
3. On the days that you drank alcohol, what was the average amount of alcohol that you consumed? (In number of standard drinks, 1 standard drink=12 oz. beer, 1.5 oz. liquor, or 5 oz. wine)	_____ drinks
4. What was the highest amount of alcohol that you consumed in a single drinking day? (In number of standard drinks)	_____ drinks
5. On how many days did you experience significant cravings for alcohol or urges to drink?	_____ days

The Leeds Dependence Questionnaire

On this page there are questions about the importance of alcohol and/or other drugs in your life.

Think about your drinking/other drug use in the last week and answer each question ticking the closest answer to how you see yourself.

	Never	Sometimes	Often	Nearly always
1. Do you find yourself thinking about when you will next be able to have another drink or take more drugs?				
2. Is drinking or taking drugs more important than anything else you might do during the day?				
3. Do you feel that your need for drink or drugs is too strong to control?				
4. Do you plan your days around getting and taking drink or drugs?				
5. Do you drink or take drugs in a particular way in order to increase the effect it gives you?				
6. Do you take drink or other drugs morning, afternoon and evening?				
7. Do you feel you have to carry on drinking or taking drugs once you have started?				
8. Is getting the effect you want more important than the particular drink or drug you use?				
9. Do you want to take more drink or drugs when the effect starts to wear off?				
10. Do you find it difficult to cope with life without drink or drugs?				

Clinical Institute Withdrawal Assessment of Alcohol Scale, Revised (CIWA-Ar)

Patient:_____ Date: _____ Time: _____ (24 hour clock, midnight = 00:00)

Pulse or heart rate, taken for one minute:_____ Blood pressure:_____

Nausea and Vomiting – Ask "Do you feel sick to your stomach? Have you vomited?" Observation.
0 No nausea and no vomiting
1 Mild nausea with no vomiting
2
3
4 Intermittent nausea with dry heaves
5
6
7 Constant nausea, frequent dry heaves and vomiting

Tactile Disturbances – Ask "Have you any itching, pins and needles sensations, any burning, any numbness, or do you feel bugs crawling on or under your skin?" Observation.
0 None
1 Very mild itching, pins and needles, burning or numbness
2 Mild itching, pins and needles, burning or numbness
3 Moderate itching, pins and needles, burning or numbness
4 Moderately severe hallucinations
5 Severe hallucinations
6 Extremely severe hallucinations
7 Continuous hallucinations

Tremor – Arms extended and fingers spread apart. Observation.
0 No tremor
1 Not visible, but can be felt fingertip to fingertip
2
3
4 Moderate, with patient's arms extended
5
6
7 Severe, even with arms not extended

Auditory Disturbances – Ask "Are you more aware of sounds around you? Are they harsh? Do they frighten you? Are you hearing anything that is disturbing to you? Are you hearing things you know are not there?" Observation.
0 Not present
1 Very mild harshness or ability to frighten
2 Mild harshness or ability to frighten
3 Moderate harshness or ability to frighten
4 Moderately severe hallucinations
5 Severe hallucinations
6 Extremely severe hallucinations
7 Continuous hallucinations

Paroxysmal Sweats – Observation.
0 No sweat visible
1 Barely perceptible sweating, palms moist
2
3
4 Beads of sweat obvious on forehead
5
6
7 Drenching sweats

Visual Disturbances – Ask "Does the light appear to be too bright? Is its color different? Does it hurt your eyes? Are you seeing anything that is disturbing to you? Are you seeing things you know are not there?" Observation.
0 Not present
1 Very mild sensitivity
2 Mild sensitivity
3 Moderate sensitivity
4 Moderately severe hallucinations
5 Severe hallucinations
6 Extremely severe hallucinations
7 Continuous hallucinations

Anxiety – Ask "Do you feel nervous?" Observation.
0 No anxiety, at ease
1 Mild anxious
2
3
4 Moderately anxious, or guarded, so anxiety is inferred
5
6
7 Equivalent to acute panic states as seen in severe delirium or acute schizophrenic reactions

Headache, Fullness in Head – Ask "Does your head feel different? Does it feel like there is a band around your head?" Do not rate for dizziness or lightheadedness. Otherwise, rate severity.
0 Not present
1 Very mild
2 Mild
3 Moderate
4 Moderately severe
5 Severe
6 Very severe
7 Extremely severe

Agitation – Observation.
0 Normal activity
1 Somewhat more than normal activity
2
3
4 Moderately fidgety and restless
5
6
7 Paces back and forth during most of the interview, or constantly thrashes about

Orientation and Clouding of Sensorium – Ask
"What day is this? Where are you? Who am I?"
0 Oriented and can do serial additions
1 Cannot do serial additions or is uncertain about date
2 Disoriented for date by no more than 2 calendar days
3 Disoriented for date by more than 2 calendar days
4 Disoriented for place/or person

Total **CIWA-Ar** Score _____
Rater's Initials _____
Maximum Possible Score 67

The CIWA-Ar is not copyrighted and may be reproduced freely. This assessment for monitoring withdrawal symptoms requires approximately 5 minutes to administer. The maximum score is 67 (see instrument). Patients scoring less than 10 do not usually need additional medication for withdrawal.

Sullivan, J.T.; Sykora, K.; Schneiderman, J.; Naranjo, C.A.; and Sellers, E.M. Assessment of alcohol withdrawal: The revised Clinical Institute Withdrawal Assessment for Alcohol scale (**CIWA-Ar**). *British Journal of Addiction* 84:1353–1357, 1989.

Short Index of Problems

Directions: Here are a number of events that drinkers sometimes experience. Read each one carefully and indicate how often each one has happened to you DURING THE PAST 3 MONTHS (0=Never, 1=Once or a few times, etc.). If an item does not apply to you, circle (0).

During the Past 3 Months, about how often has this happened to you?
Circle one answer for each item.

	Never	Once or a few times	Once or twice a week	Daily almost daily
1. I have been unhappy because of my drinking.	0	1	2	3
2. Because of my drinking, I have not eaten properly.	0	1	2	3
3. I have failed to do what is expected of me because of my drinking.	0	1	2	3
4. I have felt guilty or ashamed because of my drinking.	0	1	2	3
5. I have taken foolish risks when I have been drinking.	0	1	2	3
6. When drinking, I have done impulsive things that I regretted later.	0	1	2	3
7. My physical health has been harmed by my drinking.	0	1	2	3
8. I have had money problems because of my drinking.	0	1	2	3
9. My physical appearance has been harmed by my drinking.	0	1	2	3
10. My family has been hurt because of my drinking.	0	1	2	3
11. A friendship or close relationship has been damaged by my drinking.	0	1	2	3
12. My drinking has gotten in the way of my growth as a person.	0	1	2	3
13. My drinking has damaged my social life, popularity, or reputation.	0	1	2	3

14. I have spent too much or lost a lot of money because of my drinking.	0	1	2	3
15. I have had an accident while drinking or intoxicated.	0	1	2	3

The AWARE Questionnaire (Revised Form)

The AWARE Questionnaire (Advance WArning of RElapse) was designed as a measure of the warning signs of relapse, as described by Gorski (Gorski & Miller, 1982). In a prospective study of relapse following outpatient treatment for alcohol abuse or dependence (Miller et al., 1996) we found the AWARE score to be a good predictor of the occurrence of relapse ($r = 0.42, p < 0.001$). With subsequent analyses, we refined the scale from its 37-item original version to the current 28-item scale (version 3.0) (Miller & Harris, 2000).

The items are arranged in the order of occurrence of warning signs, as hypothesized by Gorski. In our prospective study, however, we found no evidence that the warning signs actually occur in this order in real time (Miller & Harris, 2000). Rather, the total score was the best predictor of impending relapse.

ADMINISTRATION: This is a self-report questionnaire that can be filled out by the client. Be sure that the client understands the 1–7 rating scale. When the client has finished, make sure that all items have been answered and none omitted.

SCORING: Total the numbers circled for all items, but *reverse the scoring* for the following five items: 8, 14, 20, 24, 26. For these five items only:

If the client circles this number:	1	2	3	4	5	6	7
Add this number to the total score:	7	6	5	4	3	2	1

INTERPRETATION: The higher the score, the more warning signs of relapse are being reported by the client. The range of scores is from 28 (lowest possible score) to 196 (highest possible score). The following table shows the probability of heavy drinking (not just a slip) during the *next two months*, based on our prospective study of relapse in the first year after treatment (Miller & Harris, 2000).

Probability of heavy drinking during the next two months

AWARE score	If *already* drinking in the prior 2 months (%)	If *abstinent* during the prior 2 months (%)
28–55	37	11
56–69	62	21
70–83	72	24
84–97	82	25
98–111	86	28
112–125	77	37
126–168	90	43
169–196	>95	53

This instrument was developed through research funded by the National Institute on Alcohol Abuse and Alcoholism (NIAAA, contract ADM 281-91-0006). It is in the public domain, and may be used without specific permission provided that proper acknowledgment is given to its source. The appropriate citation is Miller & Harris (2000).

References

Gorski, T. F., & Miller, M. (1982). *Counseling for relapse prevention*. Independence, MO: Herald House – Independence Press.

Miller, W. R., & Harris, R. J. (2000). A simple scale of Gorski's warning signs for relapse. *Journal of Studies on Alcohol, 61*, 759–765.

Miller, W. R., Westerberg, V. S., Harris, R. J., & Tonigan, J. S. (1996). What predicts relapse? Prospective testing of antecedent models. *Addiction, 91* (Supplement), S155–S171.

AWARE Questionnaire 3.0

Please read the following statements and for each one circle a number, from 1 to 7, to indicate *how much this has been true for you recently*. Please circle one and only one number for every statement.

	Never	Rarely	Some-times	Fairly often	Often	Almost always	Always
1. I feel nervous or unsure of my ability to stay sober.	1	2	3	4	5	6	7
2. I have many problems in my life.	1	2	3	4	5	6	7
3. I tend to overreact or act impulsively.	1	2	3	4	5	6	7
4. I keep to myself and feel lonely.	1	2	3	4	5	6	7
5. I get too focused on one area of my life.	1	2	3	4	5	6	7
6. I feel blue, down, listless, or depressed.	1	2	3	4	5	6	7
7. I engage in wishful thinking.	1	2	3	4	5	6	7
8. The plans that I make succeed.	1	2	3	4	5	6	7
9. I have trouble concentrating and prefer to dream about how things could be.	1	2	3	4	5	6	7
10. Things don't work out well for me.	1	2	3	4	5	6	7
11. I feel confused.	1	2	3	4	5	6	7
12. I get irritated or annoyed with my friends.	1	2	3	4	5	6	7
13. I feel angry or frustrated.	1	2	3	4	5	6	7
14. I have good eating habits.	1	2	3	4	5	6	7
	Never	Rarely	Some-times	Fairly often	Often	Almost always	Always

	Never	Rarely	Some-times	Fairly often	Often	Almost always	Always
15. I feel trapped and stuck, like there is no way out.	1	2	3	4	5	6	7
16. I have trouble sleeping.	1	2	3	4	5	6	7
17. I have long periods of serious depression.	1	2	3	4	5	6	7
18. I don't really care what happens.	1	2	3	4	5	6	7
19. I feel like things are so bad that I might as well drink.	1	2	3	4	5	6	7
20. I am able to think clearly.	1	2	3	4	5	6	7
21. I feel sorry for myself.	1	2	3	4	5	6	7
22. I think about drinking.	1	2	3	4	5	6	7
23. I lie to other people.	1	2	3	4	5	6	7
24. I feel hopeful and confident.	1	2	3	4	5	6	7
25. I feel angry at the world in general.	1	2	3	4	5	6	7
26. I am doing things to stay sober.	1	2	3	4	5	6	7
27. I am afraid that I am losing my mind.	1	2	3	4	5	6	7
28. I am drinking out of control.	1	2	3	4	5	6	7
	Never	Rarely	Some-times	Fairly often	Often	Almost always	Always

Scoring sheet for AWARE Questionnaire 3.0

For these items, record   For these 5 items,
the number circled   reverse the scale (* see below)

1._____
2._____
3._____
4._____
5._____
6._____   *For reverse-scaled items: 1 = 7
7._____   2 = 6
                      8._____   3 = 5
9._____   4 = 4
10._____   5 = 3
11._____   6 = 2
12._____   7 = 1
13._____
                      14._____
15._____
16._____
17._____
18._____
19._____
                      20._____
21._____
22._____
23._____
                      24._____
25._____
                      26._____
27._____
28._____

Totals: _____   +   _____   =   _____
              Subtotal   Subtotal   AWARE Score

Tiffany QSU-Brief

This questionnaire consists of ten questions about experiences you are feeling **right now**. To answer the questions, please determine and then circle the degree in which the experience described in the question applies to you.

		Very little	A little	Some	Much	Very much
1.	I have a desire for a cigarette right now.	1	2	3	4	5
2.	Nothing would be better than smoking a cigarette right now.	1	2	3	4	5
3.	If it were possible, I probably would smoke right now.	1	2	3	4	5
4.	I could control things better right now if I could smoke.	1	2	3	4	5
5.	All I want right now is a cigarette.	1	2	3	4	5
6.	I have an urge for a cigarette.	1	2	3	4	5
7.	A cigarette would taste good right now.	1	2	3	4	5
8.	I would do almost anything for a cigarette now.	1	2	3	4	5
9.	Smoking would make me less depressed.	1	2	3	4	5
10.	I am going to smoke as soon as possible.	1	2	3	4	5

Wisconsin Smoking Withdrawal Scale

To answer the questions, please determine and then circle the degree in which the experience described in the questions applies to you. Answer all the questions on the basis of your own experiences.

		Strongly disagree	Disagree	Feel neutral	Agree	Strongly agree
1	Food is not particularly appealing to me.	0	1	2	3	4
2	I am getting restful sleep.	0	1	2	3	4
3	I have been tense or anxious.	0	1	2	3	4
4	My level of concentration is excellent.	0	1	2	3	4
5	I awaken from sleep frequently during the night.	0	1	2	3	4
6	I have felt impatient.	0	1	2	3	4
7	I have felt upbeat and optimistic.	0	1	2	3	4
8	I have found myself worrying about my problems.	0	1	2	3	4
9	I have had frequent urges to smoke.	0	1	2	3	4
10	I have felt calm lately.	0	1	2	3	4
11	I have been bothered by the desire to smoke a cigarette.	0	1	2	3	4
12	I have felt sad or depressed.	0	1	2	3	4
13	I have been irritable, easily angered.	0	1	2	3	4
14	I want to nibble on snacks or sweets.	0	1	2	3	4
15	I have been bothered by negative moods such as anger, frustration, and irritability.	0	1	2	3	4
16	I have been eating a lot.	0	1	2	3	4
17	I am satisfied with my sleep.	0	1	2	3	4
18	I have felt frustrated.	0	1	2	3	4
19	I have felt hopeless or discouraged.	0	1	2	3	4
20	I have thought about smoking a lot.	0	1	2	3	4
21	I have felt hungry.	0	1	2	3	4
22	I feel that I am getting enough sleep.	0	1	2	3	4
23	It is hard to pay attention to things.	0	1	2	3	4
24	I have felt happy and content.	0	1	2	3	4
25	My sleep has been troubled.	0	1	2	3	4
26	I have trouble getting cigarettes off my mind.	0	1	2	3	4
27	It has been difficult to think clearly.	0	1	2	3	4
28	I think about food a lot.	0	1	2	3	4

Fagerström Test for Nicotine Dependence

1. How soon after you wake up do you have your first cigarette?
   - A. Within 5 minutes (3)
   - B. 6–30 minutes (2)
   - C. 31–60 minutes (1)
   - D. After 60 minutes (0)

2. Do you find it difficult to refrain from smoking in places where it is forbidden?
   - A. Yes (1)
   - B. No (0)

3. Which cigarette would you hate most to give up?
   - A. The first one in the morning (1)
   - B. All others (0)

4. How many cigarettes per day do you smoke?
   - A. 10 or fewer (0)
   - B. 11–20 (1)
   - C. 21–30 (2)
   - D. 31 or more (3)

5. Do you smoke more frequently during the first hours after waking than during the rest of the day?
   - A. Yes (1)
   - B. No (0)

6. Do you smoke even if you are so ill that you are in bed most of the day?
   - A. Yes (1)
   - B. No (0)

Total: _____

Chapter 6
Screening for Personality Disorders in Psychiatric Settings: Four Recently Developed Screening Measures

Caleb J. Siefert

Abstract Prevalence rates for Personality Disorders are higher in psychiatric settings. Nonetheless, the presence of a personality disorder may go undetected for some time during the early phases of treatment. This is problematic as a failure to detect a Personality Disorder as part of the initial evaluation can result in less beneficial treatment plans, negative outcomes, and a more difficult treatment course. Nonetheless, the benefits of early detection must be weighed against practical considerations, including time and resources. Currently gold-standard assessment measures for Personality Disorders are lengthy and time consuming which may limit their practical utility. The present chapter reviews data on the importance of assessing for personality disorders, reviews the benefits of stage I (screening for Personality Disorders) and stage II (thorough evaluation for a Personality Disorder), and then reviews four recently developed measures that can be used as part of the personality disorder screening process. Information on more detailed measures for stage II assessment is also briefly presented and clinical implications are discussed.

Keywords Personality disorder · Screening · Rating scales · Questionnaires · Assessment · Psychiatry

Mental-health clinicians have become increasingly interested in accurately identifying personality disorders (PDs) in patients presenting for psychiatric treatment. Prevalence rates for PDs are higher in psychiatric settings as compared to community settings [1, 2] and PDs significantly affect the management, course, and outcome of psychiatric treatment [3–5]. As such, it is important for clinicians to assess for PDs as part of an initial evaluation and to consider a patient's PD status in formulating a treatment plan. At this time structured clinical interviews, such as the Structured Clinical Interview for DSM-IV Personality Disorders (SCID-II)

C.J. Siefert (✉)
Department of Psychiatry, Massachusetts General Hospital and Harvard Medical School, Boston, MA 02115, USA
e-mail: csiefert@partners.org

L. Baer, M.A. Blais (eds.), *Handbook of Clinical Rating Scales and Assessment in Psychiatry and Mental Health*, Current Clinical Psychiatry, DOI 10.1007/978-1-59745-387-5_6,
© Humana Press, a part of Springer Science+Business Media, LLC 2010

[6], are typically preferred for making a PD diagnosis. These instruments, however, are lengthy, require specialized training, and are often overly burdensome for both clinician and patient [7–11]. As such, the utility of these instruments for initial evaluations is limited and a full assessment for PD with every patient is unlikely to be cost effective or time efficient. As an alternative, a two-stage approach has been suggested for assessing PDs [11]. In this approach, all incoming patients are screened for PD (stage I) and patients whose screen suggests risk for a PD can then be more thoroughly evaluated (stage II) using one of the more extensive and comprehensive PD diagnostic instruments.

The present chapter is designed to familiarize clinicians with four PD screening measures. Each of these instruments has been developed within the past decade. The four measures included are the Standardised Assessment of Personality – Abbreviated Scale (SAPAS) [12], Iowa Personality Disorder Screen (IPDS) [10], the Inventory of Interpersonal Problems – Personality Disorders – 25 (IIP-PD-25) [13], and the Five-Factor Model Rating Form (FFMRF) [14]. Though all four measures are designed to screen for the presence of PD in general, each was developed from a slightly different theoretical perspective. All of these measures can be easily incorporated into an initial diagnostic evaluation.

Why Screen for Personality Disorders?

PDs affect a number of factors associated with the management of psychiatric treatment. Patients with PDs often experience a less robust response to first-line treatments of Axis I conditions [3–5] and tend to have longer, more complicated treatment courses [15]. In addition to complicating treatment of Axis I conditions, PDs may become the focus of treatment in and of themselves. Indeed, the PDs have been shown to cause distress and impairment beyond that caused by comorbid Axis I conditions [16] and some forms of PD may require specialized adjunctive interventions (i.e., psychotherapy) for optimal outcomes [17, 18]. When a patient's PD goes undiagnosed, clinicians may fail to adequately appreciate the role of a patient's personality in their current difficulties, may develop less than optimal treatment plans, or may fail to recommend appropriate adjunctive treatments. In addition to their impact on treatment planning, there is ample evidence that patients with PDs are at higher risk for a number of maladaptive behaviors, such as substance abuse and suicidal behavior that can interfere or complicate the course of treatment [19, 20]. It is important that a clinician be aware of a patient's PD status and consider these factors when making important clinical decisions such as selecting medications or deciding to hospitalize a patient. In short, identifying the presence (or absence) of a PD is important for developing effective and comprehensive treatment plans for all patients. A patient's PD status, however, may not always be easily detected. The majority of patients with a PD also experience comorbid Axis I disorders [21]. Axis I difficulties, at times, may initially mask a patient's PD status. Additionally, some patients with PD may not view their symptoms and difficulties as related to their personality. Finally, many factors associated with PD are difficult to evaluate by clinical interview alone [22]. Indeed, structured assessment instruments have been demonstrated to improve diagnostic accuracy of PDs and increase clinicians' willingness to make an II diagnosis [22, 23]. Even when screening for PD, the use of structured screening instruments is likely to aid clinicians in accurately identifying patients who are at heightened risk and require a more thorough PD evaluation. Patients whose screen indicates risk for PD can then be more thoroughly evaluated and diagnosed.

Four Recently Developed Screening Instruments

Standardised Assessment of Personality – Abbreviated Scale (SAPAS)

Moran et al. have recently developed the SAPAS as a screen for PDs [12]. The SAPAS is a brief *interview-based instrument* that can be used to screen for PD. It focuses on eight key factors associated with PD (reproduced in the appendix to this chapter). The SAPAS was developed based on the more extensive Standardised Assessment of Personality (SAP) [24]. The SAPAS is brief taking roughly 2 min to complete. Clinicians can easily integrate the SAPAS into a standard clinical interview. Additionally, the SAPAS does not require training to administer. Initial validation research suggests that the SAPAS can adequately screen for PDs.

Measure development: The items for the SAPAS were taken from the opening section of the SAP. The eight items were selected on the basis of an exploratory analysis from a prior study [25]. In this study, these eight probe items from the SAP were highly effective in predicting PD status for 303 primary care patients when they were administered to informants who knew the patient well. Moran et al. then utilized these items to develop the SAPAS, which could be administered *directly* to patients (as opposed to informants) as part of a standard clinical evaluation. The final items included on the SAPAS are written in a descriptive fashion.

Administration and Scoring Procedures: As can be seen in the appendix to this chapter, the SAPAS contains a brief statement that can be used to introduce the measure to patients. Each item of the SAPAS can be read directly to the patient. Items are rated on a dichotomous yes–no basis. Patients are instructed to endorse items if they feel that the item accurately describes them *most of the time in most situations*. Item number 3 ("In general do you trust people?") is reverse coded. As such, it should be scored "no" only if the patient feels this is true of them most of the time in most situations. With the exception of item 3, a response of "yes" is scored (i.e., yes = 1; no = 0). For item 3 a response of "no" is scored (i.e., yes = 0; no = 1). A total score is then calculated by summing the number of items scored "1" and can range from 0 to 8. When used for screening purposes, the authors suggest that patients who receive a total score of 3 or higher on the SAPAS should be further evaluated for PD.

Table 6.1 Diagnostic efficiency statistics for the personality disorder-screening instruments

Study	Measure	Cut Score	Sensitivity	Specificity	PPV	NPV
Moran et al. [12]	SAPAS	≥3	0.94	0.85	0.89	0.92
Langbehn et al. [7]	IPDS	≥2	0.96	0.64	0.47*	0.98*
		≥3	0.79	0.86	0.65*	0.93*
Trull and Amdur [10]	IPDS	≥2	0.69	0.91	0.81	0.85
		≥3	0.36	0.99	0.93	0.74
Kim and Pilkonis [13]	IIP-PD-25	≥.70	0.93	0.27	0.61	0.75
		≥1.10	0.80	0.46	0.65	0.65
		≥1.30	0.71	0.58	0.67	0.62

PPV = positive predictive value; NPV = negative predictive value; SAPAS = Standardised Assessment of Personality – Abbreviated Scale; IPDS = Iowa Personality Disorders Screener; IIP-PD-25 = Inventory of Interpersonal Problems – Personality Disorders – 25.
*Assumes a base rate of 25%.

Previous Research: Moran et al. have presented initial validation data on the SAPAS [12]. In this study, 60 adult patients were assessed using the SCID-II and the SAPAS. Of the 60 patients included, 33 were found to have a PD as determined by SCID-II interview. As can be seen in Table 6.1, the SAPAS proved to be highly sensitive to the detection of PDs and reasonably specific. Though the authors investigated several cutoff points, a cutoff score of 3 or greater proved to provide the optimal balance between sensitivity and specificity. Further, the positive predictive value (PPV) and negative predictive value (NPV) are both strong for the SAPAS. In this case, PPV refers to the proportion of patients with an actual PD that were accurately identified by the screen. Conversely, NPV refers to the proportion of patients without an actual PD diagnosis who scored below the cutoff for the screen. Though these initial findings are strong, the authors point out several limitations of their study. Patients were included in the study on a non-random basis and the proportion of patients with a PD was high. As such, the sensitivity of the instrument may decline somewhat in settings where the base rates for PD are lower (e.g., community settings, primary care settings, non-clinical research) [12]. Thus, at this time the use of the SAPAS should be limited to clinical settings.

Summary: The SAPAS has a number of strengths that are likely to make it an appealing instrument to clinicians who wish to screen for PD as part of their initial clinical evaluation. First, it is *extremely* brief, requiring a matter of minutes to complete. Second, it can be easily incorporated into routine clinical evaluations. Third, the initial validation study found it to have excellent sensitivity and high specificity for detecting PD in a clinical population. Additionally, there are a number of advantages to using interview-based methods and clinical observation for detecting and diagnosing PDs. For example, interview-based methods allow clinicians to follow up on particular responses, ask for clarification and elaboration, and draw inference based on both a patient's overt verbal response and non-verbal behavior. As with the majority of PD-screening instruments, the SAPAS is fairly new and has not been studied in non-clinical samples and has yet to be extensively studied with clinical samples. At this time, additional studies examining the diagnostic efficiency of the SAPAS are underway.

Iowa Personality Disorder Screen *(IPDS)*

Langbehn et al. initially developed the IPDS to screen for PDs by assessing 11 key beliefs and behaviors associated with PDs [10]. After research suggested that 7 of the 11 items were most efficient discriminators of PD, a 7-item short-version of the IPDS was created (reproduced in the appendix to this chapter). Like the SAPAS, the IPDS is a brief interview-based measure requiring roughly 5 min to complete. It can be easily integrated into standard diagnostic clinical interviews and initial validation research has suggested that it is adequate in identifying patients requiring further evaluation to determine if they meet criteria for a PD.

Measure development: The IPDS was developed by drawing items from recorded structured II interviews conducted with a large clinical sample (n = 1,203) gathered from multiple research centers [10]. In the original version, 11 items were selected based on their ability to discriminate between individuals with and without PDs in the measure development sample. Subsequent pilot studies at the University of Iowa were undertaken to test the initial feasibility of the items and the ease with which various raters could score them. These resulted in small changes in the wording of some items, how they were probed, and how they were scored to increase their utility as screening items. The original version of the IPDS contained 11 items, but was shortened to 7 items after research suggested that these 7 items were most useful for detecting PDs [10].

Administration and scoring procedures: As can be seen in the appendix to this chapter, the IPDS contains a brief introduction that can be read to patients to introduce the measure. Each item of the IPDS contains one or two specific prompts that can be directly read to the patient. For example, to administer item 3 the clinician simply reads the text below item 3: "Do you find that most people will take advantage of you if you let them know too much about you?" Some items of the IPDS are scored only if the patient responds "Yes" to *both* prompts (e.g., item 1), while other items are scored if the patient responds "Yes" to *either* prompt (e.g., item 2). Given its moderate degree of complexity, it is important that clinicians familiarize themselves with the measure prior to administration. To score the IPDS, clinicians simply tally the number of items endorsed. When using the IPDS for screening purposes, a score of 2 or more is suggested as a cutoff score for determining if there is a need for a further PD evaluation [10].

Previous Research: In the initial validation study, the IPDS was used to identify PD in 52 patients currently in psychiatric treatment [10]. All participants carried an Axis I diagnosis, 24 participants were diagnosed with a PD and 28 participants did not meet criteria for a PD. PD diagnosis in this study was determined on the basis of a standardized diagnostic interview [26]. As can be seen in Table 6.1, a cutoff score of ≥ 2 on the IPDS proved fairly sensitive to PD, and showed adequate PPV and NPV in the clinical sample. Though a cutoff score of ≥ 3 improved specificity, it lowered sensitivity. Since high sensitivity is important for screening purposes, the authors suggest using a cutoff score of 2 or greater on the IPDS to screen for PD.

A subsequent study, conducted by Trull and Armdur examined the effectiveness of the IPDS in a *non-clinical* sample of 103 undergraduate students [10]. In this study all participants were administered a structured diagnostic interview as well as the IPDS. In this sample, 35% met criteria for a PD. As can be seen in Table 6.1, the results from this study suggested high PPV and NPV for the IPDS. However, in the non-clinical sample the sensitivity of the IPDS to PD was somewhat low. As such, it may not be as effective a screening instrument when used in non-clinical settings as compared to clinical settings, though this finding requires further investigation.

Summary: The IPDS has a number of strengths and should be strongly considered as part of a general screen for PD. First, as its authors note, it is easily integrated into a standard clinical evaluation interview. Second, it is a low-burden instrument requiring roughly 5 min to complete. Finally, it has been shown to be reasonably sensitive and specific in a clinical sample. Fourth, it has shown good convergence with other PD screeners [11]. In considering the IPDS, it is important to note that very few subjects in the initial validation sample were diagnosed with antisocial personality disorder. Thus, the IPDS may be less effective in screening for this particular PD diagnosis.

Inventory of Interpersonal Problems – Personality Disorders – 25 *(IIP-PD-25)*

There is ample evidence that persons with PD experience impairment in interpersonal functioning [13]. Further, interest in the use of attachment theory to conceptualize and identify PDs has increased substantially [27]. In this context, Kim and Pilkonis developed the IIP-PD-25 (reproduced in the appendix to this chapter) as a screening instrument for PD by asking respondents about problems they experience in social relationships. The IIP-PD-25 can be easily completed by patients in 10 min or less. In addition to acting as a screen for PD, the IIP-PD-25 also provides clinicians with information on the patient's interpersonal functioning in general and is often helpful in highlighting areas of difficulty that may become the target for treatment.

Measure development: The IIP-PD-25 is one of a number of measures that have been developed based on the original Inventory of Interpersonal Problems (IIP) [28]. Pilkonis et al. (1996) developed a version of the IIP, called the Inventory of Interpersonal Problems – Personality Disorders (IIP-PD) [29], that is specifically tailored for detecting PD and has proven highly effective in discriminating between patients with and without a PD [12, 29]. Kim and Pilkonis created the IIP-PD-25 as brief version of the IIP-PD that could be used for screening purposes. They utilized Item Response Theory (IRT) to determine the most effective screening items for each of the five subscales of the IIP-PD. IRT is particularly effective in determining the discriminating power of *individual items* in both high and low base rate samples [30]. As such, IRT offers a number of advantages for selecting items that are useful for screening purposes. Using six separate clinical samples (Total N = 1149) taken from different treatment sites, Kim and Pilkonis utilized IRT to determine the five most effective items of each subscale for the IIP-PD. The five best items for each of the five subscales were then used to create the IIP-PD-25. For the most part, the IIP-PD-25 subscales appear similar in content to the subscales of the IIP-PD. However, as Kim and Pilkonis note, the items of the Interpersonal Ambivalence subscale of the IIP-PD-25 appear to tap negativistic or passive–aggressive interpersonal attitudes as opposed to Interpersonal Ambivalence.

Administration and Scoring Procedures: The IIP-PD-25 can be easily administered at the beginning or end of an initial evaluation. As can be seen in the appendix to this chapter, items are broken into two sections. In the first part, respondents rate how hard it is for them to engage in a particular interpersonal behavior (e.g., It is hard for me to join in groups). In the second part, respondents rate problematic interpersonal behaviors or reactions that they experience *too much* (e.g., I get irritated or annoyed too easily). All items are rated on a 5-point Likert scale that ranges from 0 (not at all) to 4 (extremely) based on how problematic the particular interpersonal behavior or reaction is. The 25 items compose five separate scales: Interpersonal Sensitivity, Interpersonal Ambivalence, Aggression, Need for Social Approval, and Lack of Sociability. Subscale scores are determined by calculating the mean score for the items on the subscale. Items 8, 13, 15, 18, and 25 compose the Interpersonal Sensitivity subscale. Items 2, 3, 6, 7, and 9 compose the Interpersonal Ambivalence subscale. Items 12, 14, 16, 22, and 23 compose the Aggression subscale. The mean score for these first three subscales (Interpersonal Sensitivity, Interpersonal Ambivalence, and aggression) can then be calculated and used as a PD screening index. Kim and Pilkonis suggest that when an individual's PD index score falls between 0.70 and 1.10, a PD is possible and when the PD index score is above 1.10 a PD is probable. The remaining items compose the other two IIP-PD-25 subscales. Items 10, 17, 19, 20, and 21 compose the Need for Social Approval subscale. Items 1, 4, 5, 11, and 24 compose the Lack of Sociability subscale [13].

Previous Research: Initial development and investigation of the IIP-PD-25 was conducted using six large clinical samples (Total N = 1149) collected at six separate sites [13]. In addition to completing the IIP-PD, all patients were evaluated using a structured diagnostic PD interview. In this initial development and validation study, the psychometric properties of the IIP-PD-25 were examined, its agreement with the longer IIP-PD was evaluated, and its ability to screen for PD was investigated. All five subscales evidenced excellent internal consistency (alphas > 0.80). The IIP-PD-25 subscales also showed strong agreement with subscale scores obtained from the IIP-PD (Pearson product-moment correlations ranged from 0.92 to 0.97). A sample of 178 patients was utilized to examine the utility of the PD index of the IIP-PD-25 for detecting the presence of a PD. As can be seen in Table 6.1, the various suggested cutoff scores were highly sensitive to PD and showed acceptable PPV and NPV.

Summary: There are a number of reasons clinicians should strongly consider the IIP-PD-25 as a screening tool to assess for PDs. First, it was developed using IRT which makes this approach particularly well suited for identifying effective screening items [30]. Second, its brevity and high face validity make it a low-burden measure for patients to complete as part of an initial psychiatric evaluation. Third, items from the IIP-PD-25 were taken from the larger IIP-PD and subscales have initially shown a high level of agreement with this more established measure [13]. Fourth, there is considerable evidence that individuals with a wide range of PDs experience interpersonal problems; thus, the assessment of interpersonal problems may be particularly useful for screening for the presence or absence of a PD in general [13, 29]. One of the weaknesses of the IIP-PD-25 is the relatively low specificity values for the suggested cutoff scores in the initial validation research. Thus, many patients who score above the suggested cutoff scores will fail to have a PD. It should, however, be noted that in the case of screening as opposed to diagnosing, the focus in scale development is to maximize sensitivity. Thus, lower levels of specificity may be accepted in order to increase the sensitivity of an instrument. While the initial investigation into the IIP-PD-25 has been promising, its authors note that further investigation into the operating characteristics of the IIP-PD-25 will be needed in the future to better determine its full clinical utility. Thus, at this time, the IIP-PD-25 is likely to be particularly useful as a Stage-I assessment screening tool to assist in the assessment of interpersonal functioning. When patients score above the critical cutoff for the PD scale of the IIP-PD-25, it suggests that they are experiencing interpersonal problems to a degree that is commonly associated with PDs. Thus, patients scoring above this cutoff should be further evaluated (stage-II assessment) to determine if they meet criteria for a PD.

Five Factor Model Rating Form *(FFMRF)*

A number of studies utilizing clinical and non-clinical samples provide evidence that there are five broad domains of personality [14, 31, 32]. This approach to understanding personality is referred to as the Five Factor Model (FFM). The FFM is composed of the following five factors: neuroticism, extraversion, agreeableness, conscientiousness, and openness to experience. In addition to the five factors, each factor of the FFM can be further broken down into six facet areas that compose the factor. For example, the factor agreeableness is composed of the following facets: trust, straightforwardness, altruism, compliance, modesty, and tender-mindedness (for a more detailed description of the FFM factors and facets see Costa and McCrae [32]). Research suggests that the facet scores for each of the five factors are especially important for describing and identifying PDs [31, 33].

There has been growing interest in the clinical applications of the FFM, with particular focus on the utility of the FFM for diagnosing, understanding, and describing PDs [34]. A recent meta-analysis focusing on the relationship of PDs to the FFM concluded that PDs are systematically related to the five factors in meaningful and predictable ways [35]. Widiger et al. have recently produced a brief one-page 30-item FFM measure called the Five-Factor Model Rating Form (FFMRF; reproduced in the appendix to this chapter) [14]. In addition to being shorter, it also differs from previous brief FFM measures in that the FFMRF produces a score for the six facets for each factor. Since facet scores of the FFM are particularly important for understanding and diagnosing personality disorders [31, 33], the FFMRF is likely to be useful as a brief FFM measure that can be used to screen for PD.

Measure Development: The FFMRF is composed of 30 items. Items were created such that each item reflects one facet of the FFM. All items make use of bipolar dimensional rating scales that range from 1 (extremely low) to 5 (extremely high). For all items, two to four adjectives are used to describe each pole of the item. For example, to assess the neuroticism facet of anxiousness, respondents are presented with the descriptors "fearful, apprehensive" on one pole and the descriptors "relaxed, unconcerned, cool" on the opposite pole. Respondents then rate each item by indicating which pole is more descriptive of their personality. Items of the FFMRF are organized with respect to the five factors.

Administration and Scoring Procedures: The FFMRF contains instructions that can be read to the patient, or read by the patient, explaining how to complete the measure. Once the patient completes the FFMRF, it can be used to create a FFM profile for patients by calculating the mean score for the six items composing each factor. Items 1–6 compose the neuroticism factor, items 7–12 extraversion, items 13–18 openness to experience, items 19–24 agreeableness, and items 25–30 conscientiousness. Facet profiles can also be created by using the individual facet item score. Thus, each facet score of the FFMRF is determined by the individuals' response to the individual item that taps that facet.

It is important to note that unlike the previous measures discussed in this chapter, the FFMRF does not produce a single scale designed to determine the likelihood of PD. Instead, a patient's constellation of scores across each of the factors and facets of the FFM must be considered. In assessing for PD with the FFMRF, it is helpful to utilize the four-step approach suggested by Widiger et al. [36]. These authors suggest first assessing the personality traits of the FFM (such as the FFMRF). Then identifying distressing social and/or occupational impairments associated with an individual's personality traits. Next, determining if the degree of impairment reaches a clinically significant level, and finally examining the quantitative matches between the individual's FFM profile and prototypic diagnostic profiles [36]. When screening for PD, clinicians may be most interested in steps 1 and 4. For example, the FFMRF could be given and scored. Next, the patients profile could then be compared to prototypic diagnostic profiles for the various PDs. Also, unlike other screening measures, this approach may also be quite helpful in determining which specific type of PD is most likely. It should, however, be noted that steps 2 and 3 of the model may also be facilitated by the use of the FFMRF. Recently, problem checklists have been developed to guide clinicians in follow-up inquiry based on individuals factor and facet scores for the FFM. For example, an individual scoring very high in conscientiousness is unlikely to experience a sense of purposelessness or difficulties in establishing occupational goals. However, such an individual may have significant difficulties with workaholism or fears of failure, and these issues should be further investigated [37]. Recently, Widiger et al. [38] have developed a problem checklist for the FFM that identifies common problems associated with very high or very low factor and facet level scores. Checklists such as these can be used to guide subsequent inquiries related to factor and facet scores that are very high or very low [37]. Many clinicians are likely to find these checklists to be helpful in guiding follow-up questions after the patient has completed the FFMRF.

Initial investigations into the utility of the FFMRF have been promising. The validation research of the FFMRF to this point has focused on the degree to which factor and facet scores for the FFMRF converge with more lengthy measures of the FFM, agreement on PD prototypes using the FFMRF, and the ability of the FFMRF to identify individuals experiencing PDs. In five separate studies, self-report ratings made by college undergraduates using the FFMRF showed good convergent validity with longer measures of the FFM at factor level (median convergent coefficients ranged from 0.47 for openness to experience to 0.69 for extraversion), suggesting that the FFMRF accurately assesses the FFM [14]. Further, across studies, each of the FFMRF facet items was significantly correlated with its respective facet scale as assessed by a longer measure of the FFM [14]. This initial research suggests good agreement between self-report ratings using the FFMRF and longer measures of the FFM at both the factor and facet level. To examine the descriptive utility of the FFMRF for identifying prototypes for PDs, Samuels and Widiger asked 154 therapists in private practice to use the FFMRF to provide prototype descriptions of two PDs. Clinicians ratings showed high agreement for the PD prototypes (average interrater reliability correlations within each profile ranging from 0.60 for the schizotypal profile to 0.76 for the dependent profile) [39]. Further, PD prototype ratings by the clinicians in this study showed good agreement with PD prototypes ratings made by expert researchers in the area of personality (convergent correlations between researchers and clinicians ranged from 0.90 [dependent PD] to 0.97 [antisocial PD]) [31, 39]. Finally, FFM facet scores obtained using self-report ratings of the FFMRF correlate with PD scales of other widely used self-report measures of PD in a manner consistent with expert FFM prototypes for the PDs. For example, consistent with previous research [39], individuals who rated themselves high on scales tapping antisocial PD, also tended to rate themselves low on the FFM facets of trust, straightforwardness, compliance, tender-mindedness, dutifulness, and deliberation, while rating themselves high on the FFM facets of angry hostility, impulsivity, and assertiveness [14].The one exception, however, was narcissistic PD, in which the facets typically associated with it did not correlate as would be expected. Taken as a whole, these results suggest that the FFMRF is an effective tool for describing personality and suggest that patient ratings of the FFMRF can be reasonably used in screening for the presence of PDs.

Summary: The FFMRF offers a number of potential advantages in screening for PD. First, the measure is very brief, easy to complete, and easy for clinicians to score. Second, though a brief measure of the FFM, the FFMRF has shown strong convergence with longer measures at both the factor and the facet level and is the only brief FFM measure to provide facet scores. Third, the FFMRF was developed as part of an extensive literature on the FFM and its application to understanding PD [14]. In addition to these strengths, clinicians are likely to find a FFM profile useful in understanding the personalities of patients with and without PD. Extreme scores at the factor and facet level have been linked to important problems in living [37, 38]. Thus, clinicians can use FFMRF facet and factor scores to develop hypotheses about potential personality-related difficulties which may serve to guide subsequent lines of questioning. Despite these strengths, one of the drawbacks of the FFMRF is that clinicians are likely to find that some familiarity with the FFM is required to maximize the measure's benefits. Unlike the other measures discussed in this chapter, the FFMRF does not have an individual scale for screening for PD, nor does it have specific cut scores that can be used to determine if further evaluation is necessary. Instead profile analysis is required in which an individual patient's FFM profile is compared to prototypic PD FFM profiles. As such, clinicians who are inexperienced with the FFM may need to use the FFMRF in conjunction with additional screening instruments to best determine if further evaluation for PD is needed. Finally, much debate currently exists regarding if PDs are best conceptualized with categorical versus dimensional models of personality and which has more utility for clinical practice. Clinicians interested in the FFMRF may wish to consider the model of PD assessment put forth by Widiger et al. [36, 39] to best determine how they wish to integrate the FFMRF into their evaluation process. In sum, the FFMRF is likely to be useful in helping clinicians identify extreme aspects of personality and patterns of personality traits that are associated with particular types of difficulties. It can also be extremely helpful in guiding clinicians' follow-up questions during the subsequent sessions and, as compared to other screening instruments, may be more capable of indicating which specific PDs are more likely to be present. Its brevity, ease of administration, ease of scoring, and capacity to assess each of the 30 FFM facets is likely to make it highly useful in early evaluation sessions and intakes. The clinical utility of this measure is likely to increase with experience as the FFM becomes more integrated into the conceptualization of PDs.

Diagnosing Personality Disorders

When screening suggests a PD, further evaluation is needed to determine if a patient meets criteria for a specific PD. A number of instruments have been developed that can aid clinicians in making a PD diagnosis. A full discussion of these measures is beyond the scope of this chapter. Nonetheless clinicians who screen for PD should be aware of some of the most well-known diagnostic instruments. Though no "gold standard" method for diagnosing PD exists, structured clinical interview methods are the preferred approach for making a PD diagnosis at this time. Among the most widely used structured clinical interviews for diagnosing PDs are the Structured Clinical Interview for DSM-IV Personality Disorders

(SCID-II) [9], the Structured Interview for DSM-IV Personality Disorders (SIDP-R) [26], the Personality Disorder Interview-IV (PDI-IV) [40], and International Personality Disorder Examination (IPDE) [41]. In addition to structured interview approaches targeting the DSM-IV symptoms of PD, the Structured Interview for the Five-Factor Model (SIFFM) [42] has been developed to assess patient personalities. The SIFFM is an interview-based instrument that assesses the adaptive and maladaptive personality features of the FFM and is also likely to be useful in identifying PDs. In addition to structured clinical interviews, a number of multi-item multi-scale self-report measures have been developed that can also be used to further evaluate PDs. These instruments are much better suited that the PD screeners to investigate which specific types of PD a patient is experiencing. Such measures include the Personality Diagnostic Questionnaire-4 (PDQ-4) [43], the Millon Clinical Multiaxial Inventory-III (MCMI-III) [44], and the OMNI-IV Personality Inventory [45].

Conclusion

In addition to causing distress, impairing functioning, and placing patients at risk for a number of negative outcomes, PDs can significantly affect the course of treatment. The presence of PD can significantly limit the benefit of standard interventions for Axis I complaints. Further many types of PD require mixed treatments involving both psychopharmalogical interventions and psychotherapeutic interventions [46]. As such, identification and diagnosis of a patient's PD is important in providing patients with care, determining the most optimal treatment plan, and educating the patient regarding the nature of their difficulties.

Currently, interview-based methods for diagnosing PDs (e.g., SCID-II) are considered among the best practices for diagnosing PD. These methods, however, have a number of limitations. They are time consuming, require specific training, and are not cost effective for use with all patients. Given these difficulties, several authors have suggested that clinicians should first screen patients for PD to identify patients who are in need of more thorough evaluation. Though based on highly different approaches to conceptualizing PDs, the SAPAS, IPDS, IIP-PD-25, and FFMRF have all shown promise as effective Stage-I screening instruments. Of course, further validation of these instruments is necessary to more thoroughly determine their diagnostic operating characteristics and clinical utility. As such, their use at this time should be limited to Stage-I screening instruments. Further, the extent to which these measures will be effective for screening for PDs in non-clinical populations is unknown. Thus, at this time, the use of these measures should be limited to clinical settings.

The SAPAS, IPDS, and IIP-PD-25 all contain specific scales that are easy to calculate and the authors have suggested cutoff scores that can be used to determine if further PD assessment is necessary. Clinicians familiar with the FFM are likely to find the FFMRF quite helpful. Its ability to produce facet scores may make it useful as a screen for PD and it may prove particularly useful in aiding clinicians in identifying extreme traits that are associated with particular life problems. As such, it may serve to guide interview questions and queries into particular life difficulties. Conversely, clinicians unfamiliar with the FFM may find the IPDS and IIP-PD-25 more "user friendly" at this time. However, given the increasing interest in utilizing the FFM to understand, conceptualize, and assess PDs, the FFMRF is likely to become an extremely useful tool to clinicians in the future.

In conclusion, it is important to note that the formal diagnosis for a PD is ultimately a clinical decision that should be made by incorporating multiple sources of data. The screening measures reviewed in this chapter are intended to aid clinicians in making decisions with regard to identifying patients who are in need of a more thorough evaluation for PD. The four screening tools discussed are relatively low burden for both clinicians and patients to complete and require minimal time to administer, complete, and score. While scores above the critical cutoffs for the SAPAS, IPDS, or IIP-PD-25 are indicative of PD, a formal diagnosis *should not be given based exclusively on these data alone*. Instead, clinicians should use this information to guide subsequent inquiries and determine if further evaluation is necessary. Screening for PDs can greatly enhance clinicians' ability to accurately detect and diagnose a PD when present. The accurate diagnosis of a PD early in the treatment process can facilitate optimal treatment planning and can aid clinicians in making important treatment decisions with their patients.

References

1. Lewin TJ, Slade T, Andrews G, Carr VJ, Hornabrook CW. Assessing personality disorders in a national mental health survey. *Social Psychiatry and Psychiatric Epidemiology* 2005; 40: 87–98.
2. Zimmerman M, Rothschild L, Chelminski I. The Prevalence of DSM-IV Personality Disorders in Psychiatric Outpatients. *American Journal of Psychiatry* 2005; 162: 1911–1918.
3. Newton-Howes G, Tyrer P, Johnson T. Personality Disorders and the outcome of depression: meta-analysis of published studies. *British Journal of Psychiatry* 2006; 188: 13–20
4. Reich JH. The effects of Axis II disorders on the outcome of treatment of anxiety and unipolar depressive disorders: A review. *Journal of Personality Disorders* 2003; 15: 387–405.
5. Reich JH, Vasile RG. Effects of personality disorders on the treatment outcome of Axis I conditions: An update. *Journal of Nervous and Mental Disease* 1993; 181: 475–484.
6. First MB, Gibbon M, Spitzer RI, Williams JB, Benjamin LS. *Structured clinical interview for DSM-IV Axis II Personality Disorders*. Washington, DC: American Press, 1997.
7. Langbehn DR, Pfohl BM, Reynolds S, Clark LW, Battaglia M, Bellodi L, Cadoret, R, Grove W, Pilkonis P, Links P. The Iowa personality disorder screen: Development and preliminary evaluation of a brief screening interview. *Journal of Personality Disorders* 1999; 13: 75–89.
8. Morse JQ, Pilkonis PA. Screening for personality disorders. *Journal of Personality Disorders* 2007; 21: 179–198.
9. Kim Y, Pilkonis PA, Barkham M. Confirmatory factor analysis of the personality disorder subscales from the Inventory of Interpersonal Problems. *Journal of Personality Assessment* 1997; 69: 284–296.
10. Trull TJ, Amdur M. Diagnostic efficiency of the Iowa personality disorder screen items in a nonclinical sample. *Journal of Personality Disorders* 2001; 15: 351–357.

11. Dohrenwend B. "The problem of validity in field studies of psychological disorders" revisited. *Psychological Medicine* 1990; 20: 195–208.
12. Moran P, Leese M, Lee T, Walters P, Thornicroft G, Mann A. Standardised Assessment of Personality Scale (SAPAS): Preliminary validation of a brief screen for personality disorder. *British Journal of Psychiatry* 2003; 183: 228–232.
13. Kim Y, Pilkonis PA. Selecting the most informative items in the IIP scales for personality disorders: An application of item response theory. *Journal of Personality Disorders* 1999; 13: 157–174.
14. Mullins-Sweatt SN, Jamerson JE, Samuel DB, Olson DR, Widiger TA. Psychometric properties of an abbreviated instrument of the five-factor model. *Assessment* 2006; 13: 119–137.
15. Massion AO, Dyck I, Shea MT, Phillips KA, Warshaw MG, Keller MB. Personality disorders and time to remission in generalized anxiety disorder, social phobia, and panic disorder. *Archives of General Psychiatry* 2002; 59: 434–440.
16. Skodal AE, Gunderson JG, Shea MT, et al. The Collaborative Longitudinal Personality Disorders study (CLPS): Overview and implications. *Journal of Personality Disorders* 2005; 19: 487–504.
17. Clarkin JF, Yeomans FE, Kernberg OF. *Psychotherapy for borderline personality: Focusing on object relations.* Washington, DC: American Psychiatric Publishing Inc, 2006.
18. Linehan, M. *Skills training manual for treating borderline personality disorder.* New York: Guilford Press, 1993.
19. Bell SA. Personality traits, problems, and disorders: Clinical application to substance use disorders. *Journal of Research in Personality* 2005; 39: 84–102.
20. Harris EC, Barraclough B. Suicide as an outcome for mental disorders. A meta-analysis. *British Journal of Psychiatry* 1997; 170: 205–228.
21. Oldham JM, Skodal AE, Kellman HD et al. Comorbidity of Axis I and Axis II disorders. *American Journal of Psychiatry* 1995; 152: 571–578.
22. Egan S, Nathan P, Lumley M. Diagnostic concordance of ICD-10 personality and comorbid disorders: A comparison of standard clinical assessment and structured interviews in a clinical setting. *Australian and New Zealand Journal of Psychiatry* 2003; 37: 484–491.
23. Zimmerman M. Diagnosing personality disorders: A review of issues and research methods. *Archives of General Psychiatry* 1994; 51: 225–245.
24. Mann AH, Jenkins R, Cutting JC, et al. The development and use of a standardized assessment of abnormal personality. *Psychological Medicine* 1981; 11: 839–847.
25. Moran P, Rendu A, Jenkins R, et al. The impact of personality disorder in UK primary care: a 1-year follow-up of attenders. *Psychological Medicine* 2001; 31: 1447–1454.
26. Pfohl B, Blum N, Zimmerman M. *Structured interview for DSM-IV personality SIDP-IV.* Iowa City, IA. The University of Iowa, 1995.
27. Meyer B, Pilkonis PA. *An attachment model of personality disorders.* New York: Guilford Press, 2005.
28. Horowitz LM, Rosenberg SE, Baer BA, Ureño G, Villaseñor VS. Inventory of Interpersonal Problems: Psychometric properties and clinical applications. *Journal of Consulting and Clinical Psychology* 1988; 56: 885–892.
29. Pilkonis PA, Kim Y, Proietta JM, Barkham M. Scales for personality disorders developed from the Inventory of Interpersonal Problems. *Journal of Personality Disorders* 1996; 10: 355–369.
30. Embretson S. The new rules of measurement. *Psychological Assessment* 1996; 8: 341–349.
31. Lynman DR, Widiger TA. Using the Five-Factor Model to represent the DSM-IV personality disorder: An expert consensus approach. *Journal of Abnormal Psychology* 2001; 110: 401–42.
32. Costa PT, McCrae RR. Domains and facets: Hierarchical personality assessment using the revised NEO personality inventory. *Journal of Personality Assessment* 1995; 64: 21–50.

33. Miller JD, Reynolds SK, Pilkonis PA. The validity of the Five-Factor Model prototypes for personality disorders in two clinical samples. *Psychological Assessment* 2004; 16: 310–322.
34. Costa PT, Widiger TA. *Personality disorders and the five-factor model of personality.* (2nd edition). Washington DC US: American Psychological Association, 2002.
35. Saulsman LM, Page AC. The five-factor model and personality disorder empirical literature: A meta-analytic review. *Clinical Psychology Review* 2004; 23: 1055–1085.
36. Widiger TA, Costa PT, McCrae RR. A proposal for Axis II: Diagnosing personality disorders using the five-factor model. In TA Widiger & PT Costa (Eds.) *Personality disorders and the five-factor model of personality* (2nd ed., pp. 431–456). New York: Oxford University Press, 2002.
37. McCrae RR, Lockenhoff CE, Costa, PT. A step Toward DSM-V: Cataloguing personality-related problems in living. *European Journal of Personality* 2005; 19: 269–286.
38. Widiger TA, Costa PT, McCrae RR. A proposal for Axis II: Diagnosing personality disorders using the Five-Factor Model. In PT Cost & TA Widiger (Eds.), *Personality Disorders and the five-factor model of personality* (2nd edition); Washington, DC: American Psychological Association 2002; 431–456.
39. Samuel DB, Widiger TA. Clinicians' personality descriptions of prototypic personality disorders. *Journal of Personality Disorders* 2004; 16: 55–62.
40. Widiger TA, Mangine S, Corbittt EM, Ellis CG, Thomas GV. *Personality disorder interview-IV: A semistructured interview for the assessment of personality disorders.* Odessa, FL: Psychological Assessment Resources, 1995.
41. Loranger AW, Sartorius N, Andreoli A, et al. The international Personality Disorder Examination: The WHO/ADAMHA International pilot study of personality disorders. *Archives of General Psychiatry* 1994; 51: 215–224.
42. Trull TJ, Widiger TA. *Structured Interview for the five-factor model of personality (SIFFM): Professionals manual.* Odessa, FL: Psychological Assessment Resources, 1997.
43. Hyler, SE. *Personality questionnaire, PDQ-4 +.* New York, NY: New York State Psychiatric Institute, 1994.
44. Millon T, Millon C, Davis R. *Millon clinical inventory-III manual,* Minneapolis MN: National Computer Systems, 1994.
45. Loranger AW. *The OMNI personality inventories professional manual.* Odessa, FL: Psychological Assessment Resources, 2001.
46. Rivas-Vazquez, R, Blais, M. Pharmacological treatment of personality disorders, *Professional Psychology: Research and Practice,* 2002, *33,* 104–107.

Five Factor Model Rating Form

Please describe yourself on a 1–5 scale on each of the following 30 personality traits, where 1 is extremely low (i.e., extremely lower than the average person), 2 is low, 3 is neither high nor low (i.e., does not differ from the average person), 4 is high and 5 is extremely high. Use any number from 1 to 5. Please provide a rating for all 30 traits.

For example on the first trait (anxiousness), a score of 1 would indicate that you think you are extremely low in anxiousness (i.e., relaxed, unconcerned, cool). A score of 2 would indicate that you think you are low in anxiousness (lower than the average person, but not extremely low). A score of 5 would indicate that you think you are extremely high in anxiousness (i.e., fearful, apprehensive); a score of 4 would indicate you think you are higher than the average person in anxiousness, but not extremely high. A score of 3 would indicate that you think you are neither high nor low in anxiousness (does not differ from the average person) or that you are unable to decide. Circle the number that applies to the individual for each of the 30 traits.

5= Extremely high	4= High	3= Neither high nor low	2= Low	1=Extremely Low

Trait	5	4	3	2	1	Description
1. Anxiousness (fearful, apprehensive)	5	4	3	2	1	(relaxed, unconcerned, cool)
2. Angry hostility (angry, bitter)	5	4	3	2	1	(even-tempered)
3. Depressiveness (pessimistic, glum)	5	4	3	2	1	(optimistic)
4. Self-consciousness (timid, embarrassed)	5	4	3	2	1	(self-assured, glib, shameless)
5. Impulsivity (tempted, urgency)	5	4	3	2	1	(controlled, restrained)
6. Vulnerability (helpless, fragile)	5	4	3	2	1	(clear-thinking, fearless, unflappable)
7. Warmth (cordial, affectionate, attached)	5	4	3	2	1	(cold, aloof, indifferent)
8. Gregariousness (sociable, outgoing)	5	4	3	2	1	(withdrawn, isolated)
9. Assertiveness (dominant, forceful)	5	4	3	2	1	(unassuming, quiet, resigned)
10. Activity (vigorous, energetic, active)	5	4	3	2	1	(passive, lethargic)
11. Excitement-seeking (reckless, daring)	5	4	3	2	1	(cautious, monotonous, dull)
12. Positive emotions (high-spirited)	5	4	3	2	1	(placid, anhedonic)
13. Fantasy (dreamer, unrealistic, imaginative)	5	4	3	2	1	(practical, concrete)
14. Aesthetics (aberrant interests, aesthetic)	5	4	3	2	1	(uninvolved, no aesthetic interests)
15. Feelings (self-aware)	5	4	3	2	1	(constricted, unaware, alexythymic)
16. Actions (unconventional, eccentric)	5	4	3	2	1	(routine, predictable, habitual, stubborn)
17. Ideas (strange, odd, peculiar, creative)	5	4	3	2	1	(pragmatic, rigid)
18. Values (permissive, broad-minded)	5	4	3	2	1	(traditional, inflexible, dogmatic)
19. Trust (gullible, naïve, trusting)	5	4	3	2	1	(skeptical, cynical, suspicious, paranoid)
20. Straightforwardness (confiding, honest)	5	4	3	2	1	(cunning, manipulative, deceptive)
21. Altruism (sacrificial, giving)	5	4	3	2	1	(stingy, selfish, greedy, exploitative)
22. Compliance (docile, cooperative)	5	4	3	2	1	(oppositional, combative, aggressive)
23. Modesty (meek, self-effacing, humble)	5	4	3	2	1	(confident, boastful, arrogant)
24. Tender-mindedness (soft, empathetic)	5	4	3	2	1	(tough, callous, ruthless)
25. Competence (perfectionistic, efficient)	5	4	3	2	1	(lax, negligent)
26. Order (ordered, methodical, organized)	5	4	3	2	1	(haphazard, disorganized, sloppy)
27. Dutifulness (rigid, reliable, dependable)	5	4	3	2	1	(casual, undependable, unethical)
28. Achievement (workaholic, ambitious)	5	4	3	2	1	(aimless, desultory)
29. Self-discipline (dogged, devoted)	5	4	3	2	1	(hedonistic, negligent)
30. Deliberation (cautious, ruminative, reflective)	5	4	3	2	1	(hasty, careless, rash)

IIP – 25

Name_____   Todayís Date:_____

Age_____   Date of Birth:_____   ID_____

Years of Schooling_____

Instructions: here is a list of problems that people re port in relating to other people. Please read the list below, and for each item, consider whether that problem has been a problem for you with respect to any significant person in your life. Then select the number that describes how distressing that problem has been, and circle that number.

0 = Not at all
1 = A little bit
2 = Moderately
3 = Quite a bit
4 = Extremely

Part I.   The following are things you find hard to do with other people

It is hard for me to:

	Not at all	A little bit	Moderately	Quite a bit	Extremely
1. Join in groups.	0	1	2	3	4
2. Do what another person wants me to do.	0	1	2	3	4
3. Get along with people who have authority over me.	0	1	2	3	4
4. Socialize with other people.	0	1	2	3	4
5. Feel comfortable around other people	0	1	2	3	4
6. Be supportive of another person's goals in life.	0	1	2	3	4
7. Accept another person's authority over me.	0	1	2	3	4
8. Ignore criticism from other people.	0	1	2	3	4

	Not at all	A little bit	Moderately	Quite a bit	Extremely
9. Take instructions from people who have authority over me.	0	1	2	3	4
10. Be assertive without worrying about hurting the other person's feelings.	0	1	2	3	4
11. Be self-confident when I am with other people.	0	1	2	3	4

Part II. The following are things that you do too much

12. I fight with other people too much.	0	1	2	3	4
13. I am too sensitive to criticism	0	1	2	3	4
14. I get irritated or annoyed too easily.	0	1	2	3	4
15. I am too sensitive to rejection	0	1	2	3	4
16. I am too aggressive toward other people.	0	1	2	3	4
17. I try to please other people too much.	0	1	2	3	4
18. I feel attacked by other people too much.	0	1	2	3	4
19. I worry too much about other people's reactions to me.	0	1	2	3	4
20. I am influenced too much by another person's thoughts and feelings.	0	1	2	3	4
21. I worry too much about disappointing other people.	0	1	2	3	4
22. I lose my temper too easily.	0	1	2	3	4
23. I argue with other people too much.	0	1	2	3	4
24. I feel embarrassed in front of other people too much.	0	1	2	3	4
25. I feel too anxious when I am involved with another person.	0	1	2	3	4

IIP-25 Screening scales score sheet

Interpersonal sensitivity	Interpersonal ambivalence	Aggression	Need for social approval	Lack of sociaility
8.	2.	12.	10.	1.
13.	3.	14.	17.	4.
15.	6.	16.	19.	5.
18.	7.	22.	20.	11.
25.	9.	23.	21.	24.
MEAN =	MEAN =	MEAN =	MEAN =	MEAN =
	MEAN OF 3 SCALES =			

Single any single threshold is arbitrary (and is likely to be influenced by differing base rates), we tend to think more in terms of ranges: 0–0.7 as no PD, 0.7–1.1 as possible or probably, ≥ 1.1 as probable to definite (using the mean of item scores on the first 3 IIP-PD scales – interpersonal sensitivity, ambivalence, and aggression). One advantage of the measure is that it can be used continuously, of course, as well.

0–4 not likely
5–6 possible to probably
>7 definite

Standardised Assessment Of Personality – Abbreviated Scale (SAPAS)

Rater's Name _____   Date _ _ / _ _ / _ _

Patient Details

Name _____

Gender   **M / F** (circle)   **Date of Birth** _ _ / _ _ / _ _

Ethnicity _____

Main Psychiatric Diagnosis _____

Please give the following explanation before proceeding to the questions:

> *'I'd like to ask you some questions about yourself. Your answers will help me better understand what you are usually like. If the way you have been in recent weeks or months is different from the way you usually are, please look back to when you were your usual self.'*

NB. Only circle 'Yes' (or in the case of q3 'No'), if the client thinks that the description applies to them most of the time/more often than not and in most situations.

Please circle

1. *In general*, do you have difficulty making and keeping friends?   Y / N

2. Would you *normally* describe yourself as a loner?   Y / N

3. *In general*, do you trust other people?   Y / N

4. Do you *normally* loose your temper easily?   Y / N

5. Are you *normally* an impulsive sort of person?   Y / N
   (If need clarification: Do you rush into most things without thinking about the consequences?)

6. Are you *normally* a worrier?   Y / N

7. *In general*, do you depend on others a lot?   Y / N

8. *In general*, are you a perfectionist?   Y / N
   (Check that this applies to most tasks – not just isolated areas of their life?)

Chapter 7
Clinical Ratings Scales and Assessment in Eating Disorders

Jennifer L. Derenne, Christina W. Baker, Sherrie S. Delinsky, and Anne E. Becker

Abstract Eating disorders have one of the highest mortality rates among psychiatric condition. However, these conditions are difficult to detect by both primary-care physicians and mental health professionals. As a result, eating-disordered patients often go unrecognized and untreated. The utilization of standardized rating scales and structured interviews can increase the recognition of these conditions and also improve treatment planning and outcome monitoring. This chapter provides a detailed review of the available self-report instruments and semi-structured interviews for the eating disorders.

Keywords Eating disorder · Anorexia nervosa · Bulimia nervosa · Screening · Rating scales · Questionnaires · Assessment · Psychiatry

Assessment of eating disorders presents diagnostic challenges in both clinical and research settings. Indeed, the majority of individuals with bulimia nervosa (BN) and binge-eating disorder (BED) never receive specialty mental health care for their illness, and eating disorders are frequently not recognized in primary-care settings [1–3]. Difficulty detecting eating disorders can relate to an individual's reluctance to seek treatment as well as the absence or subtlety of clinical signs in many cases. Standardized assessments for eating disorders can be useful in clinical settings by eliciting a report of symptoms. However, eliciting symptoms may be difficult even when using a standardized assessment [2, 4]. Standardized psychological assessments and structured clinical interviews can also be useful in establishing a firm diagnosis for treatment planning or for evaluating inclusion criteria in treatment outcomes research. Despite considerable phenomenologic overlap among the eating disorders, there are distinctive differences in course of illness and treatment outcome among patients with anorexia nervosa, BN, and

A.E. Becker (✉)
Massachusetts General Hospital and Harvard Medical School, WACC 8th floor,
15 Parkman St., Boston, MA 02115, USA
e-mail: abecker@partners.org

L. Baer, M.A. Blais (eds.), *Handbook of Clinical Rating Scales and Assessment in Psychiatry and Mental Health*, Current Clinical Psychiatry, DOI 10.1007/978-1-59745-387-5_7,
© Humana Press, a part of Springer Science+Business Media, LLC 2010

BED, making rigorous diagnostic assessment clinically essential. Finally, response to treatment and interval change in clinical trials can be evaluated in various dimensions. This chapter describes assessments used to evaluate and monitor patients with eating disorders. We present information relating to the most commonly used self-report assessments, interview assessments, and additional assessments for related symptoms. In addition to focusing on instruments used to assess patients with anorexia nervosa (AN) and BN, the authors also discuss assessment of BED, body image, and the manner in which these tools are adapted for use in children and adolescents.

Clinical and research goals of assessment include case detection, differential diagnosis, qualitative and dimensional evaluation of symptoms, measurement of interval change, and comprehensive evaluation for clinical management. Case detection in clinical and research settings shares overlapping goals but also reflects distinct concerns.

Prevalence Estimates

The standard for detecting cases of an eating disorder for prevalence estimates is a two-stage screening approach, utilizing a shorter self-report measure in conjunction with a semi-structured interview to confirm a diagnosis [5]. Semi-structured interviews and self-report measures in routine use for this purpose are discussed below. However, Hudson et al. [2] recently discussed a different approach, in which the World Mental Health Organization (WHO) Composite International Diagnostic Interview CIDI, version 3.0 [6] was used to detect the prevalence of eating disorders in the United States. The CIDI is a fully structured lay interview that generates present and lifetime ICD-10 and DSM-IV diagnoses. Key advantages are that it can be administered by a lay interviewer, it can generate useful research and clinical data, and it is designed to be used across diverse cultural contexts. Major limitations are the duration of the full interview – 2 hours – and the fact that the fully structured format may not allow for flexibility in defining concepts that may not be understood in consistent ways [6, 7]. The current version has been revised to reduce psychological barriers that result in minimization of symptoms – specifically with respect to feelings loss of control and distress associated with eating disorders, which are now assessed indirectly. Questions used to operationalize diagnostic criteria for the eating disorders in the CIDI, version 3.0 can be found at http://www.hcp.med.harvard.edu/ncs/ftpdir/appendix_ncsr_eatingdx.pdf. [8]. One important divergence between data generated in the CIDI and DSM-IV criteria is that the CIDI assesses binge-eating behavior for 3 months rather than the full 6 months required to establish the provisional duration criterion for BED in the DSM-IV [9]. It is important to note that the CIDI, version 3 has not been validated for eating disorders and may overestimate prevalence of BED, whereas it likely provides a conservative estimate of AN and BN [2]. It also does not generate the diagnosis of eating disorder not otherwise specified (EDNOS).

Clinical Assessment of Anorexia Nervosa and Bulimia Nervosa

Major considerations in the clinical assessment of AN and BN include detection of an eating disorder, differential diagnosis, and evaluation of symptomatic manifestations and their severity. Although structured interviews are available for making a diagnosis of AN or BN, they are time-consuming, require training [10], and are rarely used in clinical settings. Both the eating disorders module of the Structured Clinical Interview for Diagnosis (SCID) and the Eating Disorders Examination (EDE) generate the data required to assess diagnostic criteria for AN and BN but are more frequently used to establish diagnostic information for research purposes.

Individuals with eating disorders may avoid clinical detection and care for a variety of reasons. A denial of medical seriousness of symptoms and an excessive concern with weight – both of which can be intrinsic to either disorder – contribute to patient ambivalence about relinquishing symptoms. Given that the majority of individuals with an eating disorder do not access care for it and the evidence that individuals may avoid disclosure, clinicians may need to rely on collateral history, physical findings, and/or weight fluctuations to raise clinical suspicion. However, many individuals with an eating disorder are careful to conceal their behaviors, attitudes, and (sometimes) their weight loss; so affirmative collateral history may be unavailable. Moreover, BN, BED, and EDNOS often present without physical signs or laboratory abnormalities, and individuals with AN occasionally drink excessive water, hide weights under clothes, and/or layer clothing to conceal weight loss. In many cases, simple direct questioning and even empathic gentle confrontation (e.g., about weight fluctuation or suggestive physical findings) may be helpful and/or necessary, but not sufficient, to elicit eating disorder symptoms and confirm a diagnosis [11].

When an eating disorder is suspected or acknowledged by a patient in a clinical setting, a directed clinical interview assessing body shape and weight concerns, dietary patterns, and inappropriate compensatory behaviors to control weight is recommended for evaluating signs or symptoms of an eating disorder and establishing a differential diagnosis. The clinical history includes information about onset of symptoms, precipitants to behaviors, treatment history and response, weight history (minimum, maximum, and desired weights), and co-morbid medical and psychiatric conditions. This information is supplemented with measurement of weight and height to evaluate nutritional status as well as to establish the weight criterion (that is, an inappropriately low weight for height and age; e.g., BMI < 17.5 kg/m^2 in an adult) for a diagnosis of AN. Physical and laboratory examination and findings supplement the clinical interview and contribute key information to diagnosis and treatment planning.

Semi-Structured Interviews

The Structured Clinical Interview for Psychiatric Diagnosis (SCID)

The SCID is a semi-structured, clinician-administered interview for making major DSM Axis I diagnoses. Ratings are achieved by following module-based diagnostic algorithms that guide the rater in determining whether diagnostic criteria are met, yielding categorical diagnostic data. Key advantages of the SCID for making a diagnosis of an eating disorder also lead to certain drawbacks. For example, an experienced clinician can apply his or her judgment to probe, clarify, expand, and/or challenge patient responses in arriving at a criteria-based diagnosis [12]. The expected enhanced validity, however, is offset by the burden of time required of respondents, investigators, and/or clinicians. Highly trained non-clinicians can administer the SCID [13], but may lack the clinical acumen to clarify and rate responses sufficiently, impacting on both validity and inter-rater reliability [14]. A comprehensive SCID performed on a patient with complex psychiatric diagnoses could take up to several hours to complete, although the completion time for a patient is reported to average 90 minutes [13]. Although some data have suggested the clinical utility (and possibly superiority) of a SCID-generated diagnosis over a routine clinical evaluation [15, 16], the SCID is optimally used with supplemental clinical information [16, 17]. Comprised of modules, the SCID uses a decision tree approach, and identifies both present state and lifetime diagnoses [12]. A major advantage of the SCID is its widespread use and translation into many languages that facilitates comparison across studies [12, 13].

The SCID-I provides a module on eating disorders that allows for a diagnosis of AN or BN, but not for EDNOS. Key advantages of the SCID are its potential brevity in asymptomatic individuals as well as its utility in probing for a lifetime history of symptoms in the absence of current symptoms. Disadvantages of the SCID specific to eating disorders include wording about symptoms that may be understood differently across respondents from different cultural or educational backgrounds, relatively less probing of complex dimensions of body image (that the EDE is able to address), and reliance on self-reported weight and height. Although the SCID can establish a diagnosis, it is not designed to capture detailed information about symptoms or severity [18]. Whereas skip-out questions add efficiency, this branched approach may be more likely to misclassify true eating disorder cases as negative, especially in populations in which symptoms present less typically (e.g., in adolescents or in non-Western populations) [19]. The screening (skip-out) questions are also inherently problematic since the screen for AN relies on an individual's awareness that he or she was underweight (as well as a candid self-report), and neither the screening questions nor the more detailed criterion-based questions to assess BN would detect individuals who routinely purge without bingeing. Moreover, the SCID does not provide specific criteria for a diagnosis of eating disorder, not otherwise specified (EDNOS), which is the most frequent presentation of an eating disorder. Notwithstanding these potential limitations, test–retest reliability kappas reported for AN and BN on the SCID-III-R ranged from 0.84 to 0.92 for lifetime diagnoses among patient samples and from 0.72 to 0.90 for current diagnoses [14].

The Eating Disorder Examination (EDE)

The Eating Disorder Examination is regarded as the best available interview for fully characterizing an eating disorder and its symptoms [19]. A key advantage of the EDE is that the interview is semi-structured and investigator-based, which allows considerable flexibility in probing the complex body and weight concern features of the eating disorders. The initial version of the EDE was developed in 1987 to overcome limitations in using self-report assessments for research in psychopathology and clinical trials [20]. The authors of the EDE have argued that an interview assessment for eating disorders is essential to elicit and describe the multiple dimensions of certain complex features of eating disorders (e.g., the phenomenology of a binge) and to provide clarity for concepts that may have varying and subjective definitions. For example, this instrument probes binge eating along the dimensions of size of the binge (relative to the social context) as well as perceived loss of control [21]. The original version of the EDE assessed attitudinal dimensions of disordered eating in five subscales – "restraint," "bulimia," "eating concern," "weight concern," and "shape concern" as well as frequencies of binge eating, purging, exercise, and fasting. The current version EDE-16.OD [22] assesses four subscales (omitting the bulimia subscale from the above). Both subscale scores and a global score may be calculated from the data.

The inter-rater reliability, test–retest reliability [20, 23, 24], and internal consistency of the subscales have been reported as satisfactory in previous versions [21, 25]. For example, Cronbach's alpha coefficient on subscales ranged from 0.68 to 0.83 and was 0.90 for the global scale in a community sample of adult women [25]. Whereas subscale scores have been shown to differentiate between patients with anorexia nervosa and healthy controls [21], overweight controls have been reported to have significantly higher weight and shape concern subscale scores than normal weight controls [26]. Eating attitudes and behaviors elicited on the EDE have also shown modest but significant correlation with corresponding behaviors assessed with self-reported food and binge/purge behavior diaries [27]. DSM diagnoses of AN, BN, BED, as well as EDNOS can also be extracted from the data. Thus, this assessment allows an evaluation of both categorical and dimensional interval change over time. A Spanish language version of the EDE (the S-EDE) has been developed and reportedly has good to excellent test–retest reliability and modest to excellent inter-rater reliability for objective binge episodes and subscales, respectively [28].

A major drawback of the EDE is the long duration of the interview (between 30 and 60 minutes). The EDE is focused on present symptoms and does not probe for history of symptoms prior to the past 3–6 months; so it is not an appropriate assessment for a history of an eating disorder. Administration of the EDE does require training, but can be performed by a non-clinician after proper training. An important limitation is apparently poor reliability for subjective (as opposed to objective) binge episodes on the EDE [23, 24, 28]. Adaptation of the EDE for assessment in children and adolescents is discussed below. Now in its 16th version [22], the EDE is preferred to the SCID in clinical trials given that greater phenomenological and severity data about cognitive symptoms can be systematically assessed. The major advantages of the capacity SCID are potential brevity and capacity to assess a lifetime history rather than just a current diagnosis.

Self-Report Assessments

Self-report measures may have multiple advantages for assessing eating disorder pathology. Chief among these are that they can be administered without a trained interviewer in a relatively short duration of time. Others have argued that a self-report assessment for eating disorders has the additional advantage of sparing the respondent from discussing with a rater the eating disorder behaviors and attitudes that he or she may perceive as socially undesirable.

Dietary Records

Nutritional behaviors are notoriously challenging to ascertain [29], and symptoms related to eating disorders may be even more problematic to characterize because of the shame and minimization of symptoms that can accompany the disorders. Prospective self-report of dietary patterns has the advantage of eliminating recall bias and may be useful for assessing behavior in patients with BED [30]. On the other hand, dietary records in real time may influence the behaviors themselves. Indeed, they are also used therapeutically for this reason. Patients' food diaries can also be used to augment patients' reports in order to assist both patient and clinicians in understanding the frequency, pattern, and scope of symptoms.

The Eating Disorder Examination Questionnaire (EDE-Q)

The EDE-Q was developed as a self-report, present-state version of the EDE. Like the EDE, it assesses the frequency of bingeing and purging behaviors and the presence of attitudes in four domains that correspond to the four EDE subscales "restraint," "eating concern," "weight concern," and "shape concern." The current version of the EDE-Q (the EDE-Q6.0) comprises 28 items that allow assessment of both presence and severity of symptoms (with either a request for frequency over the last 28 days or a response on a forced choice 7-point Likert scale) as well as self-report items about height, weight, menstruation, and oral contraceptive use. Subscale and global scores can be calculated to provide severity data. Items in each subscale are summed and averaged to calculate the score provided that more than half the items within each respective subscale have been completed. The global scale is an average of the subscale scores. A score of 4 or higher on any of the subscales or the global scale is suggestive of eating disorder pathology. The EDE-Q is designed to be completed in approximately 15 minutes [10, 31, 32]. Thus, the self-report version overcomes the EDE's disadvantages of long duration and requirement for a trained investigator to administer the assessment. Disadvantages for the EDE-Q include lack of correlation with prospective self-reported behavior on subjective binge episodes and objective overeating. Specifically, data suggest that the EDE-Q may underestimate objective overeating [30].

Several investigators have reported on psychometric properties of the various versions of the EDE-Q. Both the EDE and the EDE-Q have undergone several revisions; so further investigation of psychometric properties across diverse populations for these versions is desirable to establish their utility and limits. Internal consistency reliability has been assessed to be adequate in women without symptoms [33], as well as those with bulimic symptoms [34]. For example, Cronbach's alpha coefficient ranged from 0.73 to 0.87 on subscales and was reported as 0.93 on the global scale in a community sample [25] and from 0.70 to 0.83 on subscales and was reported as 0.90 on the global scale in a sample of women with bulimic symptoms [34]. Test–retest reliability has also been shown to be good over a period of 2 weeks. Not surprisingly, the frequency of behavioral symptoms is less stable than the subscale scores [33]. Ratings generated on the EDE-Q are significantly correlated with ratings based on the EDE among women with AN and BN from both community samples and clinical samples [7, 31, 35, 36]. Compared with the EDE, the EDE-Q has been reported to generate significantly higher subscale scores (i.e., indicative of more pathology) and significantly higher frequencies of binge episodes [7, 31, 35, 36]. In contrast, binge behaviors in one study were significantly less frequently reported on the EDE-Q, raising the possibility that BN and BED would be underestimated by use of this measure in a two-stage screening design [31]. A revision with specific written clarification of binge eating (the EDE-I) has been reported to enhance performance of the EDE-Q in the evaluation of binge eating [37].

Normative scores for the EDE-Q have been reported in adolescent and adult populations and suggest a relatively high prevalence of scores in the pathological range for the weight- and shape-concern subscales (i.e., 11–20% on the weight-concern subscale and 13–19% on the shape-concern subscale) [38, 39]. Data also suggest that the absence of a specific item assessing diet pill or naturaceutical use as a compensatory behavior may lead to an underestimation of purging [38, 40].

It is generally accepted that a clinical interview – with its detail and flexibility – would yield more valid information about disordered eating than a self-report questionnaire [7]. Discrepancies between the EDE and EDE-Q, especially with respect to binge eating and concerns about shape have been attributed to limitations in the self-report version in assessing complex behaviors [35]. However, others have suggested that a self-report questionnaire may elicit more candid disclosure with respect to stigmatized behaviors. For example, one study comparing responses on the EDE to the EDE-Q found that approximately 40% of individuals who reported purging on the EDE-Q later denied the behavior in an interview [41]. Another study reported greater agreement between the EDE-Q and telephone interviews than the EDE-Q and face-to-face EDE interviews [42].

Clinical Impairment Assessment (CIA), the Eating Disorders Quality of Life (EDQOL), and the Quality of Life for Eating Disorders (QOL ED)

The Clinical Impairment Assessment (CIA3.0) is a relatively new 16-item self-report designed for use immediately following the EDE-Q to evaluate psychosocial impairment related to the eating disorder symptoms referenced in the EDE-Q for clinical and epidemiological purposes. The items are scored on a 4-point Likert scale (anchored by a response option "not at all") which are summed (using prorated values for missing items) and averaged to calculate a global score as long as at least 12 of the items have responses [43]. Two additional disease-specific quality of life measures for individuals with eating disorders have been developed – the Quality of Life for Eating Disorders (QOLED; a 21-item self-report instrument) [44] and the Eating Disorders Quality of Life (EDQOL, a 25-item self-report instrument in addition to 6 demographic items) [45]. Psychometric studies of these are promising but further studies are necessary to establish how they perform and can be interpreted across diverse populations.

In summary, the EDE-Q is similar in content and scoring to the EDE. Data from the two assessments are highly correlated. However, the EDE-Q has been found to yield significantly higher subscale scores than the EDE in both clinical and community samples of women. Because normative data demonstrated elevated scores in weight and shape concern, the EDE-Q may miss diet pill and naturaceutical use, and there are discrepancies in binge eating between the self-report measure and the EDE, and the EDE-Q should optimally be used as part of the two-stage screening protocol rather than on its own. Supplementation of the EDE-Q and EDE with the self-report CIA provides additional data assessing impairment.

Eating Disorder Diagnostic Scale (EDDS)

The Eating Disorder Diagnostic Scale (EDDS, reproduced in the appendix to this chapter) is a one-page (22 item) self-report measure for eating disorder symptoms and diagnosis [46]. The EDDS has good reliability, sensitivity, and specificity for assessing a diagnosis of AN, BN, or BED in US adolescent and adult female populations. Evaluation of internal consistency reliability for the symptom composite has yielded Cronbach's alphas ranging from 0.89 to 0.91. Both the EDDS content and SPSS syntax for scoring it are published in the scientific literature [46, 47].

Test–retest reliability in initial investigation of this assessment ranged by diagnosis, with kappas of 0.91 for AN, 0.75 for BN, and 0.89 for BED [46]. When criterion validity was evaluated by diagnostic agreement with an interviewer-based diagnosis (i.e., the EDE or the SCID) as a gold standard, the kappa coefficient also ranged by diagnosis, being 0.93 for AN, 0.81 for BN, and 0.74 for BED. The EDDS showed a sensitivity and specificity of 93 and 1.0, respectively, for AN, 0.81 and 0.98 for BN, and 0.77 and 0.96 for BED. Subsequent examination of a large sample of adolescent and adult females (from education-based settings) showed excellent concordance with diagnoses generated by the EDE with a kappa coefficient of 0.78, a sensitivity of 0.88, and a specificity of 0.98 for the eating disorder diagnoses (which were predominantly BN in this sample) [47].

When the EDDS was translated for use in an adolescent sample of Hong Kong males and females, Cronbach's alphas reported on four subscales (identified with factor analysis) were adequate for all but one among females and for all among males, but test–retest kappa coefficients showed poor agreement over 1 month. The investigators concluded that the EDDS could not be used without corroborating information to identify cases in this study population, but that it might be useful as a screening instrument as additional data become available [48].

The EDDS symptom composite appears to be potentially useful in evaluating interval change in treatment trials but performs less well than the EDE with respect to evaluating change in eating disorder diagnosis [47]. The EDDS has not yet been evaluated as a screening instrument in a primary-care setting, although its brevity and excellent performance in US female study populations suggest its potential utility for this purpose after further investigation.

Eating Disorder Inventory (EDI)

The Eating Disorder Inventory (EDI) [49], a 64-item self-report measure originally developed in 1983, is one of the most widely used measures for diagnostic impression, treatment planning, and outcomes evaluation with female eating disorder patients and non-clinical samples. The EDI, which assesses psychological traits and symptoms relevant to the development and maintenance of eating disorders, is a staple of eating disorders research, and has been revised twice: the EDI-2 [50], published in 1991, involved the addition of three provisional scales; however, no changes were made to the original eight scales. The EDI-3 [51], published in 2004, contains 91 items, and expands on the EDI-2 with 12 scales plus six composite scores and three response style or profile validity indicators (inconsistency, infrequency, and negative impression) (see Cumella [52] for a review of the EDI-3). Notably, the EDI cannot be used in isolation to make diagnoses and must be interpreted along with clinical information derived from other sources for diagnostic and treatment planning purposes. The EDI-3 test package contains a symptom checklist to assess symptom frequency and history. Although few studies have evaluated the EDI-3, a criticism of all versions of the EDI has been that scales in which content does not concern eating and weight (i.e., "the personality scales") do not discriminate between eating disordered groups and non-eating-disordered psychiatric patients [53]. (See Espelage et al. [54] for a detailed review of the EDI's construct validity). Another criticism of the EDI is the lack of information about its use with men in clinical and non-clinical populations. Notably, the EDI has been translated and examined in Spanish [55], Arabic [56], German [57], Portuguese [58], Chinese [59], Japanese [60], and Bulgarian [61].

Eating Attitudes Test

The Eating Attitudes Test (EAT, reproduced in the appendix to this chapter) is a 26-item self-report measure that can be used to identify eating disturbances in a non-clinical population [62]. The EAT has good reliability (alpha = 0.90 for individuals with AN) and acceptable criterion validity (i.e., individuals with an eating disorder versus controls). Participants respond to statements on a six-point Likert scale: "never" (1), "rarely" (2), "sometimes" (3), "often" (4), "usually" (5), and "always" (6). Answers of 1, 2, or 3 are coded as 0; responses of 4, 5, or 6 are coded as 1, 2, 3, respectively (with the exception of one reverse coded item), and item responses are summed to obtain total or factor scores.

The EAT has three subscales called factors [63]. Factor I, "dieting," assesses negative preoccupations with shape and active avoidance of fattening foods. Sample items include: "I engage in dieting behavior" and "I feel extremely guilty after eating." A high score on factor I indicates the presence of dieting behaviors and concerns about eating. Factor II, "bulimia and food preoccupation," assesses binge eating and purging behaviors, as well as preoccupation with food. High scores are associated with bulimia and a higher body weight. Statements in this subscale include: "I find myself preoccupied with food" and "I feel that food controls my life." Factor III is labeled "oral control" and contains statements concerning self-control and social pressures about weight, i.e., "I feel that others pressure me to eat" and, "I display self-control around food." A high score on factor III is associated with lower weight and the absence of bulimia nervosa.

The total score on the EAT reflects global abnormal concerns with eating and weight, whereas the subscales assess specific aspects of eating and weight attitudes and behaviors. Individuals with eating concerns may score similarly on the total score, but have different scores on the subscales. For instance, in a sample of women with AN, patients with binge purge and restricting subtypes did not differ on the total EAT score, but did differ on factors II and III [62].

The Bulimia Test Revised (BULIT-R)

The BULIT-R is a 36-item self-report measure of bulimic symptomatology. Each item is scored 1–5 on a 5-point forced Likert scale. Scores from 28 items are summed to obtain the total score; higher scores are associated with more significant pathology [64]. The BULIT-R has high internal reliability (0.92) and high 1-week test–retest reliability. Although the authors' traditional cutoff score was 104, Welch et al. [65] found that a cutoff of 98 was actually associated with 100% sensitivity and 99% specificity. The BULIT-R has also been validated in adolescents [66], and has been shown to have excellent reliability coefficients across diverse ethnic groups (Cronbach's coefficient of 0.92 for college aged African-American women, 0.93 for Asian-American women, 0.95 for Caucasian-American women, and 0.93 for Latino-American women) [67]. Icelandic [68] and Spanish [69] language versions of the BULIT-R have also demonstrated high internal reliability, with Cronbach's coefficients of 0.96 and 0.93, respectively.

The SCOFF

The relatively high prevalence of eating disorders within some populations, their high associated mortality and co-morbidity, the substantial risk that an individual will not receive care for her illness, and the availability of effective treatment suggest the benefits of selective screening for eating disorders in primary health-care settings. The SCOFF questionnaire has been developed as a verbal screening tool for eating disorders in clinical settings. Consisting of only five questions that address core features of AN and BN, it takes only approximately 2 minutes to administer. In adult female general practice samples, setting the threshold for a positive response at $\geq$ 2 yes answers, the SCOFF had a sensitivity of 84.6% and specificity of 89.6% [70]. In a specialty clinic sample, it had a 100% sensitivity for cases of AN and BN and 87.5% specificity in healthy controls (recruited from the community) using the same cut-point [71]. However, the assessment did not perform as well outside of U.K. clinic populations, with reported sensitivity and specificity of 53.3 and 93.2%, respectively, in a US university setting [72] and 78.4 and 75.8%, respectively, in a Colombian university setting [73]. Two other studies report comparable (and somewhat less promising) results in adolescent school samples with sensitivity and specificity of 73.1 and 77.7%, respectively, in Barcelona, Spain [74] and 81.9 and 78.7%, respectively, in Colombia [75]. Limited data suggest that the SCOFF might achieve comparable results as either a written questionnaire or oral interview, but that a written form may encourage greater disclosure [76]. Notwithstanding its promise for efficient screening in primary-care settings, more research is necessary to evaluate how the SCOFF will perform in more diverse settings before it can be recommended as a screening tool [77].

Assessment of Binge-Eating Disorder

Binge eating is characterized primarily by two dimensions: eating a large amount of food in a discrete period of time and experiencing "a sense of lack" of control during the event [9]. Binge eating can be difficult to assess for a number of reasons. Determining whether a patient regularly eats what would qualify as a "large" amount of food requires clarification because this is a subjective term with quite variable interpretations. One patient could consider a single Hershey's kiss to be a large amount of food, while others might describe a long list of high-density foods, such as a stick of butter with a loaf of bread and a pint of ice cream. It is also important to clarify context, such as whether the eating occurs primarily in situations where everyone is eating a lot of food (e.g., Thanksgiving or a superbowl party) or in isolation of any social context. The assessment of binge eating is further complicated by efforts to define what is meant by "lack of control." The experience of losing control varies a great deal in nature and intensity.

Standardized measures provide a systematic and reliable way of asking patients about their experiences of binge eating, and there are a few instruments which provide the information needed to make a DSM-IV diagnosis of BN or BED (BED is currently coded under EDNOS unless the assessment is part of a research study and uses the research criteria in the DSM-IV appendix).

The Eating Disorder Examination (EDE) [78], the Questionnaire on Eating and Weight Patterns Revised (QEWP-R) [79], and the Binge Eating Scale (BES) [80] are the most widely used instruments for assessing binge eating.

The EDE and EDE-Q, already discussed above, are widely used for assessing eating disorders and specific eating disorder behaviors, including binge eating. Both of these instruments specifically assess the preceding 28 days and provide detailed information about the frequency and distribution of binge episodes. This is a unique advantage of the EDE. An individual may binge seven times a week on 2 days or seven times a week on 7 days, indicating very different patterns that would not be identified by asking only about episodes or days per week. Another advantage of the EDE is that it includes a distinction between subjective and objective binge episodes because of its careful assessment of the amount of food ingested. An eating episode involving a small or healthy amount of food and loss of control is considered a "subjective" binge, while the presence of both a large amount of food and a loss of control is rated as an "objective" binge. There are a few recent reports suggesting that the EDE-Q's assessment of binge eating, and concordance with other measures, can be improved by the addition of instructions (EDE-Q-I) that provide detailed definitions of large amount of food and loss of control [37]. The EDE-Q does assess frequency of binge eating, but because it does not elicit information beyond the past 28 days or additional diagnostic features of BED, supplementary information is necessary to determine whether the respondent has BED. The most updated version of the EDE does include questions that address DSM-IV provisional research criteria for BED.

Details of the scoring and psychometrics of the EDE and EDE-Q are described above. Studies comparing the interview-based EDE with the EDE-Q in terms of agreement of binge frequency have been generally favorable. A number of studies report correlations between binge frequencies on the measures, suggesting that the responses on the self-report EDE-Q are similar to those gathered through the interview [30, 81–83]. As noted above, previous research has reported that the EDE results in signficantly different estimates of objective binge frequency compared to the EDE-QI [37]. Concordance can be further improved, however, by the addition to the EDE-Q (EDE-Q-I) of a set of instructions with detailed definitions of a large amount of food and loss of control 37. Thus, the choice of whether to use the EDE interview or self-administered version will depend largely on available time and resources because the interview requires interviewer training and more time for administration.

The Questionnaire on Eating and Weight Patterns, Revised (QEWP-R) is a self-report questionnaire that obtains binge-eating frequency as well as other information necessary for establishing a diagnosis of BED. The questionnaire is categorical and does not yield a score, but rather provides information about the presence or absence of binge episodes, the frequency of episodes, and includes additional characterization of overeating and information required for a DSM-IV BED diagnosis. Two early reports on the use of the QEWP in field trials demonstrated its ability to distinguish binge eaters, non-binge eaters, and individuals with bulimia on a number of variables [79, 84]. Moreover, the QEWP-R has exhibited adequate agreement with interview-based assessments [85– 87]. One recent study reports that the QEWP-R had reasonable sensitivity in identifying individuals with BED, but less specificity in classifying individuals as not having BED, and the authors recommend using the measure for screening but not as the sole assessment of BED [88]. In summary, the QEWP-R is a good assessment instrument for assessing frequency of binge eating and can be used for screening and making diagnoses involving binge eating, but should ideally be supplemented with additional information when the primary goal is diagnostic. It does not provide a nuanced picture of binge episodes, cognitions, and associated distress, which are dimensions better captured by the EDE or the BES. Test–retest reliability has been found to be adequate [89].

The Binge Eating Scale (BES) is a 16-item self-report instrument that assesses binge-eating severity on a continuous scale. It was designed to identify behavioral and cognitive characteristics of binge eating in individuals with obesity. Each item has three or four weighted statements, and the respondent is directed to choose one. The final score, ranging from 0 to 46, is a sum of the weighted scores. The measure has two cut points, distinguishing three levels of severity: scores ≤ 17 indicate the absence of binge eating, scores from 18 to 26 (inclusive) indicate moderate levels of binge eating, and scores ≥ 27 reflect the presence of "severe" binge eating. The BES has demonstrated high internal consistency, good test–retest reliability, and moderate associations with binge-eating severity measured by food records [80, 90].

Compared to the QEWP-R, which focuses on assessing criteria needed for making a BED diagnosis, the BES has a greater focus on psychopathology associated with binge eating and is a good measure of cognitions and associated distress [91]. One significant limitation of the BES is that it does not measure frequency and is also not able to distinguish between subjective and objective binge eating. Both of these characteristics are essential for clinical utility [90]. There has been variability in the ability of the BES to categorize individuals as having BED using the defined cutoff scores when compared with interview-based assessment [88, 92, 93]. The BES may be most useful as a continuous measure of severity or to screen for diagnosis or distress associated with binge-eating behavior, but is inadequate to assess frequency of binge eating or to make a diagnosis of BED [88].

The more recently developed Eating Disorder Diagnostic Scale (EDDS; described) above shows promise for use in research and clinical settings for the identification of BED. Advantages of the EDDS are that it generates both composite symptom and diagnostic data in a one-page, self-report assessment [46]. It includes a clear and thorough assessment of binge-eating frequency as well as its affective/cognitive and behavioral correlates. Fewer data on performance with BED diagnoses are available than for BN, but reliability, sensitivity, and specificity appear adequate for BED in US adolescent and adult females [46, 47].

There has been a recent surge of interest in binge eating as a predictor of outcome after bariatric surgery as well as the impact of the surgery on binge-eating behavior. Findings have been equivocal, and one explanation is that existing measures may not provide accurate accounts of binge-eating behavior after surgery. As already described, one of the primary defining features of a binge is the consumption of a large amount of food. The meaning of "large amount" and the ability to eat large quantities are dramatically altered for individuals who have had a bariatric procedure and there are also changes as the body heals and adjusts to the surgery. Yet, in pre-post surgery studies, the same assessment measures have been used pre-

and post-operatively, without modification or the addition of instructions to qualify the meaning of "large." There is a need for psychometric evaluation of binge-eating measures (and adaptations of measures) in the early and later post-operative periods.

There are other self-report scales worth mentioning here because they assess dimensions of eating that are related to binge eating, specifically emotional overeating and disinhibition. The Three Factor Questionnaire (TFEQ) [94] is very widely used and includes a "disinhibition" subscale. However, the questionnaire's scales have been the focus of much scrutiny and criticism over the years, so questions remain about the meaning of the disinhibition construct. Emotional eating can be assessed with the Emotional Eating Scale (EES) [95] or with the emotional eating subscale of the Dutch Eating Behavior Questionnaire (DEBQ) [96]. In initial psychometric studies, the EES was associated with measures of binge eating, and treatment-associated changes in binge eating (assessed with the BES) were correlated with changes in the EES [95]. The DEBQ's 13-item emotional eating subscale has two factors, one related to diffuse emotions and one to very specific emotions, and the scale has shown high internal consistency and factorial validity [96]. A newer instrument, the Emotional Overeating Questionnaire (EOQ), is available for assessing emotional overeating [97]. While the DEBQ and EES assess desire to eat in response to emotions, the EOQ assesses the actual frequency of emotional overeating over the past 28 days. The EOQ exhibited good psychometric integrity [97].

Assessment of Body Image

Body image is a complex, multi-dimensional construct that involves perception, cognition, affect, and behavior. Assessment of body image along these dimensions is essential, as body image disturbance is considered to be one of the core features of AN and BN, a risk factor for the development of eating disorders, and its persistence after treatment is associated with elevated risk of relapse.

Diverse methods have been developed to assess the various aspects of body image disturbance, including optical distorting techniques, figure ratings, and self-report questionnaires. A number of these questionnaires are comprehensive measures of eating-related pathology (e.g., Eating Disorder Inventory [EDI], Eating Disorder Examination-Questionnaire [EDE-Q]) that include individual subscales to assess body image, whereas other instruments assess body image disturbance exclusively and are considered "stand-alone" (e.g., Body Shape Questionnaire [BSQ]).

Measurement of body image perception (i.e., judgment of appearance, size, and spatial boundaries of one's body) – and its theoretical and treatment implications for eating disorders – has been a controversial topic, given variability in findings and the lack of relation between body size estimation and treatment outcome [98]. As technologies have evolved, analog scales and image marking techniques have been replaced by optical distorting techniques that use actual images of an individual that are distorted to varying degrees in either direction (smaller or larger than actual size). The discrepancy between actual body size and perceived body size can be calculated using a "body perception index" (perceived size/actual size × 100) [99]. Research on body size perception using these techniques has produced inconsistent and inconclusive results, possibly related to certain conceptual and methodological problems. For example, Smeets [100] argued that most research has assessed memory for body size, rather than perception of body size, as these are related yet separate constructs. Another noted problem is with "life-size" images (i.e., images that are the same size as the participant) [101], because although these images resemble "real-life situations" such as viewing oneself in a mirror, the actual size of one's reflection in a mirror is half one's body size in real life [98]. To address these issues, a new method was developed recently that assesses perception (as opposed to memory) using projected images that are the same height as participant's reflections in the mirror [102]. This method holds potential as an ecologically valid and clinically relevant method of body size estimation.

Another method of body image assessment measures both perceptions of individuals' actual body size as well as their perceived ideals, thereby generating indices of dissatisfaction (i.e., discrepancy scores between actual and ideal figures). These figure drawings or silhouettes – of which many sets have been developed – typically contain a series of drawings of unclothed figure silhouettes, ranging from very thin to obese. Figures may be presented in ascending order from thin to obese [103], in an unordered array [104], or placed individually on cards [105], and research shows that the manner in which figures are presented influences body image ratings [106], thereby calling into question their validity. Other limitations of figure-rating scales are that the drawings are not very realistic [107], do not represent variations in body composition (i.e., adiposity versus lean muscle mass), and are not uniformly different in size comparing whole and different body regions between each adjacent figure drawing [108]. There are also questions as to their appropriate use with children and men (see Cafri & Thompson [109] for a review of body image assessment in men).

In contrast to figure ratings, the Somatomorphic Matrix is a computer program that enables systematic assessment of body muscularity and body fat dimensions of men's and women's body image (satisfaction and perceptual accuracy) [110]. In support of the measure's validity, the silhouettes correspond to particular fat-free mass indices and body fat percentages [110]. However, a recent examination indicated low test–retest reliability for a majority of the items and the self-ideal discrepancies using this measure [111].

The other measures of body image – and there are dozens of these questionnaires – are comprised of cognitive, affective, and behavioral components. Cognitions include beliefs about the appearance of one's body (e.g., parts of the body are excessively round or unattractive) as well as the meaning or value of appearance (e.g., being excessively round means being unattractive and worthless). Although often confused in the literature, body dissatisfaction (i.e., negative evaluations of appearance) is distinct from over-evaluation of shape and weight, in which individuals define their self-worth by their shape/weight. An example of a measure of body dissatisfaction is the Body Parts Satisfaction Scale [112], which assesses satisfaction with specific body parts, such as stomach, buttocks, and thighs, areas typically associated with dissatisfaction in women. Distinct from dissatisfaction, excessive valuation of shape and weight is considered to be a core feature in AN and BN, is typically associated with excessive preoccupation with weight and shape, and there is some evidence that excessive valuation is a more stable marker for body image disturbance than is body dissatisfaction [113]. This distinction is apparent in the items from the EDE-Q Weight and Shape Concern subscales assessing dissatisfaction: "How dissatisfied have you felt about your weight?" versus excessive valuation: "Has your shape influenced how you think about (judge) yourself as a person?"

Affect includes feeling fat, disgusted, ashamed, or self-conscious, especially in situations that trigger thoughts about weight/shape (e.g., seeing one's reflection, being seen by others) or after eating certain foods. The Body Shape Questionnaire (BSQ), described below, contains many affective items. Behaviors include various methods of checking one's weight or appearance, or alternatively, avoiding or preventing exposure to one's weight/appearance. There are two primary measures of behavioral manifestations of body image disturbance, the Body Checking Questionnaire (BCQ) [114] and the Body Image Avoidance Questionnaire (BIAQ) [115]. Each of these self-report measures assesses the frequency of behaviors typically associated with high levels of body image disturbance (e.g., checking behaviors such as pinching stomach to measure fatness, and avoidance behaviors such as wearing baggy clothing).

The Body Shape Questionnaire (BSQ)

The Body Shape Questionnaire (reproduced in the appendix to this chapter) is a widely used measure of body image disturbance [116]. The BSQ is a 34-item measure that assesses global concerns about body shape and appearance in both normal and clinical populations. Each item asks how often the participant has felt a particular way about her appearance during the past 4 weeks. The BSQ has high concurrent and discriminant validity [116, 117], and high test–retest reliability [117]. Shorter forms of the BSQ, containing 8 and 14 items, have also been shown to have good construct validity [118, 119]. Notably, the BSQ has been validated in Swedish [120] and French [121] samples.

The Eating Disorder Inventory (EDI)

Other widely used body image scales come from the Eating Disorder Inventory (EDI) described above. Three of the 12 EDI-3 subscales are eating/weight specific. Of these, two are specific to body image: drive for thinness (i.e., "excessive concern with dieting, preoccupation with weight, and entrenchment in an extreme pursuit of thinness", p. 17) and body dissatisfaction (i.e., "the belief that specific parts of the body associated with shape change or increased 'fatness' at puberty are too large", p. 18).

Assessment of Children and Adolescents

Assessment of eating disorders and nutritional status in children and adolescents can be particularly difficult, since there are no widely accepted "normal weight" charts for children and adolescents. While there are general guidelines for expected body weight for height in adults, normal childhood growth and development is far more variable and difficult to predict. Childhood growth expectations change on a month-by-month basis, and expected weight for height will depend on other factors such as parental size, bone age, and reproductive status. It is often most helpful for the clinicians involved to obtain pediatric records, and to plot weight for height throughout childhood on the Center for Disease Control pediatric weight charts [122]. One can then extrapolate expected weight and height at the current age based on prior trends. A plateau or decrease in height is particularly concerning, and may indicate severe malnutrition. If prior data are not available, CDC weight tables based upon age (up to age 20) and height can be used to estimate a child's ideal body weight for comparison with the actual weight. These scales use weight at the 50% percentile for gender, age, and height to calculate expected body weight [123].

Clinical and research assessment of eating-disordered behavior in this population can be particularly challenging due to cognitive and emotional developmental factors which may affect an individual's ability to accurately answer questions about symptoms.

The K-SADS-PL [124] is a semi-structured diagnostic interview designed to assess current and past episodes of psychopathology in children and adolescents according to DSM-III-R and DSM-IV criteria. It incorporates interviews of parents and child, and information obtained from the school and medical chart in making diagnoses. Interviewers screen for anorexia nervosa and bulimia nervosa using a number of probe questions; the interviewers ask more detailed supplemental questions should the initial screen indicate that further exploration is warranted.

A number of eating disorder-specific assessment tools have been psychometrically validated in children and adolescents. The Eating Disorders Evaluation for Children (EDE-Ch), the Children's Eating Attitudes Test (ChEAT), the Eating Disorder Inventory for Children (EDI-C), the Kids Eating Disorder Survey (KEDS), and the Questionnaire on Eating and Weight Patterns for adolescents (QWEP-A) have been adapted for use in children and adolescents and are widely used for research purposes. The EDE-Ch is a structured interview, while the Ch-EAT, QWEP-A, KEDS, and the EDI-C are self-report questionnaires. The EDI-C is somewhat unique in that it measures personality traits and characteristics that are thought to be associated with eating disorders. Investigation of the SCOFF and inclusion of adolescents in evaluation of the EDDS are reported above [46, 47, 75].

The challenge in adapting these research measures for use in children is that language often needs to be modified to take into account developmental understanding of the questions being asked. For example, a child may not understand the concepts of binge eating or restricting. They may also have more difficulty remembering the chronology of their symptoms, and may also have difficulty accurately expressing the effect symptoms have had on the quality of life.

The Eating Disorder Examination – Child (EDE-Ch)

In 1996, Bryant-Waugh et al. adapted the "gold standard" Eating Disorders Examination for use in children aged 8–14 [125]. Similar to the EDE used in adult populations, the EDE-Ch uses a structured interview to assess pathology over the past 28 days in the areas of eating concern, shape concern, weight concern, and dietary restraint. It identifies three types of eating episodes: objective bulimic episodes, subjective bulimic episodes, and objective overeating. It is scored on a seven-point Likert scale, with higher scores suggestive of more severe eating pathology. However, it is important to note that the summary scores do not reflect the frequency of disordered eating behaviors such as bingeing or purging. The EDE-Ch demonstrates high inter-rater reliability, internal consistency, and discriminant validity [126]. In order for the scale to be used in very young children, authors modified the language used and took great care to explain concepts that might be confusing to a latency-aged child. Both the EDE (an hour-long interview) and EDE-Q, a shorter self-report version of the EDE, have been administered to adolescents. As in adult populations, adolescents tend to over-estimate eating pathology on the self-report version as compared to the interview version [33, 127].

The Children's Eating Attitudes Test (Ch-EAT)

Maloney et al. adapted the Children's Eating Attitudes Test (Ch-EAT) in 1988 [128] from Garner and Garfinkel's Eating Attitudes Test. A self-report inventory, the Ch-EAT is composed of 26 items intended to assess dieting behaviors, food preoccupation, bulimia, and concerns about being overweight. Children (as young as 8 years old) are asked to pick one of six response alternatives ranging from "always" to "never." The "always" response is scored 3, while the "very often" response is scored 2, and the "often" response is scored 1. The other three responses for each question are scored 0. A score greater than 20 is suggestive of disordered eating. The ChEAT has adequate to good internal reliability and good test–retest reliability [129].

The Questionnaire on Eating and Weight Patterns (QEWP-A)

The adolescent version of the Questionnaire on Eating and Weight Patterns (QEWP-A) is another self-report screen, which has been modified from the original by using simpler language and compressing two of the questions [130]. Unlike the EDE-Ch, it does not use a standardized method for determining the size of eating episodes. The QEWP-A has adequate concurrent validity and good test–retest reliability over a 3-week interval [131].

Kid's Eating Disorders Survey (KEDS)

The Kid's Eating Disorders Survey (KEDS) is a 14-item self-report scale adapted from the Eating Symptoms Inventory. It is accompanied by figure drawings intended to assess body image and body dissatisfaction. Children are asked to respond "yes," "no," or "I don't know" to each question. In addition to the total score (values above 16 are considered elevated), the KEDS provides weight dissatisfaction and purging/restricting subscales [132]. Children are also asked to quantify binge-eating episodes; this is accomplished through the use of concrete examples of amounts of food consumed (e.g., two doughnuts and a cup of ice cream and five cookies). The KEDS has been validated for children aged 10–13, and has been demonstrated to have acceptable test–retest reliability [133].

Eating Disorder Inventory – Child (EDI-C)

The Eating Disorder Inventory, described above, is another multidimensional self-report measure, which has been modified for use in children and adolescents (EDI-C) [134]. Eklund et al. suggest low reliability of the original 11 factors when the EDI is used in children, and propose a modified subscale structure for the EDI-C using the five factors with high reliability in children and adolescents (drive for thinness, emotional instability, self-esteem, overeating, and maturity fears) [135].

When self-report methods (ChEAT and QWEP-A) have been compared to structured interviews (EDE-Ch) in a population of non-treatment seeking normal and overweight children, the ChEAT appeared to correlate more closely with the EDE-Ch than did the QWEP-A. The QEWP-A appeared to over-estimate eating episodes, but was not sensitive for the presence of different types of eating episodes identified by the EDE-Ch [136]. Overall, the structured interview method employed by the EDE-Ch is thought to be superior to self-report in that it minimizes the child's interpretation and personal bias in answering questions.

Conclusion

Clinicians and researchers specializing in eating disorders have a wide array of assessment instruments available to aid in diagnostic evaluation, treatment planning, and research. Some are focused on specific aspects of eating disorders, such as body image, while others focus on personality traits thought to be associated with disordered eating. Many have been adapted for use in youth populations as well. The standard for population screening is a two-stage process with a short self-report form followed by a semi-structured interview. Several measures are available for the first stage of screening, including the EAT-26, the EDE-Q, the EDI-2, and the EDDS, which have been used across diverse populations. When nested within an assessment of other psychiatric illness, items included in the CIDI – a fully structured lay interview – assess eating disorder pathology as well. The Eating Disorders Examination is widely accepted as the best available semi-structured interview for assessing diagnostic information, frequency, and severity data as well as a wide breadth of dimensional information within several relevant cognitive domains. A comprehensive clinical assessment, augmented by information from collateral sources (when necessary), as well as data from the physical and laboratory examination, is the most appropriate evaluation for treatment planning.

Eating disorders have the highest mortality rate among psychiatric disorders as well as have serious associated medical complications and psychological distress. Given the unacceptably low access to care for eating disorders, detection in primary-care settings could serve an important purpose in facilitating initiation of treatment. However, eating disorders are frequently not recognized in primary-care settings. Notwithstanding the breadth of assessments available, structured interviews are too time-consuming to be used in routine clinical practice. The SCOFF has been developed for screening within general health-care settings and shows promise for identifying individuals who may have an eating disorder for additional evaluation with a minimal burden of time.

References

1. Mond JM, Hay PJ, Rodgers B, Owen C. Health service utilization for eating disorders: findings from a community-based study. International Journal of Eating Disorders 2007; 40:399–408.
2. Hudson JI, Hiripi E, Pope HG Jr, Kessler RC. The prevalence and correlates of eating disorders in the National Comorbidity Survey Replication. Biological Psychiatry 2007; 61:348–358.
3. Whitehouse AM, Cooper PJ, Vize CV, Hill C, Vogel L. Prevalence of eating disorders in three Cambridge general practices: Hidden and conspicuous morbidity. British Journal of General Practice 1992; 42:57–60.
4. Couturier JL, Lock J. Denial and minimization in adolescents with anorexia nervosa. International Journal of Eating Disorders 2006; 39:212–216.
5. Hoek HW, van Hoeken D. Review of the prevalence and incidence of eating disorders. International Journal of Eating Disorders 2003; 34:383–396.
6. World Health Organization. CIDI. 1990.
7. KesslerRC, Ustun TB. The World Mental Health (WMH) Survey Initiative Version of the World Health Organization (WHO) Composite International Diagnostic Interview (CIDI). The International Journal of Methods in Psychiatric Research 2004; 13:93–121.
8. www.Hcp.Med.harvard.edu/ncs/eating.php accessed December 4, 2007.
9. American Psychiatric Association. Diagnostic and Statistical Manual of Mental Disorders, 4th Edition, Text Revision, Washington DC: APA Press; 2000.
10. Fairburn CG, Beglin SJ. Assessment of eating disorders: Interview or self-report questionnaire? International Journal of Eating Disorders 1994; 16:363–370
11. Becker AE, Thomas JJ, Franko DL, Herzog DB. Disclosure patterns of eating and weight concerns to clinicians, educational professionals, family, and peers. International Journal of Eating Disorders 2005; 38:18–23.
12. Spitzer RL, Williams JB, Gibbon M, First MB. The structured clinical interview for DSM-III-R (SCID). I: History, rationale, and description. Archives of General Psychiatry 1992; 49:624–629.
13. http://www.scid4.org/faq/scidfaq.html; accessed December, 2007

14. Williams JB, Gibbon M, First MB, Spitzer RL, Davies M, Borus J, Howes MJ, Kane J, Pope HG Jr, Rounsaville B, et al. The structured clinical interview for DSM-III-R (SCID). II. Multisite test-retest reliability. Archives of General Psychiatry 1992; 49:630–636.

15. Shear MK, Greeno C, Kang J, Ludewig D, Frank E, Swartz HA, Hanekamp M. Diagnosis of nonpsychotic patients in community clinics. American Journal of Psychiatry 2000; 157: 581–587.

16. Basco MR, Bostic JQ, Davies D, Rush AJ, Witte B, Hendrickse W, Barnett V. Methods to improve diagnostic accuracy in a community mental health setting. American Journal of Psychiatry 2000; 157:1599–1605

17. Steiner JL, Tebes JK, Sledge WH, Walker ML. A comparison of the Structured Clinical Interview for DSM-III-R and clinical diagnoses. Journal of Nervous and Mental Disease 1995; 183:365–369.

18. Pike KM, Loeb K, Walsh BT. Binge Eating and Purging. In Allison DB (ed.) Handbook of Assessment Methods for Eating Behaviors and Weight-related Problems. Thousand Oaks: Sage 1995 pp. 303–346.

19. Striegel-Moore RH, Franko DL, Ach EL. Epidemiology of eating disorders: An update. In Wonderlich S, Mitchel JE, de Zwaan M, Steiger H (eds.) Annual Review of Eating Disorders, Part 2. 2006, Oxford: Radcliffe Publishing; pp. 65–80.

20. Cooper Z, Fairburn C. The Eating Disorder Examination: A semi-structured interview for the assessment of the specific psychopathology of eating disorders. International Journal of Eating Disorders 1987; 6:1–8.

21. Cooper Z, Cooper PJ, Fairburn C. The validity of the eating disorder examination and its subscales. British Journal of Psychiatry 1989; 154:807–812.

22. Fairburn CG, Cooper Z, O'Connor M. Eating Disorders Examination 16th Version. In Fairburn CG. Cognitive Behavioral Treatment for Eating Disorders. New York: Guilford Press, New York; 2008; (in press).

23. Rizvi SL, Peterson CB, Crow SJ, Agras WS. Test-retest reliability of the eating disorder examination. International Journal of Eating Disorders 2000; 28:311–316.

24. Grilo CM, Masheb RM, Lozano-Blanco C, Barry DT. Reliability of the eating disorder examination in patients with binge eating disorder. International Journal of Eating Disorders 2003; 35:80–85.

25. Mond JM, Hay PJ, Rodgers B, Owen C, Beumont PJV. Temporal stability of the Eating Disorder Examination Questionnaire. International Journal of Eating Disorders 2004; 36:195–203.

26. Wilfley DE, Schwartz MB, Spurrel EM, Fairburn CG. Using the eating disorder examination to identify the specific psychopathology of binge eating disorder. International Journal of Eating Disorders 2000; 27:259–269.

27. Rosen JC, Vara L, Wendt S, Leitenberg H. Validity studies of the eating disorder examination. International Journal of Eating Disorders 1990; 9:519–528.

28. Grilo C, Lozano C, Elder KA. Inter-rater and test-retest reliability of the Spanish language version of the Eating Disorders Examination interview: Clinical and Research Implications. Journal of Psychiatric Practice 2005; 11: 231–240.

29. Willet W. Nutritional Epidemiology, Second Edition. Oxford: Oxford University Press. 1998.

30. Grilo CM, Masheb RM, Wilson GT. A comparison of different methods for assessing the features of eating disorders in patients with binge eating disorder. Journal of Consulting and Clinical Psychology 2001; 69:317–322.

31. Mond JM, Hay PJ, Rodgers B, Owen C, Beumont PJV. Validity of the Eating Disorder Examination Questionnaire (EDE-Q) in screening for eating disorders in community samples. Behaviour Research and Therapy 2004; 42:551–567.

32. Fairburn CG, Beglin S. Eating Disorder Examination Questionnaire-EDE-Q(6.0) In: Fairburn CG. Cognitive Behavior Therapy and Eating Disorders. New York: The Guilford Press. 2008; 309–313.

33. Luce KH, Crowther JH. The reliability of the eating disorder examination—Self-report questionnaire version (EDE-Q). International Journal of Eating Disorders 1999; 25:349–351.

34. Peterson CB, Crosby RD, Wonderlich SA, Joiner T, Crow SJ, Mitchell JE, Bardone-Cone AM, Klein M, le Grange D. Psychometric properties of the eating disorder examination-questionnaire: Factor structure and internal consistency. International Journal of Eating Disorders 2007; 40: 386–389.

35. Sysko R, Walsh BT, Fairburn CG. Eating Disorder Examination-Questionnaire as a measure of change in patients with bulimia nervosa. International Journal of Eating Disorders 2005; 37:100–106.

36. Wolk SL, Loeb KL, Walsh BT. Assessment of patients with anorexia nervosa: Interview versus self-report. International Journal of Eating Disorders 2005; 37:92–99.

37. Goldfein JA, Devlin MJ, Kamanetz C. Eating Disorder Examination-Questionnaire with and without instruction to assess binge-eating in patients with binge eating disorder. International Journal of Eating Disorders 2005; 37:107–111.

38. Mond JM, Hay PJ, Rodgers B, Owen C. Eating Disorder Examination Questionnaire (EDE-Q): Norms for young adult women. Behaviour Research and Therapy 2006; 44:53–62.

39. Carter JC, Stewart DA, Fairburn CG. Eating disorder examination questionnaire: Norms for young adolescent girls. Behaviour Research and Therapy 2001; 39:625–632.

40. Becker AE, Thomas JJ, Bainivualiku A, Richards L, Navare K, Roberts A, Gilman SE, Striegel-Moore R. Validity and reliability of a Fijian translation and adaptation of the Eating Disorder Examination-Questionnaire. International Journal of Eating Disorders; 2009 in press.

41. Mond JM, Hay PJ, Rodgers B, Owen C. Self-report versus interview assessment of purging in a community sample of women. European Eating Disorders Review 2007; 15:403–409.

42. Keel PK, Crow S, Davis TL, Mitchell J. Assessment of eating disorders: Comparison of interview and questionnaire data from a long-term follow-up study of bulimia nervosa. Journal of Psychosomatic Research 2002; 53:1043–1047.

43. Bohn K, Fairburn CG. The Clinical Impairment Assessment questionnaire (CIA). In Fairburn CG (ed.) Cognitive Behavior Therapy for Eating Disorders. New York: Guilford Press, pp. 315–319 2008.

44. Abraham SF, Brown T, Boyd C, Luscombe G, Russell J. Quality of life: Eating disorders. Australian and New Zealand Journal of Psychiatry 2006; 40:150–155.

45. Engel SG, Wittrock DA, Crosby RD, Wonderlich SA, Mitchell JE, Kolotkin RL. Development and psychometric validation of an eating disorder specific health-related quality of life instrument. International Journal of Eating Disorders 2006; 39:62–71.

46. Stice E, Telch CF, Rizvi SL. Development and validation of the Eating Disorder Diagnostic Scale: a brief self-report measure of anorexia, bulimia, and binge-eating disorder. Psychological Assessment 2000; 12: 123–131.

47. Stice E, Fisher M, Martinez E. Eating Disorder Diagnostic Scale: Additional evidence of reliability and validity. Psychological Assessment 2004; 16: 60–71.

48. Lee SW, Stewart SM, Striegel-Moore RH, Lee S, Ho S-Y, Lee PWH, Katzman MA, Lam T-H. Validation of the Eating Disorder Diagnostic Scale for use with Hong Kong adolescents. International Journal of Eating Disorders 2007; 40:569–574.

49. Garner DM, Olmstead MP, Polivy J. Development and validation of a multidimensional eating disorder inventory for anorexia nervosa and bulimia. International Journal of Eating Disorders 1983; 2: 15–34.

50. Garner DM. Eating Disorders Inventory—2: Professional manual. 1991. Odessa, FL: Psychological Assessment Resources.

51. Garner DM. Eating Disorders Inventory—3: Professional manual. 2004. Odessa, FL: Psychological Assessment Resources.

52. Cumella EJ. Review of the Eating Disorder Inventory-3. Journal of Personality Assessment 2006; 87: 116–117.

53. Hurley JB, Palmer RL, Stretch D. The specificity of the Eating Disorders Inventory: A reappraisal. International Journal of Eating Disorders 1990; 9: 419–424.
54. Espelage DL, Mazzeo SE, Aggen SH, et al. Examining the construct validity of the Eating Disorder Inventory. Psychological Assessment 2003: 15: 71–80.
55. Guimera E, Torrubia R. Adaptacion Espanola del "Eating disorder inventory" (EDI) en una muestra de pacientes anorexicas. Anales Psiquiatria 1987; 3:185–190.
56. Al-Subaie AS, Bamgboye E, Al-Shummari S, et al. Validity of the Arabic version of the eating disorder inventory. British Journal of Psychiatry 1996; 168: 636–640.
57. Thiel A, Jacobi C, Horstmann S, et al. A German version of the Eating Disorder Inventory EDI-2. Psychotherapy Psychosomatic and Medical Psychology 1997; 47: 365–376.
58. Machado PPP, Gonçalves S, Martins C, et al. The Portuguese version of the Eating Disorders Inventory: Evaluation of its psychometric properties. European Eating Disorders Review 2001; 9: 43–52.
59. Lee S, Lee AM, Leung, et al. Psychometric properties of the Eating Disorders Inventory (EDI-1) in a nonclinical Chinese population in Hong Kong. International Journal of Eating Disorders 1997; 21: 187–194.
60. Nakano K. Confirmatory factor analysis of the eating disorder inventory. Psychological Reports 2005; 97: 337–338.
61. Boyadjieva S, Steinhausen H-C. The eating attitudes test and the eating disorders inventory in four Bulgarian clinical and nonclinical samples. International Journal of Eating Disorders 1996; 19: 93–98.
62. Garner DM, Garfinkel PE. The eating attitudes test: An index of the symptoms of anorexia nervosa. Psychological Medicine 1979; 9: 273–279.
63. Garner DM, Olmsted MP, Bohr Y, Garfinkel PE. The eating attitudes test: Psychometric features and clinical correlates. Psychological Medicine 1982; 12: 871–878.
64. Thelan MH, Farmer J, Wonderlich S, Smith M. A revision of the Bulimia test: the BULIT-R. Psychological Assessment 1991; 3:119–124.
65. Welch G, Thompson L, Hall A. The BULIT-R: It's reliability and clinical validity as a screening tool for DSM III-R bulimia nervosa in a female tertiary education population. International Journal of Eating Disorders. 1993; 14(1):93–105.
66. Vincent MA, McCabe MD, Ricciardelli LA. Factorial validity of the BULIT-R in adolescent boys and girls. Behavioral Research and Therapy. 1999; 37:1129–1140.
67. Fernandez F, Malacrne VL, Wilfley DE, McQuaid J. Factor structure of the Bulimia test-revised in college women from four ethnic groups. Cultural Diversity and Ethnic Minority Psychology. 2006; 12(3):403–419.
68. Jonsdottir SM, Thornorsteindottir G, Smari J. Reliability and validity of the Icelandic version of the Bulimia test- revised. Laeknabladid 2005; 91(12):923–928.
69. Velasquez AJ, Garcia R, Jiminez R. Psychometric characteristics of Spanish adaptation of a test for bulimia (BULIT). Actas Espanolas de Psiquiatria 2007; 35(5): 309–314.
70. Luck AJ, Morgan JF, Reid F, O'Brien A, Brunton J, Price C, Perry L, Lacey JH. The SCOFF questionnaire and clinical interview for eating disorders in general practice: comparative study. British Medical Journal 2002; 325:755–756.
71. Morgan JF, Reid F, Lacey JH. The SCOFF questionnaire: Assessment of a new screening tool for eating disorders. British Medical Journal 1999; 319:1467–1468.
72. Parker SC. Lyons J. Bonner J. Eating disorders in graduate students: Exploring the SCOFF questionnaire as a simple screening tool. Journal of American College Health 2005; 54: 103–107.
73. Rueda GE, Diaz LA, Campo A, Barros JA, Avila GC, Orostegui LT, Osorio BC, Cadna L del P. Validation of the SCOFF questionnaire for screening of eating disorders in university women. Biomedica 2005; 25:196–202.
74. Muro-Sans P, Amador-Campos JA, Morgan JF. The SCOFF-c: Psychometric properties of the Catalan version in a Spanish adolescent sample. Journal of Psychosomatic Research 2008; 64:81–86.

75. Rueda GE, Diaz Martinez LA, Ortiz Baraja DP, Pinzon Plata C, Rodriquez Martinez J, Cadnea Afanador LP. Validation of the SCOFF questionnaire for screening the eating behaviour disorders of adolescents in school. Atencion Primaria 2005; 35: 89–94.

76. Perry L. Morgan J. Reid F. Brunton J. O'Brien A. Luck A. Lacey H. Screening for symptoms of eating disorders: reliability of the SCOFF screening tool with written compared to oral delivery. International Journal of Eating Disorders 2002; 32:466–472.

77. Crosby RD, Mitchell, JE. SCOFF- a promising instrument, but more research is needed. Western Journal of Medicine 2000; 172:164–165.

78. Fairburn CG, Cooper Z. The Eating Disorder Examination (12th ed.). In Fairburn CG, Wilson GT (eds.), Binge eating: Nature, assessment, and treatment. New York, NY: Guilford Press, 1993.

79. Spitzer RL, Yanovski SZ, Marcus MD. The Questionnaire on Eating and Weight Patterns – Revised (QEWP-R, 1993). (Available from the New York State Psychiatric Institute, 722 West 168th Street, New York, NY 10032).

80. Gormally J, Black S, Daston S, Rardin D. The assessment of binge eating severity among obese persons. Addictive Behaviors, 1982; 7:47–55.

81. Black CMD, Wilson GT. Assessment of eating disorders: Interview versus questionnaire. International Journal of Eating Disorders, 1996; 20(1):43–50.

82. Grilo CM, Masheb RM, Wilson GT. Different methods for assessing the features of eating disorders in patients with binge eating disorder: A replication. Obesity Research 2001; 9(7): 418–422.

83. Kalarchian MA, Wilson GT, Brolin RE, Bradley L. Assessment of eating disorders in bariatric surgery candidates: self-report questionnaire versus interview. International Journal of Eating Disorders, 2000; 28: 465–469.

84. Spitzer RL, Devlin M, Walsh BT, Hasin D, Wing R, Marcus M, Stunkard A, Wadden T, Yanovski S, Agras S, Mitchell J, Nonas C. Binge eating disorder: A multisite field trial of the diagnostic criteria. International Journal of Eating Disorders, 1992; 11:191–203.

85. Borges MBF, Morgan CM, Claudino AM, da Silveira DX . Validation of the Portuguese version of the Questionnaire on Eating and Weight Patterns – Revised (QEWP-R) for the screening of binge eating disorder. Revista Brasileira de Psiquiatria 2005; 27: 319–322.

86. De Zwaan M, Mitchell JE, Specker SM, Pyle RL, Mussell MP, Seim HC. Diagnosing binge eating disorder: Level of agreement between self-report and expert rating. International Journal of Eating Disorders, 1993; 14: 289–295.

87. Spitzer RL, Yanovski S, Wadden T, Wing R, Marcus MD, Stunkard A, Devlin M, Mitchell J, Hasin D, Horne RL. Binge eating disorder: Its further validation in a multi-site study. International Journal of Eating Disorders, 1993; 3:137–153.

88. Celio AA, Wilfley DE, Crow SJ, Mitchell J, Walsh BT. A comparison of the Binge eating scale, questionnaire for eating and weight patterns-revised, and eating disorder examination questionnaire with instructions with the eating disorder examination in the assessment of binge eating disorder and its symptoms. International Journal of Eating Disorders 2004; 36: 434–444.

89. Nangle DW, Johnson WG, Carr-Nangle RE, Engler LB. Binge eating disorder and the proposed DSM-IV criteria: Psychometric analysis of the questionnaire of eating and weight patterns. International Journal of Eating Disorders 1994; 16(2):147–157.

90. Timmerman GM. Binge eating scale: Futher assessment of validity and reliability. Journal of Applied Biobehavioral Research, 1999; 4:1–12.

91. Gladis MM, Wadden TA, Foster GD, Vogt RA, Wingate BJ. A comparison of two approaches to the assessment of binge eating in obesity. International Journal of Eating Disorders 1998; 23:17–26.

92. Brody ML, Walsh BT, Devlin MJ. Binge eating disorder: Reliability and validity of a new diagnostic category. Journal of Consulting and Clinical Psychology 1994; 62: 381–386.

93. Greeno CG, Marcus MD, Wing RR. Diagnosis of binge eating disorder: Discrepancies between a questionnaire and clinical interview. International Journal of Eating Disorders 1995;17:153–160.

94. Stunkard A, Messick S. The three factor eating questionnaire to measure dietary restraint, disinhibition, and hunger. Journal of Psychosomatic Research 1985; 29:71–83.

95. Arnow B, Kenardy J, Agras WS. The emotional eating scale: The development of a measure to assess coping with negative affect by eating. International Journal of Eating Disorders 1995; 17: 79–90.

96. van Strein T, Frijters J, Bergers G, Defares, P. The dutch eating behavior questionnaire (DEBQ) for assessment of restrained, emotional, and external eating behavior. International Journal of Eating Disorders 1986; 5:295–315.

97. Masheb RM, Grilo CM. Emotional overeating and its associations with eating disorder psychopathology among overweight patients with binge eating disorder. International Journal of Eating Disorders 2006; 39:141–146.

98. Farrell C, Lee M, Shafran R. Assessment of body size estimation: A review. European Eating Disorders Review 2005;13: 75–88.

99. Smeets MAM, Smit F, Panhuysen GEM, Ingleby JD. Body perception index: Benefits, pitfalls, ideals. Journal of Psychosomatic Research 1998; 44: 457–464.

100. Smeets MAM. The rise and fall of body size estimation research in anorexia nervosa: A review and reconceptualization. European Eating Disorders Review 1997; 5: 75–95.

101. Probst M, Van Coppenolle H, Vandereycken W, Kampman M, Goris M. Body-size estimation in eating disorder patients: Testing the video-distorting mirror on a life-size screen. Behaviour Research and Therapy 1995; 33: 985–990.

102. Shafran R, Fairburn CG. A new ecologically valid method to assess body size estimation and body size dissatisfaction. International Journal of Eating Disorders 2002; 32: 458–465.

103. Fallon AE, Rozin P. Sex differences in perceptions of desirable body shape. Journal of Abnormal Psychology 1985; 94: 102–105.

104. Beebe DW, Holmbeck GN, Greskiewicz C. Normative and psychometric data on the Body Image Assessment-Revised. Journal of Personality Assessment 1999; 73: 374–394.

105. Gardner RM, Stark K, Jackson NA, Friedman BN. Development and validation of two new scales for assessment of body image. Perceptual& Motor Skills 1999; 89:981–993.

106. Doll M, Ball GDC, Willows ND. Rating of figures used for body image assessment varies depending on the method of figure presentation. International Journal of Eating Disorders 2004; 35: 109–114.

107. Cullari S, Vosburgh M, Shotwell A, Inzodda J, Davenport W. Body-image assessment: A review and evaluation of a new computer-aided measurement technique. North American Journal of Psychology 2002; 4: 221–232.

108. Gardner RM, Friedman BN, Jackson NA. Methodological concerns when using silhouettes to measure body image. Perceptual & Motor Skills 1998; 86: 387–395.

109. Cafri G, Thompson JK. Measuring male body image: A review of the current methodology. Psychology of Men & Masculinity 2004; 5: 18–29.

110. Gruber AJ, Pope HG, Borweicki J, Cohane G. The development of the Somatomorphic Matrix: A bi-axial instrument for measuring body image in men and women. In Olds TS, Dollman J, Norton KI (eds.) Kinanthropometry VI 1999; (217–232). Sydney: International Society for the Advancement of Kinanthropometry.

111. Cafri G, Roehrig M, Thompson JK. Reliability assessment of the Somatomorphic Matrix. International Journal of Eating Disorders 2004; 35: 597–600.

112. Berscheid E, Walster E, Bohrnstedt G. The happy American body: A survey report. Psychology Today 1973; 7: 119–131.

113. Masheb RM, Grilo CM, Burke-Martindale CH, Rothschild BS. Evaluating oneself by shape and weight is not the same as being dissatisfied about shape and weight: A longitudinal examination in severely obese gastric bypass patients. International Journal of Eating Disorders 2006; 39: 716–720.

114. Reas DL, Whisenhunt BL, Netemeyer R, Williamson DA. Development of the body checking questionnaire: A self-report measure of body checking behaviors. International Journal of Eating Disorders 2002; 31: 324–333.
115. Rosen JC, Srebnik D, Saltzberg E, Wendt, S. Development of a body image avoidance questionnaire. Psychological Assessment 1991; 3, 32–37.
116. Cooper P, Taylor M, Cooper Z, Fairburn C. The development and validation of the body shape questionnaire. International Journal of Eating Disorders 1987; 6: 485–494.
117. Rosen JC, Jones A, Ramirez E, Waxman S. Body shape questionnaire: Studies of validity and reliability. International Journal of Eating Disorders 1996; 20: 315–319.
118. Evans C, Dolan B. Body shape questionnaire: Derivation of shortened "alternate forms". International Journal of Eating Disorders 1993; 315–321.
119. Dowson J, Henderson L. The validity of a short version of the Body Shape Questionnaire. Psychiatry Research 2001; 263–271.
120. Ghaderi A, Scott B. The reliability and validity of the Swedish version of the body shape questionnaire. Scandinavian Journal of Psychology 2004; 45: 319–324.
121. Rousseau A, Knotter A, Barbe P, et al. Validation of the French version of the body shape questionnaire. L'Encéphale 2005; 31: 162–173.
122. American Academy of Pediatrics Policy Statement: Identifying and Treating Eating Disorders. Pediatrics 111(1):204–211, 2003.
123. http://www.cdc.gov/nccdphp/dnpa/bmi/childrens_BMI/about_childrens_BMI   accessed 4/5/07
124. http://www.wpic.pitt.edu/ksads/ accessed 4/4/07
125. Bryant-Waugh RJ, Cooper PJ, Taylor CL, Lask BD. The use of the eating disorder examination with children: A pilot study. International Journal of Eating Disorders 1996; 19:391–397.
126. Watkins B, Framptom I, Lask B, Bryant-Waugh R. Reliability and validity of the child version of the eating disorder examination: A preliminary investigation. International Journal of Eating Disorders 2005; 38:183–187.
127. Passi VA, Bryson SW, Lock J. Assessment of eating disorders in adolescents with anorexia nervosa: self-report questionnaire versus interview. International Journal of Eating Disorder 2003; 33:45–54.
128. Maloney M, McGuire J, Daniels S. Reliability testing of a children's version of the Eating Attitude Test. Journal of American Acadey of Child & Adolescent Psychiatry 1988; 28: 541–543.
129. Smolak L, Levine MP. Psychometric properties of the children's eating attitudes test. International Journal of Eating Disorders 1994; 16:275–282.
130. Johnson WG, Grieve FG, Adams CD, Sandy J. Measuring binge eating in adolescents: Adolescent and parent version of the questionnaire of eating and weight patterns. International Journal of Eating Disorders 1999; 26:301–314.
131. Johnson WG, Kirk AA, Reed AE. Adolescent version of the questionnaire of eating and weight patterns: Reliability and gender differences. International Journal of Eating Disorders 2001; 29:94–96.
132. Childress AC, Brewerton TD, Hodges EL, Jarrell MP. The kids' eating disorder survery (KEDS): A study of middle school students. Journal of American Academy Child & Adolescent Psychiatry 1993; 32(4):843–850.
133. Epstein LH, Paluch RA, Saelens BE, Ernst MM, Wilfley DE. Changes in eating disorder symptoms with pediatric obesity treatment. Journal of Pediatrics 2001; 139:58–65.
134. Garner DM. Eating Disorders Inventory-C. Lutz, FL: Psychological Assessment Resources; 1991.
135. Eklun K, Paavonen EJ, Almqvist F. Factor structure of the eating disorder inventory-C. International Journal of Eating Disorders 2005; 37:330–341.
136. Tanovsky-Kraff M, Morgan CM, Yanovski SZ, Marmarosh C, Wilfley DE, Yanovski JA. Comparison of assessments of children's eating-disordered behaviors by interview and questionnaire. International Journal of Eating Disorders 2003; 33:213–224.

Eating Attitudes Test (EAT-26)

Eating Attitudes Test (EAT-26)©

Instructions: This is a screening measure to help you determine whether you might have an eating disorder that needs professional attention. This screening measure is not designed to make a diagnosis of an eating disorder or take the place of a professional consultation. Please fill out the below form as accurately, honestly and completely as possible. There are no right or wrong answers. All of your responses are confidential.

Part A: Complete the following questions:

1) Birth Date   Month: ___   Day: ___   Year: ___   2) Gender: Male ☐   Female ☐

3) Height   Feet: ___   Inches: ___

4) Current Weight (lbs): ___   5) Highest Weight (excluding pregnancy): ___

6) Lowest Adult Weight: ___   7) Ideal Weight: ___

Part B: Please check a response for each of the following statements:	Always	Usually	Often	Some times	Rarely	Never
1. Am terrified about being overweight.	☐	☐	☐	☐	☐	☐
2. Avoid eating when I am hungry.	☐	☐	☐	☐	☐	☐
3. Find myself preoccupied with food.	☐	☐	☐	☐	☐	☐
4. Have gone on eating binges where I feel that I may not be able to stop.	☐	☐	☐	☐	☐	☐
5. Cut my food into small pieces.	☐	☐	☐	☐	☐	☐
6. Aware of the calorie content of foods that I eat.	☐	☐	☐	☐	☐	☐
7. Particularly avoid food with a high carbohydrate content (i.e. bread, rice, potatoes, etc.)	☐	☐	☐	☐	☐	☐
8. Feel that others would prefer if I ate more.	☐	☐	☐	☐	☐	☐
9. Vomit after I have eaten.	☐	☐	☐	☐	☐	☐
10. Feel extremely guilty after eating.	☐	☐	☐	☐	☐	☐
11. Am preoccupied with a desire to be thinner.	☐	☐	☐	☐	☐	☐
12. Think about burning up calories when I exercise.	☐	☐	☐	☐	☐	☐
13. Other people think that I am too thin.	☐	☐	☐	☐	☐	☐
14. Am preoccupied with the thought of having fat on my body.	☐	☐	☐	☐	☐	☐
15. Take longer than others to eat my meals.	☐	☐	☐	☐	☐	☐
16. Avoid foods with sugar in them.	☐	☐	☐	☐	☐	☐
17. Eat diet foods.	☐	☐	☐	☐	☐	☐
18. Feel that food controls my life.	☐	☐	☐	☐	☐	☐
19. Display self-control around food.	☐	☐	☐	☐	☐	☐
20. Feel that others pressure me to eat.	☐	☐	☐	☐	☐	☐
21. Give too much time and thought to food.	☐	☐	☐	☐	☐	☐
22. Feel uncomfortable after eating sweets.	☐	☐	☐	☐	☐	☐
23. Engage in dieting behavior.	☐	☐	☐	☐	☐	☐
24. Like my stomach to be empty.	☐	☐	☐	☐	☐	☐
25. Have the impulse to vomit after meals.	☐	☐	☐	☐	☐	☐
26. Enjoy trying new rich foods.	☐	☐	☐	☐	☐	☐

Part C: Behavioral Questions: In the past 6 months have you:	Never	Once a month or less	2–3 times a month	Once a week	2–6 times a week	Once a day or more
A Gone on eating binges where you feel that you may not be able to stop?	☐	☐	☐	☐	☐	☐
B Ever made yourself sick (vomited) to control your weight or shape?	☐	☐	☐	☐	☐	☐
C Ever used laxatives, diet pills or diuretics (water pills) to control your weight or shape?	☐	☐	☐	☐	☐	☐
D Exercised more than 60 minutes a day to lose or to control your weight?	☐	☐	☐	☐	☐	☐
E Lost 20 pounds or more in the past 6 months	Yes ☐		No ☐			

*Defined as eating much more than most people would under the same circumstances and feeling that eating is out of control

EAT-26: Garner et al, 1982, *Psychological Medicine*, 12, 871-878); adapted by D. Garner with permission.

Body Shape Questionnaire (BSQ)

Body Shape Questionnaire (BSQ)
BSQ

We should like to know how you have been feeling about your appearance over the *past four weeks.* Please read each question and circle the appropriate number to the right. Please answer all the questions.

Over the past four weeks:

	Never	Rarely	Some-times	Often	Very often	Always
1. Has feeling bored made you brood about your shape?	1	2	3	4	5	6
2. Have you been so worried about your shape that you have been feeling you ought to diet?	1	2	3	4	5	6
3. Have you thought that your thighs, hips, or bottom are too large for the rest of you?	1	2	3	4	5	6
4. Have you been afraid that you might become fat (or fatter)?	1	2	3	4	5	6
5. Have you worried about your flesh being not firm enough?	1	2	3	4	5	6
6. Has feeling full (e.g., after eating a large meal) made you feel fat?	1	2	3	4	5	6
7. Have you felt so bad about your shape that you have cried?	1	2	3	4	5	6
8. Have you avoided running because your flesh might wobble?	1	2	3	4	5	6
9. Has being with thin women made you feel self-concious about your shape?	1	2	3	4	5	6
10. Have you worried about your thighs spreading out when sitting down?	1	2	3	4	5	6
11. Has eating even a small amount of food made you feel fat?	1	2	3	4	5	6
12. Have you noticed the shape of other women and felt that your own shape compared unfavorably?	1	2	3	4	5	6
13. Has thinking about your shape interfered with your ability to concentrate (e.g., while watching television, reading, listening to conversations)?	1	2	3	4	5	6
14. Has being naked, such as when taking a bath, made you feel fat?	1	2	3	4	5	6
15. Have you avoided wearing clothes which make you particularly aware of the shape of your body?	1	2	3	4	5	6

continued

	Never	Rarely	Some-times	Often	Very often	Always
16. Have you imagined cutting off fleshy areas of your body?	1	2	3	4	5	6
17. Has eating sweets, cakes, or other high-calode food made you feel fat?	1	2	3	4	5	6
18. Have you not gone out to social occasions (e.g., parties) because you have felt bad about your shape?	1	2	3	4	5	6
19. Have you felt excessively large and rounded?	1	2	3	4	5	6
20. Have you felt ashamed of your body?	1	2	3	4	5	6
21. Has worry about your shape made you diet?	1	2	3	4	5	6
22. Have you felt happiest about your shape when your stomach has been empty (e.g., in the morning)?	1	2	3	4	5	6
23. Have you thought that you are in the shape you are because you lack self-control?	1	2	3	4	5	6
24. Have you worried about other people seeing rolls of fat around your waist or stomach?	1	2	3	4	5	6
25. Have you felt that it is not fair that other women are thinner than you?	1	2	3	4	5	6
26. Have you vomited in order to feel thinner?	1	2	3	4	5	6
27. When in company have you worried about taking up too much room (e.g., sitting on a sofa, or a bus seat)?	1	2	3	4	5	6
28. Have you worried about your flesh being dimply?	1	2	3	4	5	6
29. Has seeing your reflection (e.g., in a mirror or shop window) made you feel bad about your shape?	1	2	3	4	5	6
30. Have you pinched areas of your body to see how much fat there is?	1	2	3	4	5	6
31. Have you avoided situations where people could see your body (e.g., communal changing rooms or swimming pools)?	1	2	3	4	5	6
32. Have you taken laxatives in order to feel thinner?	1	2	3	4	5	6
33. Have you been particularly self-conscious about your shape when in the company of other people?	1	2	3	4	5	6
34. Has worry about your shape made you feel you ought to exercise?	1	2	3	4	5	6

Eating Disorder Diagnostic Scale (EDDS)

EDDS

Please carefully complete all questions.

Over the past 3 months...	Not at all		Slightly		Moderately		Extremely
1. Have you felt fat?...................	0	1	2	3	4	5	6
2. Have you had a definite fear that you might gain weight or become fat?..........	0	1	2	3	4	5	6
3. Has your weight influenced how you think about (judge) yourself as a person?.........	0	1	2	3	4	5	6
4. Has your shape influenced how you think about (judge) yourself as a person?.........	0	1	2	3	4	5	6

5. During the past **6 months** have there been times when you felt you have eaten what other people would regard as an unusually large amount of food (e.g., a quart of ice cream) given the circumstances?........   Yes   No

6. During the times when you ate an unusually large amount of food, did you experience a loss of control (feel you couldn't stop eating or control what or how much you were eating)?.....   Yes   No

7. How many **DAYS per week** on average over the **past 6 MONTHS** have you eaten an unusually large amount of food and experienced a loss of control?   0   1   2   3   4   5   6   7

8. How many **TIMES per week** on average over the **past 3 MONTHS** have you eaten an unusually large amount of food and experienced a loss of control?   0   1   2   3   4   5   6   7   8   9   10   11   12   13   14

During these episodes of overeating and loss of control did you...

9. Eat much more rapidly than normal?...................................	Yes	No
10. Eat until you felt uncomfortably full?.................................	Yes	No
11. Eat large amounts of food when you didn't feel physically hungry?.............	Yes	No
12. Eat alone because you were embarrassed by how much you were eating?........	Yes	No
13. Feel disgusted with yourself, depressed, or very guilty after overeating?.........	Yes	No
14. Feel very upset about your uncontrollable overeating or resulting weight gain?...	Yes	No

15. How many **times per week** on average over the past **3 months** have you made yourself vomit to prevent weight gain or counteract the effects of eating?   0   1   2   3   4   5   6   7   8   9
         10   11   12   13   14

16. How many **times per week** on average over the past **3 months** have you used laxatives or diuretics to prevent weight gain or counteract the effects of eating?   0   1   2   3   4   5   6   7   8   9
         10   11   12   13   14

17. How many **times per week** on average over the past **3 months** have you fasted (skipped at least 2 meals in a row) to prevent weight gain or counteract the effects of eating?   0   1   2   3   4   5   6   7
         8   9   10   11   12   13   14

18. How many **times per week** on average over the past **3 months** have you engaged in excessive exercise specifically to counteract the effects of overeating episodes?   0   1   2   3   4   5   6   7   8
         9   10   11   12   13   14

19. How much do you weigh? If uncertain, please give your best estimate. _____ lbs.

20. How tall are you? _Please specify in inches (5 ft.= 60 in.)_____ in.

21. Over the past **3 months**, how many menstrual periods have you missed?   0   1   2   3   n/a

22. Have you been taking birth control pills during the past **3 months**?............. Yes   No

Chapter 8
The Use of Rating Scales to Measure Outcomes in Child Psychiatry and Mental Health

Gwyne W. White, Michael S. Jellinek, and J. Michael Murphy

Abstract *Objective.* To help clinicians and administrators select among rating scales in common use in child and adolescent psychiatry.

Background. In Massachusetts, many insurers now require the use of standardized scales to rate child and adult mental health patients. With literally hundreds scales available, clinicians and administrators who have to choose a rating scale may find the vast assortment of instruments bewildering. This chapter brings a theoretical framework to bear on a review of some of the most commonly used scales and provides a case study example of a recent set of decisions in Massachusetts.

Results. We conducted a PubMed search using the term 'Rating scales' combined with 'Child psychiatry' and came up with over 700 papers. Restricting our search to the years from 2002-present reduced the list to 149 articles and 103 named scales in current use. Further restricting our search to those measures mentioned in three or more publications resulted in a list of 11 commonly and recently used measures, only three of which were broadband scales. Since a number of scales commonly used in clinical practice were not on the above list, we added the ten recommended child and adolescent instruments named on the website of a large mental health carve-out insurance company as well as two of the most widely used scales that were not on either of these two lists. We then reviewed the resultant list of 15 scales in terms of a sixteen dimensions that are important to consider in making selection decisions.

Conclusions. Results from the current review identified hundreds of instruments that potentially meet the requirements of insurers but just over a dozen broadband scales which appear to be in common recent use in child psychiatry. All of these rating scales have been used to establish profiles at intake and although all have been used as pre-post measures, none have been expressly validated as measures of clinically significant change. Thus, although there appears to be growing pressure to use standardized rating scales at intake in psychiatry, there is no evidence to support

J.M. Murphy (✉)
Department of Psychiatry, Massachusetts General Hospital and Harvard Medical School,
Yawkey 6a, Boston, MA 02114, USA
e-mail: mmurphy6@partners.org

L. Baer, M.A. Blais (eds.), *Handbook of Clinical Rating Scales and Assessment in*
Psychiatry and Mental Health, Current Clinical Psychiatry, DOI 10.1007/978-1-59745-387-5_8,
© Humana Press, a part of Springer Science+Business Media, LLC 2010

the validity of any available scale as a 'gold standard' yardstick to demonstrate diagnostic or treatment efficacy, let alone for using any scale to restrict access to care or length of treatment. Too little is known about the real world reliability and true clinical predictive validity of such measures to allow them to replace the judgment of experienced clinicians in these matters at this time.

Keywords Child psychiatry · Adolescent psychiatry · Rating scales · Questionnaires · Assessment · Psychiatry

The objective of this chapter is to help clinicians and administrators select among rating scales in common use in child and adolescent psychiatry. Many insurers now require the use of standardized scales to rate child and adult mental-health patients. With literally hundreds of scales available, clinicians and administrators who have to choose a rating scale may find the vast assortment of instruments bewildering. This chapter brings a theoretical framework to bear on a review of some of the most commonly used scales and provides a case study example of a recent set of decisions in Massachusetts. Using a comprehensive methodology outlined in the chapter, we identified 15 scales in terms of 16 dimensions that are important to consider in making selection decisions. Results from the review suggest that while there is growing pressure to use standardized rating scales at intake in psychiatry, there is no evidence showing any available scale to be a "gold standard" yardstick for demonstrating diagnostic or treatment efficacy. At present it seems too little is known about the real world reliability and true clinical predictive validity of such measures to allow them to replace the judgment of experienced clinicians in these matters.

Increasingly, governmental agencies and individual insurers are requiring mental-health clinicians to use standardized instruments as a part of clinical care. In Massachusetts, Medicaid, Blue Cross Blue Shield, PacifiCare, and other health-insurance carriers now require the use of standardized scales to rate child and adult mental-health patients. Although these mandates may be motivated as much by a desire to contain costs as to improve care, there is nevertheless a sense among some authorities that the routine use of quality and outcome measures could improve clinical care, for example, by providing important additional information for diagnosis, quality monitoring [1], or tracking outcomes. In some cases, insurers mandate a particular instrument (as Blue Cross Blue Shield now does in Massachusetts with the TOP [2, 3]), while in other circumstances the individual clinician or treatment agency is free to choose among validated instruments as the Massachusetts Behavioral Health Partnership allows for Medicaid patients in that state [4].

Deciding upon a specific measure presents a serious challenge. In child psychiatry, treatment is directed not just at symptom reduction, but also at improved functioning, returning the child to his/her developmental trajectory, enhancing self-esteem, reinforcing resiliency, and usually influencing a child's caretakers as well. To obtain a truly valid assessment of treatment efficacy, all of these areas might need to be assessed and the time frame might need to be measured in months or even years. Although one focus of treatment is often short-term symptom relief (and this narrow view may be favored by those paying for care), the most necessary and meaningful changes may be harder – and take longer – to measure. For clinicians who wish to select a standardized rating scale that is sensitive to these issues, the choices can be difficult. The review that follows therefore is meant to provide guidance based on a review of published studies, guidelines provided by a large public insurer in one state, and the experience of a large and diverse children's mental-health system of care, which recently had to make such a choice.

Focus of This Review

The sheer number of available instruments can make the choice of a rating scale quite perplexing. For example, a recent series of seven articles (see Winters et al. [5] for these references) in the *Journal of the American Academy of Child and Adolescent Psychiatry* lists nearly 100 instruments. One website that lists rating scales for "quality of life and outcomes" [6] names over 500 measures.

In preparation for this chapter, we conducted a PubMed search using the term "Rating scales" combined with "Child psychiatry" and came up with 751 published papers. Restricting the search to just the past five and one half years (2002 through 2007) reduced the list of articles was to a "mere" 149. We reviewed the abstracts of these papers and found that 103 unique instruments were mentioned. Seventy-seven of these instruments were mentioned in just one study, an additional 15 were mentioned in only two papers. Four scales were mentioned in three papers each, one in four papers, and six in five or more papers. One of these was not available in English, so it was dropped.

To restrict our search to the most commonly used scales, we limited the current review to only the instruments which were cited in at least three papers in our literature review and were available in English. The result was a list of 11 instruments. Eight of these were narrowband screens (devoted to a single specific condition or problem-like depression) and were thus not appropriate for general use, although they could be appropriate as secondary assessments for patients with these problems. The following measures will not be further reviewed in this chapter: Young Mania Rating Scale (YMRS) [7], Children's Depression Rating Scale-Revised (CDRS-R) [8], Child PTSD-Reaction Index (CPTSD-RI) [9], Revised Children's Manifest Anxiety Scale (RCMAS) [10], Dimensional Yale-Brown Obsessive-Compulsive Scale (DY-BOCS) [11], Children's Depression Inventory (CDI) [12], Screen for Child Anxiety Related Emotional Disorders (SCARED) [13], and State-Trait Anxiety Inventory for Children (STAIC) [14].

Three of the measures identified in the literature review did appear to be useful as broadband rating scales and are included as the first three rows of Table 8.1: Child Behavior Checklist (CBCL) [15]/Youth Self Report (YSR) [16], Schedule for Affective Disorders and Schizophrenia for School-Age Children (K-SADS) [17], and the Strengths and Difficulties Questionnaire (SDQ) [18]. Since many of the instruments, which in our experience are most commonly used in *clinical* settings,

Table 8.1 Child psychiatry rating scales compared according to dimensions relevant to selection

Measure	Acronym	Age focus[a]	Age range	Level of care[b]	Global vs. subscales?[c]	Type rater[d]	# of items	Time (min)	Hand vs. Comp[e]	Other Lang[f]	web $[g] site	Qualifications[h]	Training[i]	# of cites
1 Child behavior checklist/youth self-report [16]	CBCL/YSR	c, t	1.5–18	O,I,N	gs + ss	y, z, t	118/112	20–30	H, C	S+	$ Y	MA	m	6000
2 Schedule for affective disorders and schizophrenia [17]	K-SADS	c, t	6–18	O,I	ss	y, z, t	82 pp	90–120	H	dk	0 Y	CL	n	167
3 Strengths and Difficulties Qst [18]	SDQ	c, t	3–17	O, N	gs + ss	y, z, t	25	5	H, C	S+	0 Y	NC	m	249
4 Adolescent Treatment Outcomes Module [19]	ATOM	t	11–19	O, I.	ss	x, y, z	156	27	C	dk	0 Y	NC	m	10
5 Behavior and Symptom Identification Scale 32 [20]	BASIS-32	t, a	14+	O, I	gs + ss	z	32	10–20	H, C	S+	$ Y	NC	m	36
6 Behavioral and Emotional Rating Scale 2 [21]	BERS-2	c, t	5–18	N	ss	x, y, t	52	10	H	dk	$ Y	NC	m	46
7 Brief Psychiatric Rating Scale – Children [22]	BPRS-C	c, t	13–18	O, I	gs + ss	x	24	5	H	na	0 N	CL	n	7
8 Symptom Checklist-90-Revised [23]/Brief Symptom Inventory [24]	SCL-90R/BSI	t, a	13+	O, I, N	gs + ss	z	90/53	15/10	H, C	S+	$ Y	SD	m	865
9 Child-Adolescent Functional Assessment Scale [25]/Preschool Functional Assessment Scale [26]	CAFAS/PECFAS	c, t	4–17	O	gs + ss	x		10–20	H, C	na	$ Y	NC	ws/tm	18

Table 8.1 (continued)

Measure	Acronym	Age focus[a]	Age range	Level of care[b]	Global vs. subscales?[c]	Type rater[d]	# of items	Time (min)	Hand vs. Comp[e]	Other Lang[f]	$[g]	web site	Qualifications[h]	Training[i]	# of cites
10 Connors Rating Scales – REV [27]	CRS-R	c, t	3–17	O, I, N	gs + ss	y, z, t	27–87	5–20	H	dk	$	Y	BA	m	494
11 Short Form 8 [28], 12 [29], 36 [30]	SF8-36	t, a	14+	O, I, N	gs + ss	z	8–36	5–10	H, C	S+	$	Y	NC	m	412
12 Treatment Outcome Package [3]	TOP	c, t, a		O	ss	y, z	48–58	30	C	S	$	Y	NC	m	6
13 Youth Outcome Questionnaire [31]	YOQ	c, t	4–17	O, I, N	gs + ss	z	64	10	H, C	S	$	Y	NC	m	40
14 Children's Global Asmnt Scale [32]	CGAS	c, t	0–18	O, I	gs	x	1	2	H	na	0	N	NC	n	84
15 Pediatric Symptom Checklist [33]	PSC	c, t	3–18	O, N	gs + ss	y, z	35	5	H	S+	0	Y	NC	m	61

Notes: Qst=questionnaire; Asmnt=Assessment.

[a] Age focus: c = child, t = teen, a = adult;

[b] Level of care: O = outpatient, I = inpatient, NP = non-patient population;

[c] Global vs. subscales: gs = global scale, ss = subscales,;

[d] Type of rater: x = clinician, y = parent, z = patient, t = teacher;

[e] Hand vs. computer: H = hand, C = computer;

[f] Other languages: S = Spanish, + = languages other than Spanish and English; na = not available, dk=do not know ;

[g] Cost: $ = cost, 0 = available free;

[h] Qualifications: administered by – NC = non-clinician, SD = specialized degree, CL = clinician, MA = masters degree;

[i] Training: m = manual, ws = workshop, tm = training manual evaluated, n=none.

were not listed at all in the above search – which focused more on *research scales* – we supplemented this list with another provided by the company which manages mental-health benefits for Massachusetts Medicaid.

The Massachusetts Behavioral Health Partnership (MBHP) provides a list of 23 recommended instruments for use in its Outcomes Rating initiative, 10 of them (listed below in Table 8.1) aimed at or validated for use with children or adolescents: Adolescent Treatment Outcomes Module (ATOM;) [19], Behavior and Symptom Identification Scale-32 (BASIS 32) [20], Behavioral and Emotional Rating Scale 2 (BERS-2) [21], Brief Psychiatric Rating Scale – Children (BPRS-C) [22], Symptom Checklist-90-Revised (SCL-90-R) [23]/Brief Symptom Inventory (BSI) [24], Child-Adolescent Functional Assessment Scale (CAFAS) [25]/Preschool and Early Childhood Functional Assessment Scale (PECFAS) [26], Connors Rating Scales – Revised (CRS-Rev) [27], Short Form 8, 12, 36 (SF-8 [28]; SF-12 [29]; SF-36 [30]), Treatment Outcome Package (TOP) [3], and Youth Outcome Questionnaire (YOQ) [31].

Even this list of 10 scales left out two measures that are among the most widely used in clinical practice and/or research trials – the Children's Global Assessment Scale (CGAS) [32] and the Pediatric Symptom Checklist (PSC) [33] – so we added them to our list too and came up with a final set of 15 mental-health rating scales that are widely used in research and/or clinical practice with children and adolescents. These 15 measures are reviewed in terms of 16 dimensions which will be important to consider in making selection decisions. Although the resultant 240-cell matrix is still relatively complex, the needs of a given practice will probably cut down the number of possible choices to a less perplexing number, if these dimensions are given some consideration.

As noted above, the focus of this chapter will be on rating scales that may be used clinically in psychiatry or in other mental-health agencies. Community programs, schools, and outpatient pediatric sites also make use of psychological questionnaires, some of which are the same as those reviewed here but their needs are not the focus here. Research uses of rating scales are also not the focus, although they certainly count for as many or more of the published studies. The published literature on scales that can be used in clinical practice is much smaller.

Sixteen Dimensions of Rating Scales

Before focusing on specifics within the clinical problem domain, some general points are in order. First of all, the single biggest question for any potential user of rating scales in child psychiatry is intended use. If it is just to meet an external mandate, then a clear understanding of the mandate is in essential. In Massachusetts, MBHP's mandate was that all providers "will measure the effects of behavioral health treatment by using standardized outcomes measurement instruments" [4].

According to these criteria, almost any standardized instrument could suffice and a scale that was easier to use, less expensive, and/or more acceptable to clinicians and clients might be preferable to a more comprehensive instrument that was more difficult to use, more costly, or more burdensome. Therefore, when the Partners Psychiatry and Mental Health (PPMH) system of care, a major multi-agency health system, had to choose an instrument for the MBHP mandate, it made its selection according to these criteria, choosing scales which had published validation studies across a wide range of types of disorders and age groups, were easy to use and to provide training on, and were available without cost. For a full description of the PPMH outcomes rating project, see paper by Gold et al. [34]. Lessons learned from the PPMH child outcomes group will be used to illustrate points throughout this chapter.

Even when the requirements of the insurer have been taken into account, the concerns of other stakeholders should be carefully considered to be certain that they have been adequately provided for. Use of rating scales takes a fair amount of time and energy: administrative time for handing out and retrieving the forms, clerical time to score and/or keypunch them, clinician time to interpret them and use them in treatment planning, and other time for assessing the data they provide overall. Unless these issues are taken into account, the effort may not be sustainable over the long term. One way to improve the sustainability of rating scale use is to make sure that it serves the real world needs of the main stakeholder groups (clinicians, administrators, and patients at the least).

Rating scales can vary in many respects. The 16 dimensions highlighted in this review are intended to focus on the issues relevant to selecting a rating scale.

Focus on Child vs. Adult Patients – Two Different Worlds

Since respondents' problems, literacy levels, and the clinicians who treat them often differ for child vs. adult patients, two relatively distinct sets of instruments and research literatures have evolved. There are probably even more rating scales for adults than there are for children, but most of these scales cannot properly be used with children because they have not been validated for this population. The current review will focus only on rating scales validated for children and/or adolescents.

That being said, since some of these scales were originally designed for adults but have had additional validation with adolescents, we have noted adult and/or teen and/or child focus for each rating scale in the first column of Table 8.1. Although age cutoffs are somewhat arbitrary, 17 is usually used as the oldest age for children (adolescents) and 18 as the youngest age for adults. Some of the rating scales (BPRS-C, CGAS) use the same form for patients of all ages while other scales may use a modified or completely different form for children or teens (CBCL/YSR). The age range specified for each scale by its authors is listed in the next column of the table.

Individual Patient vs. Other Focus

This review will focus on scales that rate the identified (child/adolescent) patient, although there are validated scales that rate family functioning (Family APGAR)

[35], resources (HOME) [36] or parent–child interaction (NCAST rating) [37] to name just a few of the other foci possible.

Clinical Assessment vs. Other Types of Scales

Most – but not all – psychiatric rating scales are concerned with symptoms or functioning; so this review will focus primarily on this area. Only one scale listed in Table 8.1, the BERS-2 [21], does not, since it assesses a child's strengths. But it bears mention that there are dozens if not hundreds of scales that focus on other dimensions of individual patients like personality, resilience, emotional strength, demographics, or satisfaction with care. Some of the rating scales mentioned here are packaged along with components that assess these non-clinical domains as well as symptoms or functioning.

Broad- vs. Narrow-Band of Symptoms

As noted earlier in this paper, eight of the eleven most commonly mentioned rating scales had a focus on specific narrowband areas like anxiety, depression, or mania. All three of the remaining measures from the literature review and all 13 of the other recommended scales reviewed here are broadband measures covering the full range of problem areas. In most clinical settings, a broadband rating would be used at intake, possibly followed at a later time with a diagnosis-specific narrow band scale for patients who had a high level of problems in a given area. For example, if the T score on the anxiety scale of the broadband CBCL were in the clinical range (typically placed at a T-score of > 69), then the RCMAS scale might be used as a secondary rating to provide a fuller picture of anxiety symptoms and/or a better target for the assessment of change.

Outpatient vs. Inpatient or Other Level of Care

Although all but one of the rating scales reviewed can be used with clinical populations, some are targeted toward less restrictive settings like schools (BERS-2) [21] or outpatient pediatrics (PSC) [38] while other scales target patients with more serious impairments or more restrictive levels of care like partial- or full psychiatric hospitals (CAFAS [25], BPRS-C [22]). For systems like PPMH which encompass the full range of care from outpatient through inpatient and which want to use a common instrument across the full range of care, this consideration may dictate a selection from a more limited set of rating scales. The fifth column in the table lists the levels of care in which each rating scale has been used.

Single Total Score vs. Multiple Subscales

Another decision to be made is whether there is a need for a single overall rating – usually for total symptoms or global/overall functioning – and/or for subscale scores. The sixth column in Table 8.1 indicates the availability of global vs. subscale scores for each measure. As noted above, the CBCL and most of the other scales provide both. In contrast, however, the TOP and the K-SADS provide only subscale scores and the CGAS provides only a global score. Since the CGAS score is essentially the same as Axis V of DSM, it, unlike the other scales, has a 0–100 score that is readily understood by many clinicians. The CBCL, CGAS, and PSC provide cut points for total scores that allow them to be reduced to high vs. lower risk categories (outside or within the normal range).

Most of the subscale scores concern specific problem areas, with depression, anxiety, and attention being the most commonly measured. But some instruments have subscale scores in other areas. As noted earlier, the CBCL has a social competence subscale as does the YOQ. Two of the measures (YOQ and TOP) have ratings of suicide risk and four (ATOM, BERS, CRS-R and CAFAS/PECFAS) have subscales for family relationships. Role functioning is measured by the BASIS-32, PECFAS, and ATOM. School functioning is assessed via subscales on the TOP, BERS, and CAFAS. In the PPMH sites, a combination of two rating scales was used. This combination included one instrument with subscales (BPRS-C) and one with a readily understood global score (CGAS).

Who Completes the Scale

Who completes the scale varies from measure to measure and sometimes within a given measure. Some scales (CAFAS/PECFAS, CGAS, BPRS-C) are meant to be filled out by clinicians only, giving a clinician's view of the patient. Other scales are completed by parents only (YOQ) or an adult who knows that patient (BERS-2) or patients only (BASIS, SCL, SF). One of the measures (ATOM) must be filled out by a combination of raters (patient, parent, clinician). Many of these measures also have comparable or complementary scales that can be filled out by (older) children/teens (CBCL, CTRS, SDQ, K-SADS, YOQ, TOP, PSC) as well as parents. Some of these scales also have comparable teacher rating forms (CTRS, CBCL, SDQ) that can be used as supplementary sources of data.

In some of the PPMH child sites (and all of the adult sites), a combination of rating scales was used so that both clinician- (CGAS, BPRS-C) and parent-report scales (PSC) are used, providing multiple views of each patient's functioning.

Standalone or Part of a Larger System

All of the measures listed in Table 8.1 can be meaningfully used as standalone measures, but some are part of larger and/or more comprehensive systems rating many domains and/or different raters. For example, as already noted, the CBCL for 6–16 year olds contains both problem scales and a social competence scale making it a larger "problem + competence system" from the parent's perspective. As noted above, a Youth Self Report and or a Teacher Report Form could also be filled out for each case to add these perspectives. And a Semistructured Clinical Interview for Children & Adolescents (SCICA) [39], which is also available from the Achenbach group, could be added for more clinical/diagnostic information.

The aptly name SDQ has a strength (pro-social) as well as difficulty (problem) scales. The ATOM and the YOQ are full evaluation systems with required modules assessing social competence and satisfaction with treatment as well as problems from the parent's and youth's perspectives. The K-SADS is a comprehensive system of all possible DSM [40] (and also incorporates a clinician-rated CGAS).

Time Needed to Complete Ratings

As might be expected based on the previous section, rating scales can take varying amounts of time to complete and to score, anywhere from 1 minute to 1 hour or more. The CGAS is a single overall score that can be rated by a clinician in less than a minute. The mental-health component of the SF8 is just three items. The SF 36 has a five-item mental-health scale. Most of the other scales can be printed on one page or just a few pages and typically have 30–150 items and a completion time of 5–20 min. Several of the comprehensive scales like the ATOM and K-SADS take a half hour, an hour, or more.

Time should be a major consideration in selecting a scale, since adding even 5–10 min more work for each rating can put a significant burden on clinicians and/or patients. As of this writing, the impact of this kind of change in practice has not been well studied. Asking teachers or others outside the immediate family to fill out additional rating scales may seem like a good idea in principle, but it often meets with poor return rates and/or resentment on the part of the people who are asked to fill out the ratings.

Validated for Longitudinal Use

As will be discussed below, none of the scales has been expressly validated as a measure against a gold standard of clinical change or against the multiple domains of change that could be of importance. This distinction is as invisible as it is essential. Although *all* of the scales have been used in at least one published paper to assess change over time in the domains they measure, *none* can claim to be a measure of valid, reliable, and essential clinical change. The authors of one of the newest measures acknowledge the importance of this point [3], although they believe that their measure should be used anyway.

We believe that it is essential to understand that for now, the presence of a positive change score on one of these ratings scales does not mean that the patient has truly gotten better in the most important senses, and the absence of a positive change on one of these measures does not mean that the patient has not progressed in the most important ways.

Hand vs. Computer Scored

A dimension that has taken on increased importance in recent years is computerization. Up until a few years ago, all scales were completed via paper and pencil and all were scored in the same way. Things have changed now, and although all of the scales in Table 8.1 can still be *filled out* the old way (some for later keypunching), some of these scales can no longer be *scored* by hand. The TOP can only be scored by computer (either web-based or fax-back entry). The CGAS, CGI, and BPRS-C can only be *scored* by hand.

Each method of data entry, scoring, and output has advantages and disadvantages. The hand-scored scales can often be completed in minutes if not seconds, providing instant feedback. For clinicians or patients who are not computer literate, hand scoring may create fewer barriers and/or less anxiety for patients or staff. Computer-scored output often looks more authoritative, thus adding more *gravitas* to intake or follow-up routines. Computerized data entry through kiosks, electronic tablets, or digital ("smart") pens can automate some of the clerical work generated by rating scales and/or shift this burden to patients, parents, or teachers, thus saving clinician time.

Free vs. Pay for Use

A number of the scales are available for free in the public domain including the K-SADS, BPRS-C, CGAS, PSC, and SDQ. Some of the other scales (like the YOQ) are available for less than one hundred dollars to start off with, while for others costs can run into thousands of dollars. One can order a starter set of CBCL 6–16 forms, scoring templates, and a manual for about $150. Ordering computer versions of this and the CBCL forms for all of available age groups and respondents could easily cost several thousand dollars.

Has a Website

Websites can make rating scale materials more easily accessible and provide additional items and support for users of a scale. All of the scales that are offered commercially have websites as do all of the free scales except the CGAS and BPRS-C. The lack of a website and support for these scales can make them somewhat more difficult to implement and use, although these two scales are so simple that the published papers about them can provide this information.

Requires Specialized Degree and/or Training

Several of the scales can only be sold to clinicians with master's degrees (CBCL) or courses in test administration (CRS). Other scales can only be used accurately or at all by trained clinicians (K-SADS, BPRS-C). Although all of the measures provide training through a manual of some sort, this training can be more or less time consuming or intensive. The CAFAS for example requires the scoring of sample case material to demonstrate mastery of the system, which is often provided through a full day training which must be purchased. Conversely, other scales like the CGAS should be almost instantly useable by most clinicians, since it is virtually identical with Axis V in the DSM system. In addition descriptive anchors are provided for each major decile level [41]. Some forms like the TOP require no training for use, although they cannot be self-scored at all since the scoring algorithms are proprietary.

Available in Spanish or Other Languages Other than English

If English is the only language spoken by patients or their families, any of the scales listed in the Table 8.1 can be used. If patients speak other languages, either a clinician-rated measure like the CGAS, BPRS-C, or CAFAS can be used or a measure that has been translated into the required language would be needed. As indicated in the table, about half of the rating scales listed are available at least in Spanish. The CBCL, SDQ, PSC, and SF instruments have all been translated into a dozen or more languages.

Quality of Validation

The final dimension covered in the table concerns the quality of the validation work. A preliminary level of quality can be approached simply from the point of view of the number of studies that have been conducted using the scale. As noted above, the CBCL has been used in thousands of studies, the SCL-90/BSI, SF, CRS, and SDQ in hundreds, the K-SADS, CGAS, CAFAS, and PSC in dozens. Conversely, some scales like the TOP for adolescents and adults have been used in just a few published studies, and one version of the TOP, the form specifically for children, has not been used in any published studies. The use of rating scales that have not been well validated carries the obvious risk of unknown reliability and validity.

A second level of quality may be even more important and even more difficult to measure. All of the scales covered in the table were validated against diagnoses or other measures at a single point in time. The measures reviewed here probably can reflect accurately differences in overall symptomatology and possibly differences in clusters of symptoms. Most studies find moderate to high levels of correlations among similar measures (see Gardner et al. 2007 for a recent example [42]). All of the measures except the TOP for children have been used in at least once intervention study. But, as suggested earlier, none of the scales reviewed here has been validated as measures of clinically relevant or important change.

The issue of what should, and what actually does, change over the course of outpatient therapy has been explored in general by Ablon and Jones [43] but not in terms of specific rating scales. As far as we can tell, this kind of research has not yet been done but it needs to be. It seems possible if current trends continue that in the near future, insurers will try to use the psychiatric rating scales to restrict or shape care. It is imperative that independent researchers and clinicians conduct their own studies in order to determine how much or how little meaningful clinical change in therapy corresponds to change scores on measures like these and the degree to which such measures should be used to guide decisions about care.

As noted earlier, at Partners Psychiatry and Mental Health, a steering committee of senior clinicians selected the BPRS-C and CGAS to provide a rating scale that could be used with patients at all levels of care, of all ages, across a relatively large, geographically, ethnically, and economically diverse system of care. Now, nearly 3 years into the initiative, rating forms continue to be filled out at all sites at intake/admission and discharge/90 day follow up, with completion rates of about two-thirds of all admissions and follow ups. A paper summarizing this work shows that scores on both rating scales are significantly worse at more and more restrictive levels of care, and that scores on both instruments get significantly better over the course of treatment [34].

The BPRS-C is the primary symptom measure and it has shown good reliability as well as validity in our PPMH study. Several papers describing the psychometric characteristics of the BPRS-C are cited below. To summarize briefly, the BPRS-C is a 21-item rating scale designed for evaluating psychiatric problems of children and adolescents.

It has been used in a number of studies of research and clinical populations including patients with bipolar disorder, schizophrenia, and psychotic disorder and in other studies requiring a multidimensional assessment of symptoms [44–48]. The measure consists of 21 discreet symptom areas, each rated for severity [49, 50] along a 7-point Likert scale ranging from "not present" to "extremely severe". The 21 items are grouped into seven major problem clusters (depression, psychosis, etc.), each represented by 3 items. The BPRS-C is intended to be completed by a mental-health professional, most often following a clinical interview and thus presupposes a knowledge of childhood psychopathology [22].

A total score for all 21 items may be used when evaluating pre- to post-treatment change [49]. The reliability and consistency of the BPRS-C have been tested over time and it has become an integral measure in diverse psychiatric venues [50–53]. Published data on reliability show good inter-rater reliability, with the majority of scales showing evidence of substantial of internal consistency [22]. The 2001 Lachar study also showed the BPRS-C to have high concurrent validity across diagnostic groups for item and scale measurements. A version of the BPRS-C with descriptive anchors illustrating the range of severity for each item has shown even better reliability and validity [48, 54].

Since it is a public domain instrument, there is no cost, which is a major savings in this large system of care that routinely collects several thousand forms a year. A copy of the anchored version is appended to this chapter.

Conclusions

Results from the current review identified hundreds of rating scales but only about 15 broadband scales that are currently being used to measure outcomes in child psychiatry. Published papers show that all but one of these measures have been used in at least one study and may be valid for use at intake in clinical settings. Information available at this time suggests that such uses can provide a wide range of data especially regarding symptom/diagnostic clusters at a specific point in time but little that is definitive about the degree of change that can or should be expected. Clearly, further research is needed before any of these scales can be used with complete confidence. Hopefully the information contained in this chapter will allow interested clinicians and mental-health agencies to make informed choices about outcomes scales while also spurring much needed research.

References

1. Busch AB, Sederer LI. Assessing outcomes in psychiatric practice: Guidelines, challenges, and solutions. Harvard Review of Psychiatry 2000;8:323–7.
2. Blue Shield of MA B. Provider advisory; 2007.
3. Kraus DR, Seligman DA, Jordan JR. Validation of a behavioral health treatment outcome and assessment tool designed for naturalistic settings: The treatment outcome package. Journal of Clinical Psychology 2005;61:285–314.
4. Massachusetts Behavioral Health Partnership M. Clinical outcomes management protocol: Performance specifications and phase-in timelines; 2004.
5. Winters NC, Collett BR, Myers KM. Ten-year review of rating scales, VII: Scales assessing functional impairment. Journal of American Academy of Child and Adolescent Psychiatry 46(5):611–8 2005;44:309–38.

6. PROQOLID: Patient-reported outcome and quality of life instruments database. Mapi Research Trust (MRT), 2007. (Accessed at http://www.proqolid.org/.)
7. Youngstrom EAG, Danielson BL, Findling CK, Robert L. Calabrese J. Toward an integration of parent and clinician report on the Young Mania Rating Scale. Journal of Affective Disorders 2003;77:179–90.
8. Jain S, Carmody TJ, Trivedi MH, et al. A psychometric evaluation of the CDRS and MADRS in assessing depressive symptoms in children. Journal of American Academy of Child and Adolescent Psychiatry 46(5):611–8 2007;46:1204–12.
9. Zatzick DF, Grossman DC, Russo J, et al. Predicting posttraumatic stress symptoms longitudinally in a representative sample of hospitalized injured adolescents. Journal of the American Academy of Child and Adolescent Psychiatry 2006;45:1188–95.
10. White KS, Farrell AD. Structure of anxiety symptoms in urban children: competing factor models of the Revised Children's Manifest Anxiety Scale. Journal of Consulting & Clinical Psychology 2001;69:333–7.
11. Rosario-Campos MC, Miguel EC, Quatrano S, et al. The dimensional yale – brown obsessive-compulsive scale (DY-BOCS): an instrument for assessing obsessive-compulsive symptom dimensions. Molecular Psychiatry 2006;11:495–504.
12. Twenge JM, Nolen-Hoeksema S. Age, gender, race, socioeconomic status, and birth cohort difference on the children's depression inventory: A meta-analysis. Journal of Abnormal Psychology 2002;111:578–88.
13. Hale WW, Raaijmakers Q, Muris P, Meeus W. Psychometric properties of the Screen for Child Anxiety Related Emotional Disorders (SCARED) in the general adolescent population. Journal of the American Academy of Child and Adolescent Psychiatry 2005;44: 283–90.
14. Seligman LD, Ollendick TH, Langley AK, Baldacci HB. The utility of measures of child and adolescent anxiety: a meta-analytic review of the Revised Children's Manifest Anxiety Scale, the State-Trait Anxiety Inventory for Children, and the Child Behavior Checklist. Journal of Clinical Child & Adolescent Psychology 2004;33:557–65.
15. ASEBA Bibliography: Bibiliography of Published Studies Using the Achenbach System of Empirically Based Assessment (ASEBA): 2007 Edition. Research Center for Children, Youth, & Families, 2007. (Accessed at http://www.aseba.org/products/bibliography.html.)
16. Abad J, Forns M, Gomez J. Emotional and behavioral problems as measured by the YSR: Gender and age differences in Spanish adolescents. European Journal of Psychological Assessment 2002;18:149–57.
17. Ambrosini PJ. Historical development and present status of the schedule for affective disorders and schizophrenia for school-age children (K-SADS). Journal of American Academy of Child and Adolescent Psychiatry 46(5):611–8 2000;39:49–58.
18. Vostanis P. Strengths and difficulties questionnaire: research and clinical applications. Current Opinion in Psychiatry 2006;19:367–72.
19. Robbins JM, Taylor JL, Rost KM, et al. Measuring outcomes of care for adolescents with emotional and behavioral problems. Journal of American Academy of Child and Adolescent Psychiatry 46(5):611–8 2001;40:315–24.
20. Jerrell JM. Behavior and symptom identification scale 32: sensitivity to change over time. Journal of Behavioral Health Services & Research 2005;32:341–6.
21. Buckley JA, Ryser G, Reid R, Epstein MH. Confirmatory factor analysis of the behavioral and emotional rating scale 2 (BERS-2) parent and youth rating scales. Journal of Child & Family Studies 2006;15:27–37.
22. Lachar D, Randle SL, Harper RA, et al. The brief psychiatric rating scale for children (BPRS-C): Validity and reliability of an anchored version. American Academy of Child and Adolescent Psychiatry 2001;40:333–40.
23. Elliott R, Fox CM, Beltyukova SA, Stone GE, Gunderson J, Zhang X. Deconstructing therapy outcome measurement with Rasch analysis of a measure of general clinical distress: the symptom checklist-90-Revised. Psychological Assessment 2006;18:359–72.

24. Long JD, Harring JR, Brekke JS, Test MA, Greenberg J. Longitudinal construct validity of Brief Symptom Inventory subscales in schizophrenia. Psychological Assessment 2007;19:298–308.
25. Bates MP. The child and adolescent functional assessment scale (CAFAS): review and current status. Clinical Child & Family Psychology Review 2001;4:63–84.
26. Murphy JM, Pagano ME, Ramirez A, Anaya Y, Nowlin C, Jellinek MS. Validation of the preschool and early childhood functional assessment scale (PECFAS). Journal of Child and Family Studies 1999;8:343–56.
27. Conners K, Sitarenios G, Parker JDA, Epstein JN. The revised Conners' parent rating scale (CPRS-R): factor structure, reliability, and criterion validity. Journal of Abnormal Child Psychology 1998;26:257–68.
28. Lefante JJJ, Harmon GN, Ashby KM, Barnard D, Webber LS. Use of the SF-8 to assess health-related quality of life for a chronically ill, low-income population participating in the Central Louisiana Medication Access Program (CMAP). Quality of Life Research 2005;14:665–73.
29. Franks P, Lubetkin EI, Gold MR, Tancredi DJ. Mapping the SF-12 to preference-based instruments: convergent validity in a low-income, minority population. Medical Care 2003;41:1277–83.
30. Ware JEJ. SF-36 health survey update. Spine 2000;25:3130–9.
31. Wells MG, Burlingame GM, Lambert MJ, Hoag MJ, Hope CA. Conceptualization and measurement of patient change during psychotherapy: development of the outcome questionnaire and youth outcome questionnaire. Psychotherapy: Theory, Research, Practice, Training 1996;33:275–83.
32. Green B, Shirk S, Hanze D, Wanstrath J. The Children's global assessment scale in clinical practice: an empirical evaluation. Journal of American Academy of Child and Adolescent Psychiatry 46(5):611–8 1994;38:1158–64.
33. Stoppelbein L, Greening L, Jordan SS, Elkin TD, Moll G, Pullen J. Factor analysis of the Pediatric Symptom Checklist with a chronically ill pediatric population. Journal of Developmental & Behavioral Pediatrics 2005;26:349–55.
34. Gold J, Buonopane R, Caggiano R, Picciotto M, Vogeli C, Kanner N, Li Zhonghe, Babcock R, Jellinek MS, Drubner S, Sklar K, Murphy JM. Assessing outcomes in child psychiatry 2009; American Journal of Managed Care; 15:210–216.
35. Murphy JM, Kellher K, Pagano ME, et al. The family APGAR and psychosocial problems in children: A report from ASPN and PROS. Journal of Family Practice 1998;46:54–64.
36. Holditch-Davis D, Tesh EM, David Goldman B, Miles MS, D'Auria J. Use of the HOME inventory with medically fragile infants. Children's Health Care 2000;29:257–77.
37. Morisset C, ed. What the NCAST teaching scale measure. Seattle: NCAST Publications, University of Washington; 1994.
38. Jellinek MS, Murphy JM, Little M, Pagano ME, Comer DM, Kelleher KJ. Use of the Pediatric Symptom Checklist to screen for psychosocial problems in pediatric primary care: a national feasibility study. Archives of Pediatrics & Adolescent Medicine 1999;153:254–60.
39. ASEBA Achenback System of Empirically Based Assessment. Research Center for Children, Youth, & Families, 2007. (Accessed at http://www.aseba.org/index.html.)
40. APA. Diagnostic and Statistical Manual of Mental Disorders, Fourth Edition – Text Revision (DSMIV-TR) 4th ed: American Psychiatric Press; 2000.
41. Wagner A, Lecavalier L, Arnold LE, et al. Developmental disabilities modification of the children's global assessment scale. Biological Psychiatry 2007;61:504–11.
42. Gardner W, Lucas A, Kolko DJ, Campo JV. Comparison of the PSC-17 and alternative mental health screens in an at-risk primary care sample. Journal of the American Academy of Child & Adolescent Psychiatry 2007;46:611–8.

43. Ablon SJ, Jones EE. Psychotherapy process in the national institute of mental health treatment of depression collaborative research program. Journal of Consulting and Clinical Psychology 1999;67:64–75.
44. Ross RG, Novins D, Farley GK, Adler LE. A 1-year open-label trial of olanzapine in school-age children with schizophrenia. Journal of Child and Adolescent Psychopharmacology 2003;13:301–9.
45. Zalsman G, Carmon E, Martin A, Bensason D, Weizman A, Tyano S. Effectiveness, safety, and tolerability of risperidone in adolescents with schizophrenia: an open-label study. Journal of Child and Adolescent Psychopharmacology 2003;13:319–27.
46. Stayer C, Sporn A, Nitin G, et al. Multidimensionally impaired: the good news. Journal of Child and Adolescent Psychopharmacology 2005;15:510–9.
47. DelBello MP, Findling RL, Kushner S, et al. A pilot controlled trial of topiramate for mania in children and adolescents with bipolar disorder. Journal of the American Academy of Child and Adolescent Psychiatry 2005;44:539–47.
48. Lachar D, Randle SL, Harper R, et al. The brief psychiatric rating scale for children (BPRS-C): Validity and reliability of an anchored version. Journal of the American Academy of Child & Adolescent Psychiatry 2001;40:333–40.
49. Overall JE, Pfefferbaum B. Brief reports and reviews – the brief psychiatric rating scale for children. Psychopharmacology Bulletin 1982;18:10–6.
50. Overall JE, Pfefferbaum B. The brief psychiatric rating scale for children. 1982:10–6, 1982 Apr.
51. Gabbard GO, Coyne L, Kennedy LL, Beasley C, et al. Interrater reliability in the use of the brief psychiatric rating scale. Bulletin of the Menninger Clinic 1987;51:519–31.
52. Rufino AC, Uchida RR, Vilela JA, Marques JM, Zuardi AW, Del-Ben CM. Stability of the diagnosis of first-episode psychosis made in an emergency setting. General Hospital Psychiatry 2005;27:189–93.
53. Overall JE, Gorham DR. The brief psychiatric rating scale. Psychological Reports 1962;10:799–812.
54. Hughes CW, Rintelmann J, Emslie GJ, Lopez M, MacCabe N. A revised anchored version of the BPRS-C for childhood psychiatric disorders. Journal of Child and Adolescent Psychopharmacology 2001;11:77–93.

Brief Psychiatric Rating Scale for Children*

BPRS-C Rating: Please enter the score for the term which best describes the patient's condition

0= not present, 1= very mild, 2= mild, 3= moderate, 4= moderately severe, 5= severe,   Score
6= extremely severe

---

1. **Uncooperativeness** *Negative, uncooperative, resistant, difficult to manage.*
   0=Cooperative, pleasant; 2=Occasionally refuses to comply with rules/expectations in only one setting; 4=Persistent failure to comply with rules/expectations in more that one setting. Causes frequent impairment in functioning; 6=Constantly refuses to comply with rules and expectations, delinquent behaviors, running away. Causes severe impairment in functioning in most situations/settings.

2. **Hostility** *Angry or suspicious affect, belligerence, accusations, and verbal condemnations of others.* 0=Cooperative, pleasant; 2=Occasionally sarcastic, loud guarded, quarrelsome. Causes mild dysfunction in one situation or setting; 4=Causes frequent impairment in several situations/settings; 6=Assaultive, destructive. Causes severe impairment in functioning in most situations/settings.

3. **Manipulativeness** *Lying, cheating, exploitive of others.* 0=Not at all; 2=Occasionally gets in trouble for lying, may cheat on occasions; 4=Frequently lies/cons/manipulates people they know. Causes frequent impairment in functioning in several situations/settings; 6=Constantly relates to others in an exploitive/manipulative manner, cons strangers out of money/situations. Causes severe impairment in functioning in most situations/settings.

4. **Depressive Mood** *Sad, tearful, depressive demeanor.* 0=Occasionally/quickly disappears; 2=Sustained periods/excessive for event; 4=Unhappy most time/no precipitant; 6=Unhappy all time/psychic pain. Causes severe impairment in functioning.

5. **Feelings of Inferiority** *Lacking self-confidence, self-depreciatory, feeling of personal inadequacy.* 0=Feels good/positive about self; 2=Occasionally feels not as good as others/deficits in one area; 4=Feels others are better than they are. Gives negative, bland answers, can't think of anything good about themselves; 6=Constantly feels others are better. Feels worthless/not lovable.

6. **Suicidal Ideation** *Thoughts, threats, or attempts of suicide.* 0=Not at all; 2=Thoughts when angry; 4=Recurrent thoughts suicide/plans; 6=Attempt within last month/actively.

7. **Peculiar Fantasies** *Recurrent, odd, unusual, or autistic ideations.* 0=Not at all; 2=Occasionally has elaborate fantasies, imaginary companions; 4=Frequently has elaborate fantasies (exclude imaginary friends). Interferes occasionally with perception of reality; 6=Often absorbed in elaborate fantasies, has a difficult time distinguishing reality from fantasy.

8. **Delusions** *Ideas of reference, persecutory or grandiose delusions.* 0=No delusions or ideas of reference; 2=Occasionally feels strangers may be looking/talking/laughing about them; 4=Frequent distortion of thinking, mistrust; suspicious of others; 6=Mistrusts/suspicious of everyone/everything. Can't distinguish from reality.

9. **Hallucinations** *Visual, auditory, or other hallucinatory experiences or perceptions.* 0=No visual, auditory, sensory experiences; 2=Hears name called, experiences after an event, active/vivid imagination; 4=Definite experienced auditory (voices either comment or command), visual (daytime, or several incidences), sensory (specific odors); 6=Constantly experiences auditory (commanding voices), visual (images are present during interview), or other experiences or perceptions.

---

*Anchored version of BPRS-C from Lachar et al. 2001

10. **Hyperactivity** *Excessive energy expenditure, frequent changes in posture, perpetual motion.* 0=Slight restlessness, fidgeting. No impact on functioning; 2=Occasional restlessness, fidgeting, frequent changes of posture. Noticeable, but does not cause impairment in functioning; 4=Excessive energy, movement, cannot stay still or seated. Causes dysfunction on numerous occasions/situations. Guardian seeks help for behaviors; 6=Continuous motor excitement, cannot be stilled. Causes major interference in functioning on most occasions/situations.

11. **Distractibility** *Poor concentration, shortened attention span, reactivity to peripheral stimuli.* 0=Performance consistent with ability; 2=Occasionally daydreams, easily distracted. Is able to focus with prompting; 4=Frequently has trouble concentrating, avoids mental tasks, disruptive. Needs frequent assistance to stay focused. Causes decreased performance; 6=Constant, needs 1:1 assistance to stay focused.

12. **Speech or Voice Pressure** *Loud, excessive, or pressured speech.* 0=Not at all; 2=Noticeably more verbose than normal, conversation is not strained; 4=Very verbose or rapid, making conversation strained or difficult to maintain; 6=Talks rapidly, continuously and cannot be interrupted. Conversation is extremely difficult or impossible.

13. **Underproductive Speech** *Minimal, sparse inhibited verbal response pattern or weak low voice.* 0=Not at all; 2=Occasionally conveys little information because of minimal speech, vague, sparse, low or weak voice; 4=Persistently the client is vague, low or weak voice, in which at least $\frac{1}{4}$ to $\frac{1}{2}$ of the conversation comprehension is impaired; 6=On numerous occasions/situations conversation is severely impaired.

14. **Emotional Withdrawal** *Unspontaneous relations to examiner, lack of peer interaction, hypoactivity.* 0=Not at all; 2=Occasionally is unresponsive, sometimes refuses peer interactions; 4=Frequently unresponsive, lacks peer interaction, hypoactive. Interferes with relationships; 6=Constantly oblivious to those around. Preoccupied facial expressions, does not respond to questions or look at interviewer.

15. **Blunted Affect** *Deficient emotional expression, blankness, flatness of affect.* 0=Not at all or explainable by depressed mood; 2=Some flattening of affect. Occasionally shows emotional response during interview (smiles, laughs, tearful); 4=Considerable flattening. Frequently the client does not show emotional response (does not smile, laugh, look, cry); 6=Constantly flat. The client does not show emotional response (does not smile, laugh, look, cry).

16. **Tension** *Nervousness, fidgetiness, nervous movements of hands or feet.* 0=Not at all; 2=Occasionally feels nervous or fidgets. Can be relaxed or reassured; 4=Most days/time feels nervous/fidgety; 6=Pervasive and extreme nervousness, fidgeting, nervous movements of hands/feet.

17. **Anxiety** *Clinging behavior, separation anxiety, preoccupation with anxiety topics, fears, or phobias.* 0=Not at all; 2=Occasionally worries (at least three times a week) about anticipated/current events, separation, fears or phobias. Worries appear excessive for situation; 4=Most days/times worries about at least two life circumstances, or anticipated/current events; 6=Pervasive and extreme worry about most everything real or imagined.

18. **Sleep Difficulties** *Inability to fall asleep, intermittent awakening, shortened sleep time.* 0=Not at all; 2=Some difficulty (at least 1-hour initial, no middle or terminal insomnia); 4=Definitely has difficulty (at least 2 hours initial insomnia, any middle, or terminal lasting up to 1/2 1 hour). Feelings of unrestorative sleep, evidence or mild circadian reversal; 6=Claims to never sleep, feels exhausted the rest of the day, or severe circadian reversal.

---

19. **Disorientation** *Confusion over persons, places, or things.* 0=Not at all; 2=Occasionally appears confused or puzzled. Easily reacquainted with surrounding when prompted; 4=Frequently appears puzzled, confused, baffled regarding familiar surroundings, people or things; 6=Constantly confused. Perplexed.

20. **Speech Deviance** *Inferior level of speech development, underdeveloped vocabulary, mispronunciations.* 0=Not at all; 2=Occasional instances of distorted and idiosyncratic speech. Little impairment of understandability; 4=Frequent instances with definite impairment in understandability; 6=Constant speech distortion, almost incomprehensible.

21. **Stereotypy** *Rhythmic, repetitive, manneristic movements or posture.* 0=Not at all; 2=Occasionally displays rhythmic, repetitive, manneristic movements or posture; 4=Frequent rhythmic, repetitive, manneristic movements or posture; 6=Most of the time (>50%) displays rhythmic, repetitive, manneristic movement/posture

---

Total Score → _____ [Sum of scores for all 21 items]

Factor Scores: [For Internalization, Externalization, and Developmental Maladjustment, Sum of scores for indicated items]

*Internalization: 4, 5, 6, 7, 8, 9, 16, 17, 18=*_____ *Externalization: 1, 2, 3, 10, 11, 12=*_____ *Developmental Maladjustment: 13, 14, 15, 19, 20, 21:*_____

Scale Scores:

*Behavior Problem: 1, 2, 3=*_____ *Depression: 4, 5, 6=*_____ *Thinking Disturbance: 7, 8, 9=*_____
*Psychomotor Excitation: 10,11,12=*_____

*Withdrawal-Retardation: 13, 14, 15=*_____ *Anxiety: 16, 17, 18=*_____
*Organicity: 19, 20, 21=*_____

Chapter 9
Adult Attention-Deficit Hyperactivity Disorder

Laura E. Knouse and Steven A. Safren

Abstract Attention-Deficit Hyperactivity Disorder (ADHD) in adults is a valid and impairing disorder for which psychopharmacological and psychosocial treatments are recommended. Self-report ratings scales for adult ADHD can serve several functions in clinical work with this population including screening, providing information in a comprehensive assessment, and tracking treatment-related change. The use of two symptom-based ratings scales for screening and tracking treatment progress – the Current Symptoms Scale (CSS) [5] and the Adult ADHD Self-Report Scale (ASRS) [6] – is outlined for the practicing clinician. Key issues in the assessment of adult ADHD are briefly discussed, highlighting the role of rating scales within a comprehensive assessment.

Keywords Attention-Deficit/Hyperactivity Disorder · ADHD · Adults · Assessment · Rating scales

Attention-Deficit Hyperactivity Disorder (ADHD) is a developmental disorder characterized by symptoms of inattention, hyperactivity, and impulsivity that causes significant impairment in multiple domains of functioning [1]. Nearly two decades of research support the idea that ADHD continues to affect a substantial proportion of patients into adulthood [2, 3]. A recent population-based survey estimated the prevalence of ADHD in the adult population at 4.4%, which is consistent with previous estimates [4], and adults are now specifically seeking services for ADHD in mental health-care settings.

While the validity of ADHD in adulthood has been empirically established, evidence concerning the accurate assessment and appropriate treatment of the disorder in adults lags behind the knowledge base for children. Even for an experienced

S.A. Safren (✉)
Department of Psychiatry, Massachusetts General Hospital and Harvard Medical School, One Bowdoin Square, 7th Floor, Boston, MA 02114, USA
e-mail: ssafren@partners.org

Some of the investigator time to complete this project was supported by National Institute of Mental Health grant 5R01MH69812 to Dr. Steven Safren and Dr. Susan Sprich.

clinician, adult ADHD is often difficult to diagnose. Self-report rating scales can generate useful information to guide clinical decision making throughout the process of assessment and treatment. Ratings collected over time can be a source of data to guide treatment-related decision making and improve communication between provider and patient.

Rating scales can play three distinct roles in clinical work with adults with ADHD:

(1) Rating scales can be used as a general screening for patients in a variety of settings, with the goal of identifying adults who might require more comprehensive evaluation and follow-up.
(2) Rating scales can be used as part of an evaluation to obtain data pertaining to several of the diagnostic criteria for ADHD.
(3) Rating scales can be used to repeatedly assess the effects of treatment on symptom severity.

In this chapter, we focus primarily on the use of rating scales in the first and third roles – screening and tracking treatment-related change – because a comprehensive discussion of the role of rating scales in a multifaceted adult ADHD assessment is beyond the scope of this chapter. We wish to emphasize that the establishment of a diagnosis of ADHD in adults cannot be accomplished using rating scales alone (see Conclusions). However, later in this chapter, we briefly address how evidence for *Diagnostic and Statistical Manual of Mental Disorders – Fourth Edition* (*DSM-IV*) [1] criteria could be gleaned from a rating scale.

Suggested Rating Scales for ADHD

> *Current Symptoms Scale (CSS)* [5]
> *Adult ADHD Self-report Scale (ASRS)* [6]

Current Symptoms Scale (CSS)[1]

Our research program at Massachusetts General Hospital develops and tests cognitive-behavioral interventions for adults who, despite medication treatment for

---

[1] The CSS is protected by copyright and therefore is not reproduced here. It is available in *Attention-Deficit Hyperactivity Disorder: A Clinical Workbook—3rd Edition* (Barkley and Murphy, 2006). The workbook also includes self-report scales assessing childhood symptoms retrospectively. Other-report forms for both current and past symptoms can be used to collect collateral information for assessment and treatment tracking. Normative data tables are also provided along with instructions on how to administer, score, and interpret results. Scales assessing other areas including medication side effects, risky driving behavior, and work performance are also provided, as are forms for use with children. Barkley and Murphy encourage clinicians to photocopy and use these forms in their practice.

their ADHD, continue to display residual symptoms. We use the self-report Current Symptoms Scale [5] both to assess treatment-related change in symptoms over time and as part of our baseline evaluations because of its widespread use in research and clinical settings and the close correspondence of its items to *DSM-IV* criterion symptoms.

The *CSS* consists of the 18 *DSM-IV* inattentive and hyperactive-impulsive symptom items, worded in the first person and with some wording modified to fit adults (e.g., "playing" changed to "engaging in leisure activities"). Patients begin by rating their behavior over the past 6 months with respect to each item on a 4-point Likert scale (*never or rarely, sometimes, often,* or *very often*) scored 0–3. Thus, severity scores on the CSS can range from 0 to 54 across all symptoms. Next, they indicate the age of onset for endorsed symptoms. Finally, they rate how often these symptoms have interfered with functioning in ten areas of life.

Application of Scale: The *CSS* is administered throughout our treatment outcome studies. Patients first complete the measure at their baseline assessment to establish an initial level of symptom severity. Importantly, the *CSS* is only one measure in a large battery of baseline assessments – both self-report and clinician-administered – that we use in establishing the ADHD diagnosis and assessing its associated features. We use total scores on the *CSS* as baseline data. Separate totals from inattentive versus hyperactive-impulsive symptom clusters are useful in follow-up analyses of our data. The *CSS* is also completed at post-treatment and at 6- and 12-month follow-up assessments.

During our treatment studies, the *CSS* is used to track symptoms on a weekly basis. Patients are instructed to complete the 18 *DSM-IV* items of the scale at the beginning of each treatment session and to try to rate the past week only. When the patient finishes the scale, his or her therapist totals the score and also looks over each item individually. They briefly discuss which items appear to be improving and which are still problematic for the patient. Importantly, the therapist directs the patient to talk about which skills the patient used successfully over the past week and how this may have impacted his or her ratings. This is important because we have found that patients with ADHD sometimes complete the scale with a "trait-like" attitude toward their ratings rather than considering behavioral changes that may have occurred more recently. Each week, the *CSS* helps us to track changes in symptoms and also serves as an important forum for patients and therapists to discuss how treatment is progressing. When patients are able to see even small gains as a result of their work in treatment, it can sustain their motivation to continue to practice their new skills until the skills become less effortful.

The *CSS* could also be useful to clinicians as part of a comprehensive evaluation of ADHD in adults. The scale yields data for *DSM-IV* Criterion A (symptom counts, developmental deviance via norms), Criterion B (symptom onset), and Criterion C (impairment across settings). Barkley and Murphy [5] suggest that clinicians can score items rated as *often* or more as an indicator of *DSM-IV* symptom counts, although we have heard of using items rated as *sometimes* to be counted as a half symptom. Accordingly, a person would need two of these within the domain

(inattention or hyperactivity – impulsivity) to "count" toward the six-symptom criterion for diagnosis. Published deviance cutoffs for the scale enable the clinician
to gauge symptom deviance compared to a general population sample (Criterion
A). The scale collects information about symptom onset (Criterion B) and information about functional impairment across domains (Criterion C). However, during
our evaluations, we augment rating scale data using structured diagnostic interviews,
clinician ratings, and other self-report scales (e.g., quality of life, symptoms of other
disorders).

Scoring Key: In our work, we have primarily used a simple sum of patient's self-
report symptom ratings of the 18 *DSM-IV* ADHD items as an indication for ADHD
symptom severity (0–54 range). The clinician can also obtain totals for inattentive
versus hyperactive–impulsive symptoms separately – odd numbered items for inattentive and even numbered items for hyperactive–impulsive symptoms with a range
of 0–27 for each symptom cluster. See above section for how the CSS could be used
to obtain symptom counts.

Cutoff Scores: The clinical workbook in which the CSS is published [5] contains
age-based deviance thresholds (1.5 standard deviations above the mean) for inattentive symptoms, hyperactive–impulsive symptoms, and total ADHD symptoms.
These can be used as clinical cutoff scores.

Clinically Significant Change: We compare total scores on this measure at
follow-up to those obtained at the baseline assessment. Medication treatment trials often consider a 30% reduction in scores from baseline response to treatment
[7]. While the symptom ratings of a clinician blinded to treatment condition serve
as our primary outcome measure in the research setting, we believe that self-report
ratings capture aspects of treatment-related change that are not reflected in the ratings of others. For example, the patient may be in the best position to sensitively rate
changes in outcomes such as improvements in sustained attention. Thus, self-report
data collected via rating scales continue to be an important part of the measurement
of change in our research and clinical work.

Adult ADHD Self-report Scale (ASRS)

The *ASRS* (*ASRS-v1.1*) [6, 8] is reproduced in the appendix to this chapter. It is
an 18-item self-report scale developed and copyrighted by the World Health Organization as a screening tool for ADHD in adults that contains items similar to
those of the *CSS*. There are two versions of the ASRS: a short screening version
of six items (contained in Part A of the scale) and a full 18-item version containing content from all *DSM-IV* symptoms (Parts A and B). The ASRS has a
growing body of literature supporting its reliability and validity and is available
online at no cost, with links to various language versions and background data
available at http://www.hcp.med.harvard.edu/ncs/asrs.php. The full scale is available in English, Chinese (traditional), Danish, French, Hebrew, Norwegian, and
Swedish. The six-question screening version, Part A of the scale reproduced here,

is also available in Chinese (Mandarin), Dutch, German, Japanese, Portuguese, Russian, and Spanish (both for use in Mexico/United States and Spain). Note, however, that no research on the properties of these translated instruments has been conducted.

The *ASRS* was developed for use in World Health Organization (WHO) Mental Health Initiative surveys, designed to collect data from over 200,000 respondents in 28 countries. Kessler et al. [6] developed this new self-report measure covering all 18 *DSM-IV* symptoms with items reworded to be more appropriate for adults. For each item of the ASRS, patients rate the frequency with which each symptom occurred over the past 6 months on a 0–4 scale with points labeled as *never*, *rarely*, *sometimes*, *often*, or *very often*. The scale was focused on frequency of symptoms rather than severity to make scale instructions easier for participants to understand.

Application of the Scale: We describe using the ASRS-v1.1 for two purposes: as a screening tool and as a way to track changes in adult ADHD symptoms in response to treatment. As a screening tool, the clinician should follow the scale instructions (see also updated information on scoring of Part A in Scoring Key and Cutoff Points section) and refer patients who exceed these cutpoints for further evaluation for possible adult ADHD. Clinicians should keep in mind, however, that this screening threshold still fails to identify a substantial portion (about 35%) of adults who meet criteria for adult ADHD using diagnostic interviews [6]. Therefore, following up with individual patients who display elevated scores on this measure (but who do not meet or exceed the threshold) may be warranted.

Based on our experience with the 18 *DSM-IV* items of the Current Symptoms Scale, we suggest that the *ASRS* could be used as often as weekly to track treatment-related changes in adult ADHD symptoms. Recent adult ADHD medication trials have used symptom-based self-report measures, and these scales appear to be sensitive to treatment-related change [9–12]. Self-reports are often used in conjunction with clinician ratings in medication studies. Importantly, the clinician-rated version of the *ASRS*, the *AISRS*, has been sensitive to treatment-related change in three recent studies [13–15]. While far fewer studies exist on tracking the efficacy of psychosocial treatment in treating adult ADHD, our own work using the *CSS* supports the sensitivity of this type of measure. For example, our group found that adults receiving a cognitive-behavioral treatment package reported, on average, a 50% reduction in total scores on the *CSS* from baseline assessment to post-treatment [16]. Solanto and colleagues [17] recently found that their Metacognitive Therapy group treatment was associated with significant reductions on the *DSM-IV*-based inattentive items of the self-report *Conners' Adult ADHD Rating Scale (CAARS)* [18]. Because items on the *ASRS-v1.1* also parallel the *DSM-IV* symptoms, total scores on this measure are likely to be sensitive to treatment-related changes. In addition, the expanded range of total scores on this measure (0–72 vs. 0–54) and its increased face validity for ADHD symptoms in adults may increase its sensitivity to change, but this possibility has not yet been investigated empirically.

Clinicians can administer the *ASRS-v1.1* at their initial evaluation visit with a patient to establish a baseline level of total symptom scores on the measure. At each subsequent treatment session or follow-up visit, the patient should complete the measure *with respect to the time period since the last session* prior to his or her discussion with the clinician during that session. (This will avoid biasing the patient's ratings in the direction of the clinician's impressions.) We find it important to remind the patient frequently regarding the time frame of the symptoms to maximize the chances that his or her ratings reflect behavior during the previous week rather than his or her behavior in general. The clinician should then total the patient's score on the measure and keep a record. For example, a computerized spreadsheet containing a record for each patient's weekly measures is an excellent way to organize and track scores. Later, these scores can be easily plotted on a chart and used in discussions of treatment effectiveness. During a particular appointment, the clinician should note the pattern of change from the previous visit and discuss with the patient whether this pattern reflects the patient's subjective impression of changes in symptoms. If the treatment in question is a psychosocial treatment, the clinician can note individual symptoms that have improved and those that continue to be problematic and use this in a discussion of which skills and strategies the patient has been able to implement successfully. This process can help both patient and clinician to more efficiently direct their time and efforts toward the most severe symptoms.

The screening thresholds previously mentioned could also be used as targets below which it is less likely that the patient would meet criteria for adult ADHD upon clinical interview. Importantly, symptom scales should always be used to track progress in conjunction with evidence of improvement in functional domains based on the patient's report and other measures. In addition, rating scales appropriate for tracking symptoms of comorbid disorders (e.g., depression or anxiety) should also be administered during treatment if a patient's evaluation indicates that these symptoms are prominent.

Current Symptoms Scale (CSS) [5]
Adult ADHD Self-report Scale (ASRS) [6]

Scoring Key and Cutoff Points: Kessler et al. [6] identified thresholds for each item with maximum concordance with interview results. For 7 items, a rating of *sometimes* (score of 2) best differentiated a positive symptom on the interview, and for the remaining 11 items a rating of *often* or higher (score of 3) was most appropriate. These thresholds correspond to the gray boxes on the form reprinted here. While the authors point out that a clinician could use a *DSM-IV* threshold of 6+ symptoms on either list to define diagnosis, they tested several scoring methods to determine which method best predicted diagnosis.

Using the 6-item screening scale contained in Part A, a recent article by the authors recommends adding up the total score (of items rated 0-4) rather than counting responses in the gray boxes as suggested in the instructions included with the scale [19]. Clinicians should follow up with patients whose total scores for these six items are 14 or higher. If a clinician wishes to examine cutoffs for the entire scale (parts A and B), he or she should count up the number of items the patient endorses that fall in the gray shaded boxes. A count of 9 or greater was most indicative of positive screen in this full scale [6], though the scale instructions clearly recommend using only the 6-item Part A for screening purposes.

Reliability and Validity: A subsample of 154 participants age 18–44 in the National Comorbidity Survey Replication (NCSR) was the test sample for the *ASRS*. Participants in four representative subgroups (no childhood ADHD, some symptoms in childhood, diagnosis in childhood but deny current symptoms, diagnosis in childhood and endorse current symptoms) completed a structured, clinician-administered interview of current ADHD symptoms and the *ASRS*. The authors found a significant correlation of 0.43 between total scores on the *ASRS* (0–72) and current clinical symptom severity and suggest that this finding may support the use of the *ASRS* in charting clinical improvement among treatment cases. Providing further evidence for the use of this scale in the clinical population, data from 60 adult ADHD clinic patients who completed the *ASRS* and clinician interview were analyzed to assess concurrent validity and internal consistency [20]. Internal consistency for the *ASRS* (alpha = 0.88) was very good. Interclass correlation coefficients between the ASRS and clinician-administered interview were high (0.84) with significant kappa coefficients for each item.

More recently, data using the 6-item screening version of the *ASRS* were collected from a representative sample of 668 health plan members to assess its psychometric properties and to cross-validate this brief screening scale [19]. Internal consistency for continuous scores ranged from 0.63 to 0.72 and test–retest reliability ranged from 0.58 to 0.77. Note, however, that these values apply only to the 6-item screener and not the full 18-item scale.

Clinically Significant Change: Changes in total scores on the *ASRS-v1.1* or any other symptom-based measure of adult ADHD can provide information to aid in decision making about treatment course. A 30% reduction in overall scale scores can be used as a guideline for treatment response. This threshold is often employed in ADHD medication treatment studies [7] and was used in a medication treatment study that employed the clinician-report version of the *ASRS* [14]. However, patient and clinician may decide to set a lower (or higher) threshold of symptoms severity as the goal of treatment, depending on a patient's level of functioning and baseline severity.

Comment on Symptom-Based Scales: Brief comment on the strengths and weaknesses of symptom-based scales such as the *ASRS* is warranted. A growing body of literature supports the *ASRS*, particularly as a screening tool. Its item wording appears to be face valid and appropriate for tapping the expression of *DSM-IV* ADHD symptoms in adults. The scale is widely available and has numerous non-English translations available. There is evidence that similarly constructed scales are sensitive to change in medication and psychosocial treatment studies. The weaknesses of symptom-based scales highlight the need to augment the assessment and treatment process with other measures and procedures. The *ASRS* and

some other adult rating scales do not provide information on childhood symptoms, which is critical to making an ADHD diagnosis. Symptom-based scales do
not generate corroborating evidence from others of either current or childhood
symptoms. The scale assesses only the frequency – not the functional impact –
of symptoms. For these reasons, it is critical that scales like the *ASRS-v1.1* be
used for screening or tracking symptom frequency and not used as the sole basis
of clinical diagnosis. As discussed previously, rating scales are only one tool in
a comprehensive evaluation of adult ADHD that should also include diagnostic
interview, detailed history, evidence of functional impact of ADHD, other report
of symptoms, review of documentation, and thorough assessment of comorbid
conditions.

Conners' Adult ADHD Rating Scales

Though a comprehensive review of rating scales available for adults with ADHD
is beyond the scope of this chapter, we briefly mention one other widely available
set of rating scales that a clinician working with this population might consider –
Conners' Adult ADHD Rating Scales (CAARS) [18]. Detailed reviews of a much
wider range of adult ADHD rating scales are available [21, 22]. Notably, the
CAARS can be used to partially bolster some of the weaknesses of a simpler scale
like the *ASRS-v1.1*.

Involving a wide normative base and strong psychometric properties, the *CAARS*
are self- and other-report measures of current adult ADHD symptoms. The *CAARS*
items were derived from a pool of 93 items thought to be related to the manifestation of ADHD in adults and carefully selected based on exploratory factor analysis
[23]. The final 66-item self-report scale includes the DSM-IV based items with
adult-appropriate wording and non-DSM items loading on four dimensions: inatten-
tion/memory problems, hyperactivity/restlessness, impulsivity/emotional lability,
and problems with self-concept. Reliability and validity for this scale are well documented [24]. Norms for all subscales are available with respect to age and gender.

The properties of the *CAARS* demonstrate its suitability for all three functions of
a rating scale in work with adults with ADHD in clinical practice. First, the *CAARS*
can be used for screening. The entire scale shows good discriminant validity [24]
and also contains an ADHD Index which the authors describe as producing the best
discrimination between ADHD and non-ADHD patients [25]. Short (26 items) and
screening (30 items) versions of the *CAARS* contain this index and thus are suitable
for use in screening for ADHD in adults. Second, the *CAARS* would be useful as
part of a comprehensive assessment of adult ADHD. DSM-IV symptom counts can
be derived (from items rated *often* or above), and norms can be used to establish
developmental deviance. Other-report forms can provide corroborating evidence of
current symptoms – a critical element of the assessment of ADHD symptoms in
adults. (Note, however, that the *CAARS* does not assess symptoms in childhood
or age of onset.) Third, the full *CAARS* or one of the shortened versions could be

used to track treatment progress over time and the full scales show good test–retest reliability (0.88–0.91; [24]).

The *CAARS* suite of products is available from Multi-Health Systems and appears to be the most comprehensive package of rating scale products currently available to a clinician working with adults with ADHD. Hand-scoring and computer-scoring packages are available. Computer-scoring software generates two types of detailed reports from the measure. The *CAARS* scales would be an excellent addition to the assessment library of a clinician who often provides comprehensive assessment and treatment of adults with ADHD with cost and time of administration/scoring being perhaps the most prohibitive factors.

Conclusions

Although this chapter describes how rating scales are used in our research group at Massachusetts General Hospital, a clinician wishing to assess ADHD in adults must collect multiple types of data from multiple sources to address each of the criteria in *DSM-IV* and to rule out alternative explanations for the patient's presenting problems. Other authors [26, 27] address the complexities inherent in this process, and readers should refer to these resources for a full discussion of assessment issues in adult ADHD. Brief consideration of several issues in the assessment of adult ADHD helps to define the role of rating scales in clinical practice.

First, the symptom criteria for the disorder as outlined in *DSM-IV* have been criticized as not developmentally appropriate for capturing the expression of ADHD symptoms in adults, and symptom thresholds for diagnosis may be too stringent [28]. Items must reflect adult symptoms while keeping content consistent with research-based conceptualizations of the disorder. Second, a patient's symptoms must be in excess of those exhibited by individuals of similar developmental level, requiring some ability to compare patient's symptom severity with other adults. Third, onset of symptoms and at least some impairment must occur in childhood, highlighting the need for retrospective reporting and review of documentation. Fourth, corroborating evidence of both current and past symptoms via other-report is essential to accurate diagnosis, and the extent to which these sources of data converge is often variable [29–31]. Finally, assessment of comorbid disorders is critical, given that adults with ADHD report significantly more comorbid disorders than their non-ADHD counterparts [32]. The clinician must rule out that other disorders account for symptoms and must assess the influence of other disorders on impairment and their possible impact on treatment of ADHD. Because of these complexities, expert clinicians emphasize that the assessment process must be comprehensive and multi-method [26]. Thus, rating scales are only one element in a comprehensive assessment of adult ADHD.

In summary, assessment of ADHD in adults is a challenging process with a growing, but still limited, base of empirically derived knowledge. Rating scales based on DSM-IV symptoms appear to be an efficient way to collect self-report data on current symptoms for use in screening, as part of a comprehensive ADHD assessment, and in tracking treatment progress. The *Adult ADHD Self-Report Rating Scale* [6] is a widely available scale that can be used by busy clinicians for screening or in tracking treatment progress. Several other scales are available based on a clinician's needs and resources, including the *Current Symptoms Scale* [5] and the *Conners' Adult ADHD Rating Scale* [18]. Although the benefits of incorporating rating scales for adult ADHD into clinical practice certainly outweigh the costs, more research is needed on their application in the three roles outlined in this chapter.

References

1. American Psychiatric Association (2000). *Diagnostic and statistical manual of mental disorders* (4th ed., text rev.). Washington, DC: Author.
2. Barkley, R.A., Murphy, K.R., and Fischer, M. (2008). *ADHD in adults: What the science says.* New York: Guilford Press.
3. Weiss, G., and Hechtman, L. (1993). *Hyperactive children grow up* (2nd ed.). New York: Guilford Press.
4. Kessler, R.C., Adler, L., Barkley, R.A., Biederman, J., Conners, C.K., Demler, O. et al. (2006). The prevalence and correlates of adult ADHD in the United States: Results from the National Comorbidity Survey Replication. *American Journal of Psychiatry*, 163, 716–723.
5. Barkley, R.A., and Murphy, K.R. (2006). *Attention-deficit hyperactivity disorder: A clinical workbook.* New York: Guilford Press.
6. Kessler, R.C., Adler, L., Ames, M., Demler, O., Faraone, S., Hiripi, E. et al., (2005). The World Health Organization adult ADHD self-report scale (ASRS): A short screening scale for use in the general population. *Psychological Medicine*, 35, 245–256.
7. Steele, M., Jensen, P.S., and Quinn, D.M. (2006). Remission versus response as the goal of therapy in ADHD: A new standard for the field? *Clinical Therapeutics*, 28, 1892–1908.
8. World Health Organization. (n.d.). *Adult ADHD Self-Report Scale (ASRS-v1.1) Symptoms Checklist.* Retrieved February 18, 2008, from http://www.hcp.med.harvard.edu/ncs/ftpdir/adhd/18%20Question%20ADHD-ASRS-v1-1.pdf
9. Fallu, A., Richard, C., Prinzo, R., and Binder, C. (2006). Does OROS-methylphenidate improve core symptoms and deficits in executive functioning? Results of an open-label trial in adults with Attention-deficit hyperactivity disorder. *Current Medical Research and Opinion*, 22, 2557–2566.
10. Jain, U., Hechtman, L., Weiss, M., Ahmed, T.S., Reiz, J.L., Donnelly, G.A., Harsanyi, Z. et al. (2007). Efficacy of a novel biphasic controlled-release methylphenidate formula in adults with attention-deficit/hyperactivity disorder: Results of a double-blind, placebo-controlled crossover study. *Journal of Clinical Psychiatry*, 68, 268–277.
11. Reimherr, F.W., Williams, E.D., Strong, E.R., Mestas, R., Soni, P., and Marchant, B.K. (2007). A double-blind, placebo-controlled, crossover study of osmotic release oral system methylphenidate in adults with ADHD with assessment of oppositional and emotional dimensions of the disorder. *Journal of Clinical Psychiatry*, 68, 93–101.
12. Weisler, R.H., Biederman, J., Spencer, T.J., Wilens, T.E., Faraone, S.V., Chrisman, A.K., et al. (2006). Mixed amphetamine salts extended-release in treatment of adult ADHD: A randomized, controlled trial. *CNS Spectrums*, 11, 625–639.
13. Biederman, J., Mick, E., Surman, C., Doyle, R., Hammerness, P., Harpold, T., et al. (2006). A randomized, placebo-controlled trial of OROS methylphenidate in adults with Attention-deficit/hyperactivity disorder. *Biological Psychiatry*, 59, 829–835.

14. Biederman, J., Mick, E., Spencer, T., Surman, C., Hammerness, P., Doyle, R. et al. (2006). An open-label trial of OROS methylphenidate in adults with late-onset ADHD. *CNS Spectrums*, 11, 390–396.
15. Spencer, T., Biederman, J., Wilens, T., Doyle, R., Surman, C., Prince, J. et al. (2005). A large, double-blind, randomized clinical trial of methylphenidate in the treatment of adults with Attention-deficit/hyperactivity disorder. *Biological Psychiatry*, 57, 456–463.
16. Safren, S.A., Otto, M.W., Sprich, S., Winett, C.L., Wilens, T.E., and Biederman, J. (2005). Cognitive-behavioral therapy for ADHD in medication-treated adults with continued symptoms. *Behavior Research and Therapy*, 43, 831–842.
17. Solanto, M.V., Marks, D.J., Mitchell, K.J., Wasserstein, J., and Kofman, M.D. (2008). Development of a new psychosocial treatment for adult ADHD. *Journal of Attention Disorders*, 11(6), 728–736.
18. Conners, C.K., Erhardt, D., and Sparrow, E. (1999). *Adult AD/HD rating scales: Technical manual.* Toronto: Multi-Health Systems.
19. Kessler, R.C., Adler, L.A., Gruber, M.J., Sarawate, C.A., Spencer, T., and Van Brunt, D.L. (2007). Validity of the World Health Organization adult ADHD self-report scale (ASRS) screener in a representative sample of health plan members. *International Journal of Methods in Psychiatric Research*, 16, 52–65.
20. Adler, L.A., Spencer, T., Faraone, S.V., Kessler, R., Howes, M.J., Biederman, J., and Secnik, K. (2006). Validity of pilot adult ADHD self-report scale (ASRS) to rate adult ADHD symptoms. *Annals of Clinical Psychiatry*, 18, 145–148.
21. Murphy, K.R., and Adler, L.A. (2004). Assessing Attention-Deficit/Hyperactivity Disorder in adults: Focus on rating scales. *Journal of Clinical Psychiatry*, 65[suppl 3], 12–17.
22. Rösler, M., Retz, W., Schneider, M., Stieglitz, R.D., and Falkai, P. (2006). Psychopathological rating scales for diagnostic use in adults with attention-deficit/hyperactivity disorder (ADHD). *European Archives of Psychiatry and Clinical Neuroscience*, 25, 3–11.
23. Conners, C.K., Erhardt, D., Epstein, J.N., Parker, D.A., Sitarenios, G., and Sparrow, E. (1999). Self-ratings of ADHD symptoms in adults I: Factors structure and normative data. *Journal of Attention Disorders*, 3, 141–151.
24. Erhardt, D., Epstein, J.N., Conners, C.K., Parker, D.A., and Sitarenios, G. (1999). Self-ratings of ADHD symptoms in adults II: Reliability, validity, and diagnostic sensitivity. *Journal of Attention Disorders*, 3, 153–158.
25. Macey, K.D. (2003). Book review: Conners' Adult ADHD Rating Scales (CAARS). *Archives of Clinical Neuropsychology*, 18, 431–437.
26. Murphy, K.R., and Gordon, M. (2006). Assessment of adults with ADHD. In R.A. Barkley (Ed.), *Attention-deficit hyperactivity disorder: A handbook for diagnosis and treatment* (3rd ed., pp. 425–450). New York: Guilford Press.
27. Adler, L.A., Barkley, R.A., Wilens, T.E., and Ginsberg, D.L. (2006). Differential diagnosis of attention-deficit/hyperactivity disorder and comorbid conditions. *Primary Psychiatry*, 13, 1–14.
28. McGough, J.J., and Barkley, R.A. (2004). Diagnostic controversies in adult ADHD. *American Journal of Psychiatry*, 161, 1948–1956.
29. Kooij, J.J.S., Boonstra, A.M., Swinkels, S.H.N., Bekker, E.M., de Noord, I., and Buitelaar, J.K. (2008). Reliability, validity, and utility of instruments for self-report and informant report concerning symptoms of ADHD in adult patients. *Journal of Attention Disorders*, 11, 445–458.
30. Murphy, P., and Schachar, R. (2000). Use of self-ratings in the assessment of symptoms of attention-deficit hyperactivity disorder in adults. *American Journal of Psychiatry*, 157, 1156–1159.
31. Zucker, M., Morris, M.K., Ingram, S.M., Morris, R.D., and Bakeman, R. (2002). Concordance of self- and informant ratings of adults' current and childhood Attention-Deficit/Hyperactivity Disorder symptoms. *Psychological Assessment*, 14, 379–389.
32. Miller, T.W., Nigg, J.T., and Faraone, S.V. (2007). Axis I and II comorbidity in adults with ADHD. *Journal of Abnormal Psychology*, 116, 519–528.

Adult ADHD Self-Report Scale (ASRS-v1.1) Symptom Checklist
Instructions

The questions on the back page are designed to stimulate dialogue between you and your patients and to help confirm if they may be suffering from the symptoms of attention-deficit/hyperactivity disorder (ADHD).

Description: The Symptom Checklist is an instrument consisting of the eighteen DSM-IV-TR criteria. Six of the eighteen questions were found to be the most predictive of symptoms consistent with ADHD. These six questions are the basis for the ASRS v1.1 Screener and are also Part A of the Symptom Checklist. Part B of the Symptom Checklist contains the remaining twelve questions.

Instructions:

Symptoms

1. Ask the patient to complete both Parts A and B of the Symptom Checklist by marking an X in the box that most closely represents the frequency of occurrence of each of the symptoms.

2. Score Part A. If four or more marks appear in the darkly shaded boxes within Part A then the patient has symptoms highly consistent with ADHD in adults and further investigation is warranted.

3. The frequency scores on Part B provide additional cues and can serve as further probes into the patient's symptoms. Pay particular attention to marks appearing in the dark shaded boxes. The frequency-based response is more sensitive with certain questions. No total score or diagnostic likelihood is utilized for the twelve questions. It has been found that the six questions in Part A are the most predictive of the disorder and are best for use as a screening instrument.

Impairments

1. Review the entire Symptom Checklist with your patients and evaluate the level of impairment associated with the symptom.

2. Consider work/school, social and family settings.

3. Symptom frequency is often associated with symptom severity, therefore the Symptom Checklist may also aid in the assessment of impairments. If your patients have frequent symptoms, you may want to ask them to describe how these problems have affected the ability to work, take care of things at home, or get along with other people such as their spouse/significant other.

History

1. Assess the presence of these symptoms or similar symptoms in childhood. Adults who have ADHD need not have been formally diagnosed in childhood. In evaluating a patient's history, look for evidence of early-appearing and long-standing problems with attention or self-control. Some significant symptoms should have been present in childhood, but full symptomology is not necessary.

Adult ADHD Self-Report Scale (ASRS-v1.1) Symptom Checklist

Patient Name		Today's Date					
Please answer the questions below, rating yourself on each of the criteria shown using the scale on the right side of the page. As you answer each question, place an X in the box that best describes how you have felt and conducted yourself over the past 6 months. Please give this completed checklist to your healthcare professional to discuss during today's appointment.			Never	Rarely	Sometimes	Often	Very Often
1. How often do you have trouble wrapping up the final details of a project, once the challenging parts have been done?							
2. How often do you have difficulty getting things in order when you have to do a task that requires organization?							
3. How often do you have problems remembering appointments or obligations?							
4. When you have a task that requires a lot of thought, how often do you avoid or delay getting started?							
5. How often do you fidget or squirm with your hands or feet when you have to sit down for a long time?							
6. How often do you feel overly active and compelled to do things, like you were driven by a motor?							
							Part A
7. How often do you make careless mistakes when you have to work on a boring or difficult project?							
8. How often do you have difficulty keeping your attention when you are doing boring or repetitive work?							
9. How often do you have difficulty concentrating on what people say to you, even when they are speaking to you directly?							
10. How often do you misplace or have difficulty finding things at home or at work?							
11. How often are you distracted by activity or noise around you?							
12. How often do you leave your seat in meetings or other situations in which you are expected to remain seated?							
13. How often do you feel restless or fidgety?							
14. How often do you have difficulty unwinding and relaxing when you have time to yourself?							
15. How often do you find yourself talking too much when you are in social situations?							
16. When you're in a conversation, how often do you find yourself finishing the sentences of the people you are talking to, before they can finish them themselves?							
17. How often do you have difficulty waiting your turn in situations when turn taking is required?							
18. How often do you interrupt others when they are busy?							
							Part B

The Value of Screening for Adults with ADHD

Research suggests that the symptoms of ADHD can persist into adulthood, having a significant impact on the relationships, careers, and even the personal safety of your patients who may suffer from it.[1-4] Because this disorder is often misunderstood, many people who have it do not receive appropriate treatment and, as a result, may never reach their full potential. Part of the problem is that it can be difficult to diagnose, particularly in adults.

The Adult ADHD Self-Report Scale (ASRS-v1.1) Symptom Checklistwasdeveloped in conjunction with the World Health Organization (WHO), and the Workgroup on Adult ADHD that included the following team of psychiatrists and researchers:

- **Lenard Adler, MD**
  Associate Professor of Psychiatry and Neurology
  New York University Medical School, New York, NY, USA

- **Ronald C. Kessler, PhD**
  Professor, Department of Health Care Policy
  Harvard Medical School, Boston, MA, USA

- **Thomas Spencer, MD**
  Associate Professor of Psychiatry
  Harvard Medical School, Boston, MA, USA

As a healthcare professional, you can use the ASRS v1.1 as a tool to help screen for ADHD in adult patients. Insights gained through this screening may suggest the need for a more in-depth clinician interview. The questions in the ASRS v1.1 are consistent with DSM-IV criteria and address the manifestations of ADHD symptoms in adults. Content of the questionnaire also reflects the importance that DSM -IV places on symptoms, impairments, and history for a correct diagnosis.[4]

The checklist takes about 5 minutes t o complete and can provide information that is critical to supplement the diagnostic process.

References
1. Schweitzer JB, et al. Med Clin North Am. 2001;85(3):10–11, 757–777.
2. Barkley RA. Attention Deficit Hyperactivity Disorder: A Handbook for Diagnosis and Treatment. 2nd ed. New york, Guilford 1998.
3. Biederman J, et al. Am J Psychiatry.1993;150:1792–1798.
4. American Psychiatric Association: Diagnostic and Statistical Manual of Mental Disorders, 4th Ed., Text Revision. Washington, DC, American Psychiatric Association. 2000: 85–93.

Chapter 10
Rating Scales in Schizophrenia

Jennifer D. Gottlieb, Xiaoduo Fan, and Donald C. Goff

Abstract In the field of schizophrenia treatment and research, psychiatric symptom rating scales have served to evaluate and elucidate the value of antipsychotic medications and psychosocial interventions in treating this disorder. Useful scales have also been developed to assist in measuring side effects of medications, to assess areas of cognitive functioning, to evaluate quality of life, and to monitor medication treatment compliance. In this chapter, the following commonly used "gold standard" scales to assess important domains of schizophrenia are described: the Positive and Negative Syndrome Scale (PANSS), the Psychotic Symptom Rating Scales (PSYRATS), the Quality of Life Scale (QLS), the Schizophrenia Cognition Rating Scale (SCoRS), the Drug Attitude Inventory (DAI), and the Abnormal Involuntary Movement Scale (AIMS). Additional important domains to assess are also discussed, and scales to evaluate these areas are recommended.

The authors posit that utilizing a combination of these useful assessment tools will allow for a thorough evaluation of patients with schizophrenia, which in turn can significantly improve clinical care and outcome.

Keywords Schizophrenia · Psychosis · Rating scales · Assessment · Psychotic symptoms · Negative symptoms · Quality of life · Antipsychotic medication · Side effects · Cognitive functioning

The discovery of antipsychotic medications, the development of effective psychosocial interventions, and the growth of randomized clinical trials in schizophrenia research produced the need for instruments that could assign numerical values based upon observations of patients' thoughts, feelings, and behaviors. Psychiatric symptom rating scales were created to serve this purpose and demonstrate the value of these medications and interventions in treating schizophrenia when compared to

D.C. Goff (✉)
Freedom Trail Clinic, Schizophrenia Program of the Massachusetts General Hospital,
25 Staniford Street, Boston, MA 02114, USA
e-mail: goff@psych.mgh.harvard.edu

L. Baer, M.A. Blais (eds.), *Handbook of Clinical Rating Scales and Assessment in Psychiatry and Mental Health*, Current Clinical Psychiatry, DOI 10.1007/978-1-59745-387-5_10,
© Humana Press, a part of Springer Science+Business Media, LLC 2010

placebo. Scales were also developed to assist in measuring side effects of medications, to evaluate areas of cognitive functioning, to assess quality of life, and to monitor medication treatment compliance.

In addition to being essential research tools, rating scales are important clinical tools too. They allow us to evaluate treatment outcomes, which may help in determining the efficacy of different medications or treatment modalities. The information provided by such rating scales may ultimately allow clinicians to improve patient care and patients' quality of life. In this chapter, commonly used "gold standard" scales, which the authors routinely use in their schizophrenia clinic to assess important domains of this disorder, are described.

The authors posit that utilizing a combination of these useful assessment tools will allow for a thorough evaluation of patients with schizophrenia, which in turn can significantly improve clinical care and outcome.

While it may not be feasible (or necessary) to administer every rating scale described here, it is often valuable to choose at least one scale that addresses the patient's current problem area (e.g., distress caused by psychotic symptoms – PSYRATS; attitudes about a newly prescribed antipsychotic medication – DAI; cognitive changes following a recent psychotic episode – SCoRS; mood disturbance that may precede a psychotic decompensation – PANSS or BDI-II; etc.). In these cases, a particular scale can be administered on a regular basis to assess changes and improvements in the problem areas.

Assessment of General Symptoms in Schizophrenia

Gold Standard Scale: The Positive and Negative Syndrome Scale (PANSS)

Application of Scale, Administration, and Scoring

The PANSS was developed in late 1980s to assess clinical symptoms of schizophrenia [1, 2]. (This scale is not reproduced in this chapter because it is copyrighted by Multi Health Systems. Information about purchase of the scale and its manual can be found at their website: www.mhs.com.) The scale is an adaptation from earlier psychopathology scales, including the Brief Psychiatric Rating Scale (BPRS). The PANSS includes 30 items on three subscales: 7 items covering positive symptoms (e.g., delusions and hallucinations), 7 items covering negative symptoms (e.g., social withdrawal, flat affect, lack of motivation), and 16 items covering general psychopathology (e.g., anxiety, depression). The PANSS was conceived as an operationalized instrument that provides balanced representation of positive and negative symptoms, as well as mood and anxiety symptoms.

The PANSS requires a clinician rater because considerable clinical judgment is required. The assessment consists of a semi-structured clinical interview and any available supporting clinical information, such as family member's reports or previous records. The ratings can be completed in 30–40 min. Each item is scored on a 7-point Likert scale ranging from 1 to 7. Therefore, the positive and negative sub-scales each range from 7 to 49, and the general psychopathology subscale from 16 to 112.

Psychometric Issues (Reliability and Validity)

The PANSS has high inter-rater reliabilities (0.80). The split-half reliability of the General Psychopathology subscale is 0.80. The scale has also demonstrated excellent criterion-related validity and construct validity [3].

Interpreting Results, Cut-off Scores, and Clinically Significant Change

The PANSS has become the standard tool for assessing clinical outcome in treatment studies of schizophrenia and other psychotic disorders. Its high reliability and good coverage of both positive and negative symptoms make it an excellent tool in clinical practice to assess the severity of psychopathology as well as treatment response. There are no specific cut-off scores defined. This scale, although perhaps somewhat time-consuming to use frequently, can reliably be administered regularly to assess symptom improvements or exacerbations. In addition, this scale is useful as a pre- and post-assessment of change within psychosocial interventions such as cognitive behavioral therapy.

Scales to Assess Psychotic Symptoms in Schizophrenia

Gold Standard Scale: The Psychotic Symptom Rating Scales (PSYRATS)

Application of Scale, Administration, and Scoring

As more broad-based measures assess the severity of schizophrenia symptoms on a unidimensional scale (e.g., The PANSS, see above for description and use) and have been useful to assess global outcome, these measures have been able neither to evaluate the multidimensional nature of certain prominent psychotic symptoms (e.g., hallucinations and delusions), nor to assess how specific dimensions of psychotic symptoms change over time or in response to psychopharmacological and/or psychological interventions. As a result, the Psychotic Symptoms Rating Scale (PSYRATS) [4], a brief 17-item semi-structured, clinician-administered scale, was developed in order to provide needed detail about the multiple dimensions of commonly occurring psychotic symptoms (see Appendix).

Cognitive behavioral therapy (CBT) for schizophrenia has been gaining strong empirical support in recent years [5, 6]. As one of the predominant aims of CBT is to thoroughly investigate and help the patient modify preoccupation with, and conviction about psychotic symptoms, the PSYRATS has been successfully and widely used in several CBT studies (and neurobiological studies as well).

The PSYRATS consists of two subscales: auditory hallucinations (AHS), 11 items, and delusions (DS), 6 items. The AHS subscale evaluates the frequency and duration of hallucination occurrence, and also assesses specific information about the patient's attitudes about his/her hallucinations, including level of distress associated with the symptom, as well as beliefs about controllability of voices, loudness, negative versus positive content, and beliefs about hallucination origin. These dimensions are evaluated on a 5-point Likert scale, ranging from 0 to 4. The DS subscale is similarly constructed, with specific dimensions evaluating the patients' experience with the symptom, including degree of preoccupation with the delusion, delusion duration, and conviction about the belief, distress associated with the delusion, and the amount of disruption the belief causes in the patients' life. This subscale is also scored on a 5-point Likert scale ranging from 0 to 4.

Interpreting Results, Cut-off Scores, and Clinically Significant Change

The developers of the scale have suggested that the PSYRATS be used in conjunction with a global symptom scale, in order to provide a more detailed assessment of specific symptoms to target in treatment. Given the dimensionality of hallucinations and delusions, and because this is not a diagnostic instrument, cut-off scores are not per se used with this scale. Depending on the patient, and his/her individual symptoms and functioning level, clinically significant change can be represented by a one-point increase on any given item. For example, a change from a 3 on the "amount of preoccupation with delusions" item (subject thinks about beliefs at least once an hour) to a 2 (subject thinks about beliefs at least once a day) following a medication change or a course of CBT can be considered clinically meaningful. Thus, detailed PSYRATS scores (and subsequent changes on item scores) provide the clinician with a more thorough understanding of how specific symptom dimensions change as a result of antipsychotic medication trials, and can therefore be quite useful in modifying psychopharmacological interventions based on specific patient needs. When used in assessment within CBT (or other psychological interventions for schizophrenia), therapist and patient can continuously evaluate how specific interventions affect particular dimensions of psychotic symptoms (e.g., distress levels associated with voices, or the degree of conviction or daily disruption created by a delusion). Thus, the PSYRATS can be used several times throughout a course of CBT, as a way to monitor progress and revise treatment goals as needed.

Psychometric Issues (Reliability and Validity)

Psychometric properties of the PSYRATS have been evaluated with a sample of adults (n = 71; mean age 36.6) with diagnoses of schizophrenia, paranoid type, and schizoaffective disorder, who had a duration of illness of approximately 13 years [4]. More recently, reliability and validity of this scale have been assessed with a larger sample (n = 257) of younger adults experiencing their first episode of psychosis [7]. In the initial sample, inter-rater reliability for both subscales was very high (ranging from 0.79 to 0.90 for ratings within the AH subscale and from 0.88 to 0.90 for the DS subscale), as were inter-item relationships, suggesting high internal consistency. Within the first-episode sample, inter-reliability coefficients were also very high, particularly for the AH subscale (0.99–1.00), as were internal consistency correlations.

Scale validity was assessed, initially in comparison with the Psychiatric Assessment Scale (KGV) [8], a uni-dimensional severity scale similar to the PANSS, and acceptable validity was demonstrated. In the 2007 psychometric study, concurrent validity, assessed using PANSS subscales and individual items, was high, as was sensitivity to change.

Scales to Assess Social Functioning and Quality of Life in Schizophrenia

Gold Standard Scale: The Quality of Life Scale (QLS)

Application of Scale, Administration, and Scoring

Given the unique and often prominent positive symptoms of schizophrenia, much clinical attention is given to hallucinations, delusions, and formal thought disorder. However, of perhaps even greater importance is the debilitating effect that this particular disorder has on a patient's day-to-day functioning, occupational attainment, social relationships, and overall quality of life. More recent emphasis on quality of life in psychiatry and mental health reflects a greater appreciation for the patient's overall well-being, as well as a shift toward defining successful outcome in terms of improvements in psychosocial functioning instead of symptom remission exclusively [9].

One of the most widely used instruments to assess the pernicious nature of these functional impairments is the Quality of Life Scale (QLS) (reproduced in the appendix to this chapter). Developed by Heinrichs et al. in 1984 [9], the original purpose of this scale was to closely evaluate components of the "deficit syndrome" via assessment of the patients' internal state and social role performance. Today the QLS is used as a general measure of quality of life, often in addition to scales that specifically measure negative symptoms that comprise the deficit syndrome. The QLS is a semi-structured, clinician-administered, 21-item measure, designed for use with community dwelling outpatients with schizophrenia that combines subjective patient report and objective data. The scale takes less than 45 min to complete, can be used as a component of a standard clinical interview, and assesses four domains: (1) interpersonal relations, (2) instrumental role functioning, (3) intrapsychic foundations (or cognitive-emotional functioning), and (4) common objects and activities (extent of involvement with routine daily activities).

Interpreting Results, Cut-off Scores, and Clinically Significant Change

Quality of life instruments differ in terms of the emphasis they place on subjective versus objective data: some are evaluated exclusively from the patient's perspective, and others from the standpoint of a clinician or family member, and others utilize wholly objective criteria such as number of daily social contacts or outings per week. A unique quality of the QLS, however, is that it combines the patient's perspective (e.g., "are you especially close with any of the people you currently live with or your immediate family") with that of objective assessment ("are you wearing or carrying any of the following: a wallet or purse, keys, a driver's license, etc."). This synthesis of patient perspective, clinician rating, and purely objective measurement increases the validity of the quality of life construct and the utility of the scale.

The items are each rated on a 7-point Likert scale, with the following cut-off scores: 0–1 indicating "severe impairment" on the particular domain, 2–4 a range of "moderate to mild impairment," and 5–6 "adequate, normal, or unimpaired functioning." Subscale scores, as well as a total quality of life score can be calculated, where lower scores represent more impaired functioning across the particular domains of interpersonal relations, instrumental role functioning, cognitive-emotional functioning, and extent of involvement with routine daily activities. As the QLS does not provide specific cut-off scores, clinically meaningful change is likely most usefully evaluated by attending to increases in specific domains (e.g., interpersonal relations) or even specific items (e.g., perception of number of intimate relationships). When treating severe mental illness such as schizophrenia, even small increases in specific target areas can represent clinically significant improvements. For example, for a patient who previously had not engaged in any activities apart from visiting a public park, who then, following either a medication change or psychosocial intervention, reported dining in a restaurant, reading the newspaper, and attending a social event, such a change would likely indicate meaningful functional progress. As with the PANSS and PSYRATS described above, the QLS is useful to use throughout clinical treatment, as a way to closely monitor functioning changes that may co-vary with modifications in medication or the initiation of a psychosocial intervention.

Psychometric Issues (Reliability and Validity)

The QLS was initially psychometrically evaluated with a somewhat ethnically diverse (65% African American, 34% Caucasian, 1% Asian) sample of patients with schizophrenia whose duration of illness ranged from 0 to 29 years (mean = 5 years). Within this validation sample, a factor analysis was conducted and yielded four factors comparable to the conceptual model on which the subscales were based [10].

More recent psychometric evaluation utilizing demographically distinct samples (e.g., French patients with schizophrenia) have yielded acceptable test–retest coefficients for individual items, the four subscales, and the total score. Internal consistency coefficients and convergent validity were also high with these samples [11, 12]. In a comparison of several well-known quality of life measures for use with schizophrenia, Cramer et al. [13] determined that the QLS was more sensitive to change and to the effect of treatment than other similar measures.

Scales to Assess Cognitive Functioning in Schizophrenia

Gold Standard Scale: The Schizophrenia Cognition Rating Scale (SCoRS)

Application of Scale, Administration, and Scoring

Patients with chronic schizophrenia demonstrate cognitive deficits that range between one-and-a-half and two standard deviations below healthy controls on several key domains such as verbal memory, working memory, motor speed, attention, and executive function. It has been well established that cognitive impairment is significantly correlated with poorer real life functioning in schizophrenia patients [14]. The SCoRS is an 18-item interview-based assessment of cognitive deficits and the degree to which they affect day-to-day function. (This scale is not reproduced in this chapter because it is copyrighted by Neurocog Trials, Inc. Information about training in and purchase of the scale and its manual can be found at their website: http://www.neurocogtrials.com/instrument.htm.) A global rating is also generated. The items were developed to assess the cognitive domains found to be impaired in schizophrenia patients [15].

Each item is rated on a 4-point scale. Higher ratings reflect a greater degree of impairment. Each item has anchor points for all levels of the 4-point scale. The anchor points for each item focus on the degree of impairment and the degree to which the deficit impairs day-to-day functioning. Complete administration of the ScoRS includes two separate sources of information: an interview with the patient, and an interview with an informant of the patient (family member, friend, social worker etc.). A global rating is determined by the interviewer after the 18 items are rated. The global rating is rated 1–10.

The SCoRS is still relatively new and as of now, is not commonly used by most practitioners in clinical practice at this time; therefore, official recommended guidelines for frequency of administration have not been developed. However, given the importance of cognitive deficits as both a core symptom domain and a major treatment target, this scale could be administered at least on a yearly basis to monitor patient functioning.

Psychometric Issues (Reliability and Validity)

The ScoRS has been shown to have excellent inter-rater reliability. The SCoRS global ratings are strongly correlated with cognitive performance as measured by the Brief Assessment of Cognition in Schizophrenia (BACS), a formal cognitive battery that assesses the aspects of cognition found to be most impaired in patients with schizophrenia. The ScoRS global ratings are also strongly correlated with real-world functioning as measured by the Independent Living Skills Inventory (ILSI), a standard functional assessment instrument measuring the extent to which individuals are able to competently perform a broad range of skills important for successful community living.

Interpreting Results, Cut-off Scores, and Clinically Significant Change

The SCoRS may provide a valid co-primary measure for clinical trials assessing cognitive change. It may also aid clinicians desiring to assess patients' level of cognitive impairment. Clinically meaningful cut-off scores have not been defined yet.

Scales to Assess Antipsychotic Medication Attitudes and Compliance in Schizophrenia

Gold Standard Scale: Drug Attitude Inventory (DAI)

Application of Scale, Administration, and Scoring

In the treatment of schizophrenia, medication adherence is a complicated issue. Antipsychotic medications can be difficult for patients to tolerate, given their often debilitating side effects. Coupled with cognitive impairment and compromised illness insight, which are hallmark symptoms of this disorder, adherence to antipsychotic drugs can be a tremendous challenge. Inconsistent use or discontinuation of medication can cause serious consequences (e.g., relapse and rehospitalization). It has been suggested that a patient's attitudes or perceptions about his/her antipsychotic medications reflect a weighing of perceived or actual benefits and risks associated with the medication. These attitudes may in turn determine the degree of medication adherence [9, 16–18], and are therefore crucial for the clinician to assess in patients in this population. The original Drug Attitude Inventory (DAI) was developed in 1983 [17]. This 30-item, self-report, true–false questionnaire was specifically designed for use in schizophrenia. Items were derived from clinical practice related to patients' statements about the antipsychotic medication they were receiving. A factor analysis of this measure yielded seven attitudinal factors including: (1) subjective positive experience (e.g., "medications make me feel more relaxed"), (2) subjective negative experience (e.g., "I feel weird, like a 'zombie' on medication"), (3) model of health and illness (e.g., "I take medications only when I feel sick"), (4) *and* (5) locus of control/physician's control (e.g., "I take medications of my own free choice"), (6) prevention (e.g., "by staying on medications, I can prevent getting sick"), and (7) concern about harm (e.g., "medication will damage my body").

Based upon a more detailed discriminant function analysis, the authors of the scale then shortened the measure to 10 items from the "subjective positive" and "subjective negative experience" factors and the remaining "attitude" factors described above [17]. This very brief DAI-10 (administration time is approximately 10 min) is easily used in research and practice, and has been more recently been adapted into several languages, including Chinese [19], Italian [20], and Spanish [21]. (Sample items from the DAI-10 can be found in the Appendix. However, please note that this scale is under copyright and requires permission for its use.) While there are no hard and fast guidelines for the frequency of use for this instrument, it is recommended that clinicians discuss medication adherence at every visit with their patients who have schizophrenia. The DAI is a brief tool that is appropriate for use as a helpful complement to a discussion about adherence.

Interpreting Results, Cut-off Scores, and Clinically Significant Change

The authors suggest assigning a score of −1 (representing negative subjective response to medication) or a +1 (representing positive subjective response to medication) for each of the 10 items. The items are added and adjusted to yield either a total positive numerical score (indicating general positive subjective response or "compliance") or a negative total score (indicating negative subjective response or "non-compliance").

In a study evaluating various measures of subjective response to neuroleptic medication [17], a median score on the DAI-10 was calculated, and patients were subsequently categorized as "dysphoric responders" (as applied to antipsychotic medication attitudes) and "non-dysphoric responders" based on whether or not their score fell above or below the median.

When used clinically, this scale is likely best utilized by examining the percentage of positive subjective responses versus negative subjective responses, in order to obtain an overall idea about a patient's experience with, and attitude toward, his or her antipsychotic medication. As this instrument is quite brief, individual items can also be examined to identify particular perceptions that individuals have about their medication regimen. Considerable shifts in either direction (negative or positive) should be considered clinically significant and warrant the clinician's attention.

Psychometric Issues (Reliability and Validity)

In the original validation study of the 30-item DAI [17], reliability coefficients reflecting internal consistency were quite high (Kuder Richardson-20 correlation coefficient = 0.93), as was test–retest reliability in a random sample of 27 patients drawn from the original 150. An initial discriminative validity analysis was conducted by statistically comparing the item responses of medication-adherent and non-medication adherent subgroups, and was found to be acceptable. As mentioned above, the 10-item measure was derived from a detailed discriminant function analyses and retains acceptable psychometric properties in English [17]. With samples of patients with schizophrenia from other countries, internal consistency, test–retest reliability, factor structure, and validity analyses have also yielded adequate psychometric properties for the DAI-10 [19–21] .

Scales to Assess Medication Side Effects in Schizophrenia

Gold Standard Scale: Abnormal Involuntary Movement Scale (AIMS)

Application of Scale, Administration, and Scoring

Antipsychotic-induced movement disorders are a group of diverse neurological motor disturbances associated with the use of antipsychotic medications. They may occur shortly after exposure to drug (e.g., acute dystonic reactions), or appear after a variable length of time but resolve upon drug discontinuation (e.g., tremor, chorea, myoclonus, drug-induced Parkinsonism, akathisia). For some patients, the motor symptoms (e.g., tardive dyskinesia, tardive dystonia) persist after the offending drug is discontinued. The AIMS (see Appendix) was developed in the 1970s to measure tardive dyskinesia in patients taking antipsychotic drugs [22]. Tardive dyskinesia, which comprises abnormal, persistent, repetitive, purposeless involuntary movements, is a serious concern associated with chronic antipsychotic treatment.

The AIMS has 12 items, each of which is rated on a five-point severity scale ranging from 0 to 4. Ten items assess abnormal movement in specific body regions (orofacial area, extremities, and trunk) as well as the global severity; two items concern dental conditions that can complicate the diagnosis of dyskinesia. The AIMS can be completed in less than 10 min, making it a very user friendly option for evaluating medication side effects. The AIMS should be performed at least once every 6 months with patients taking atypical antipsychotics. For those taking typical antipsychotics, it should be performed more often, approximately every 3 months.

Psychometric Issues (Reliability and Validity)

Excellent reliability has been demonstrated especially for experienced raters. Test–retest reliability at 6–8 weeks ranges from 0.40 to 0.82 for individual items and is 0.71 for overall severity. The instrument appears valid.

Interpreting Results, Cut-Off Scores, and Clinically Significant Change

Total scores are not generally reported. Instead, changes in global severity and individual body areas can be monitored over time. In the presence of extended neuroleptic exposure and the absence of other conditions causing dyskinesia, mild dyskinetic movements in two areas or moderate movements in one area suggest a diagnosis of tardive dyskinesia. The AIMS is considered standard clinical practice for patients receiving long-term antipsychotic drugs, both for monitoring the development of tardive dyskinesia and for tracking changes in tardive dyskinesia over time.

Other Useful Scales for Patients with Schizophrenia

While a discussion of every useful rating scale for patients with schizophrenia is beyond the scope of this chapter, there are several additional domains that are helpful to assess with this population. For instance, depressive symptoms are common in patients with schizophrenia, particularly those who have recently experienced their first episode of psychosis. *The Beck Depression Inventory – II* (BDI-II; [23]), a 21-item self-report measure that assesses both cognitive and neurovegetative symptoms of depression (including suicidal ideation), is the gold standard in brief, reliable assessment for this disorder, and is also sensitive to change (see detailed description of this scale in Depression chapter). Substance use and abuse are unfortunately frequently occurring problems for patients with schizophrenia, and it is recommended that these behaviors be evaluated at intake, and throughout treatment. Two complementary brief self-report instruments widely-used within this population are the *Alcohol Use Disorders Identification Test* (AUDIT) [24] and the *Drug Abuse Screening Test* (DAST) [25]. The *Barnes Akathisia Scale* (BAS) [26] has been widely used to evaluate akathisia, a possible side effect related to antipsychotic medications. The scale includes objective, subjective, and global impression ratings. Finally, the *Brief Psychiatric Rating Scale* (BPRS) [27] is a widely used 18-item scale that measures both psychotic and non-psychotic symptoms in mentally ill patients (reproduced in the appendix to this chapter). The strengths of the scale include its brevity. The limitations include the ambiguity in defining different levels of severity and its lack of sensitivity to assess negative symptoms.

Utilizing a combination of these useful assessment tools will allow for a thorough evaluation of patients with schizophrenia, which in turn can significantly improve clinical care and outcome.

References

1. Kay SR, Fiszbein A, Opler LA. The positive and negative syndrome scale (PANSS) for schizophrenia. Schizophr Bull 1987; 13:261–76.
2. Kay SR, Opler LA, Fiszbein A. Significance of positive and negative syndromes in chronic schizophrenia. Br J Psychiatry 1986; 149:439–48.
3. Kay SR, Opler LA, Lindenmayer JP. Reliability and validity of the positive and negative syndrome scale for schizophrenics. Psychiatry Res 1988; 23:99–110.

4. Haddock G, McCarron J, Tarrier N, Faragher EB. Scales to measure dimensions of hallucinations and delusions: the psychotic symptom rating scales (PSYRATS). Psychol Med 1999; 29:879–89.
5. Gould RA, Mueser KT, Bolton E, Mays V, Goff D. Cognitive therapy for psychosis in schizophrenia: an effect size analysis. Schizophr Res 2001; 48:335–42.
6. Zimmermann G, Favrod J, Trieu VH, Pomini V. The effect of cognitive behavioral treatment on the positive symptoms of schizophrenia spectrum disorders: a meta-analysis. Schizophr Res 2005; 77:1–9.
7. Drake R, Haddock G, Tarrier N, Bentall R, Lewis S. The Psychotic Symptom Rating Scales (PSYRATS): Their usefulness and properties in first-episode psychosis. Schizophrenia Research 2007; 89:119–22.
8. Krawiecka M, Goldberg D, Vaughan M. A standardized psychiatric assessment scale for rating chronic psychotic patients. Acta Psychiatr Scand 1977; 55:299–308.
9. Karow A, Naber D. Subjective well-being and quality of life under atypical antipsychotic treatment. Psychopharmacology (Berl) 2002; 162:3–10.
10. Heinrichs DW, Hanlon TE, Carpenter WT, Jr. The Quality of Life Scale: an instrument for rating the schizophrenic deficit syndrome. Schizophr Bull 1984; 10:388–98.
11. Simon-Abbadi S, Guelfi JD, Ginestet D. Psychometric qualities of the French version of the Heinrichs quality of life rating scale. Eur Psychiatry 1999; 14:386–91.
12. Kaneda Y, Imakura A, Fujii A, Ohmori T. Schizophrenia Quality of Life Scale: validation of the Japanese version. Psychiatry Res 2002; 113:107–13.
13. Cramer JA, Rosenheck R, Xu W, Thomas J, Henderson W, Charney DS. Quality of life in schizophrenia: A comparison of instruments. Department of Veterans Affairs Cooperative Study Group on Clozapine in Refractory Schizophrenia. Schizophrenia Bulletin 2000; 26:659–66.
14. Green MF, Kern RS, Braff DL, Mintz J. Neurocognitive deficits and functional outcome in schizophrenia: are we measuring the "right stuff"? Schizophr Bull 2000; 26: 119–36.
15. Keefe RS, Poe M, Walker TM, Kang JW, Harvey PD. The Schizophrenia Cognition Rating Scale: an interview-based assessment and its relationship to cognition, real-world functioning, and functional capacity. Am J Psychiatry 2006; 163:426–32.
16. Weiden PJ, Mann JJ, Dixon L, Haas G, DeChillo N, Frances AJ. Is neuroleptic dysphoria a healthy response? Compr Psychiatry 1989; 30:546–52.
17. Hogan TP, Awad AG, Eastwood R. A self-report scale predictive of drug compliance in schizophrenics: reliability and discriminative validity. Psychol Med 1983; 13:177–83.
18. Freudenreich O, Cather C, Evins AE, Henderson DC, Goff DC. Attitudes of schizophrenia outpatients toward psychiatric medications: relationship to clinical variables and insight. J Clin Psychiatry 2004; 65:1372–6.
19. Cheng HL, Yu YW. [Validation of the Chinese version of "the Drug Attitude Inventory"]. Kaohsiung J Med Sci 1997; 13:370–7.
20. Rossi A, Arduini L, De Cataldo S, Stratta P. [Subjective response to neuroleptic medication: a validation study of the Italian version of the Drug Attitude Inventory (DAI)]. Epidemiol Psichiatr Soc 2001; 10:107–14.
21. Robles Garcia R, Salazar Alvarado V, Paez Agraz F, Ramirez Barreto F. [Assessment of drug attitudes in patients with schizophrenia: psychometric properties of the DAI Spanish version]. Actas Esp Psiquiatr 2004; 32:138–42.
22. Guy W, Ban TA, Wilson WH. The prevalence of abnormal involuntary movements among chronic schizophrenics. Int Clin Psychopharmacol 1986; 1:134–44.
23. Beck AT, Steer RA, Brown GK. Manual for Beck Depression Inventory II (BDI II). San Antonio, TX, Psychology Corporation. 1996.
24. Saunders JB, Aasland OG, Babor TF, de la Fuente JR, Grant M. Development of the Alcohol Use Disorders Identification Test (AUDIT): WHO Collaborative Project on Early Detection of Persons with Harmful Alcohol Consumption-II. Addiction 1993; 88:791–804.

25. Skinner HA. The drug abuse screening test. Addict Behav 1982; 7:363–71.
26. Barnes TR. A rating scale for drug-induced akathisia. Br J Psychiatry 1989; 154:672–6.
27. Rhoades HM, Overall JE. The semistructured BPRS interview and rating guide. Psychophar-
    macol Bull 1988; 24:101–4.

Psychotic Symptom Rating Scales (PSYRATS)

Part A : Auditory hallucinations

1 - **Frequency**
- 0 - Voices not present or present less than once a week
- 1 - Voices occur for at least once a week
- 2 - Voices occur at least once a day
- 3 - Voices occur at least once an hour
- 4 - Voices occur continuously or almost continuously, i.e., stop for only a few seconds or minutes

2 - **Duration**
- 0 - Voices not present
- 1 - Voices last for a few seconds, fleeting voices
- 2 - Voices last for several minutes
- 3 - Voices last for at least 1 hour
- 4 - Voices last for hours at a time

3 - **Location**
- 0 - No voices present
- 1 - Voices sound like they are inside head only
- 2 - Voices outside the head, but close to ears or head. Voices inside the head may also be present
- 3 - Voices sound like they are inside or close to ears and outside head away from ears
- 4 - Voices sound like they are from outside the head only

4 - **Loudness**
- 0 - Voices not present
- 1 - Quieter than own voice, whispers.
- 2 - About same loudness as own voice
- 3 - Louder than own voice
- 4 - Extremely loud, shouting

5 - **Beliefs re-origin of voices**
- 0 - Voices not present
- 1 - Believes voices to be solely internally generated and related to self
- 2 - Holds <50% conviction that voices originate from external causes
- 3 - Holds ≥50% conviction (but <100%) that voices originate from external causes
- 4 - Believes voices are solely due to external causes (100% conviction)

6 - **Amount of negative content of voices**
- 0 - No unpleasant content
- 1 - Occasional unpleasant content (<10%)
- 2 - Minority of voice content is unpleasant or negative (<50%)
- 3 - Majority of voice content is unpleasant or negative (≥50%)
- 4 - All of voice content is unpleasant or negative

7 - **Degree of negative content**
- 0 - Not unpleasant or negative
- 1 - Some degree of negative content, but not personal comments relating to self or family, e.g., swear words or comments not directed to self, e.g., "the milkman's ugly"
- 2 - Personal verbal abuse, comments on behavior, e.g., "shouldn't do that or say that"
- 3 - Personal verbal abuse relating to self-concept, e.g., "you're lazy, ugly, mad, perverted"

      4 - Personal threats to self, e.g., threats to harm self or family, extreme instructions or commands to harm self or others

8 -   Amount of distress
    0 - Voices not distressing at all
    1 - Voices occasionally distressing, majority not distressing (<10%)
    2 - Minority of voices distressing (<50%)
    3 - Majority of voices distressing, minority not distressing ($\geq$50%)
    4 - Voices always distressing

9 -   Intensity of distress
    0 - Voices not distressing at all
    1 - Voices slightly distressing
    2 - Voices are distressing to a moderate degree
    3 - Voices are very distressing, although subject could feel worse
    4 - Voices are extremely distressing, feel the worst he/she could possibly feel

10 -   Disruption to life caused by voices
    0 - No disruption to life, able to maintain social and family relationships (if present)
    1 - Voices causes minimal amount of disruption to life, e.g., interferes with concentration, although able to maintain daytime activity and social and family relationships and be able to maintain independent living without support
    2 - Voices cause moderate amount of disruption to life causing some disturbance to daytime activity and/or family or social activities. The patient is not in hospital although may live in supported accommodation or receive additional help with daily living skills
    3 - Voices cause severe disruption to life so that hospitalization is usually necessary. The patient is able to maintain some daily activities, self-care, and relationships while in hospital. The patient may also be in supported accommodation but experiencing severe disruption of life in terms of activities, daily living skills and/or relationships
    4 - Voices cause complete disruption of daily life requiring hospitalization. The patient is unable to maintain any daily activities and social relationships. Self-care is also severely disrupted.

11 -   Controllability of voices
    0 - Subject believes they can have control over the voices and can always bring on or dismiss them at will
    1 - Subject believes they can have some control over the voices on the majority of occasions
    2 - Subject believes they can have some control over their voices approximately half of the time
    3 - Subject believes they can have some control over their voices but only occasionally. The majority of the time the subject experiences voices which are uncontrollable
    4 - Subject has no control over when the voices occur and cannot dismiss or bring them on at all

Part B: Delusions

1 -   Amount of preoccupation with delusions
    0 - No delusions, or delusions which the subject thinks about less than once a week
    1 - Subject thinks about beliefs at least once a week
    2 - Subject thinks about beliefs at least once a day
    3 - Subject thinks about beliefs at least once an hour
    4 - Subject thinks about delusions continuously or almost continuously

2 - **Duration of preoccupation with delusions**
  0 - No delusions
  1 - Thoughts about beliefs last for a few seconds, fleeting thoughts
  2 - Thoughts about delusions last for several minutes
  3 - Thoughts about delusions last for at least 1 hour
  4 - Thoughts about delusions usually last for hours at a time

3 - **Conviction**
  0 - No conviction at all
  1 - Very little conviction in reality of beliefs, <10%
  2 - Some doubts relating to conviction in beliefs, between 10 and 49%
  3 - Conviction in belief is very strong, between 50 and 99%
  4 - Conviction is 100%

4 - **Amount of distress**
  0 - Beliefs never cause distress
  1 - Beliefs cause distress on the minority of occasions
  2 - Beliefs cause distress on <50% of occasions
  3 - Beliefs cause distress on the majority of occasions when they occur between 50 and 99% of time
  4 - Beliefs always cause distress when they occur

5 - **Intensity of distress**
  0 - No distress
  1 - Beliefs cause slight distress
  2 - Beliefs cause moderate distress
  3 - Beliefs cause marked distress
  4 - Beliefs cause extreme distress, could not be worse

6 - **Disruption to life caused by beliefs**
  0 - No disruption to life, able to maintain independent living with no problems in daily living skills. Able to maintain social and family relationships (if present)
  1 - Beliefs cause minimal amount of disruption to life, e.g., interferes with concentration, although able to maintain daytime activity and social and family relationships and be able to maintain independent living without
       support
  2 - Beliefs cause moderate amount of disruption to life causing some disturbance to daytime activity and/or family or social activities. The patient is not in hospital although may live in supported accommodation or receive additional help with daily living skills
  3 - Beliefs cause severe disruption to life so that hospitalization is usually necessary. The patient is able to maintain some daily activities, self-care, and relationships while in hospital. The patient may also be in supported accommodation but experiencing severe disruption of life in terms of activities, daily living skills and/or relationships
  4 - Beliefs cause complete disruption of daily life requiring hospitalization. The patient is unable to maintain any daily activities and social relationships. Self-care is also severely disrupted

Quality of Life Scale

Instructions: This instrument is designed to evaluate the current functioning of non-hospitalized schizophrenic persons apart from the presence or absence of florid psychotic symptomatology or need for hospitalization. It assesses the richness of their personal experience, the quality of their interpersonal relations, and their productivity in occupational roles.

It is intended to be administered as a semi-structured interview. Each item consists of three parts. First, a brief statement is provided to help the interviewer understand and focus on the parameter to be assessed. Second, a number of suggested questions are provided that may help the interviewer begin his exploration with the subject. Finally, a seven-point scale is provided for each item, with a brief description at four points to help the interviewer make his judgment and unlabeled points.

The questions provided are just suggestions. They are to be altered or supplemented as needed. Each item should be explored as much as required to allow the rater to make a good clinical judgment. The intent of the schedule is to assess limitations due to psychopathology or personality deficits. Adjustments should be made by the rater when extraneous factors are clearly and unambiguously involved (e.g., decreased social contact due to serious physical illness).

All items should be rated. Circle the appropriate number on each item scale.

---

1. RATE INTIMATE RELATIONSHIPS WITH HOUSEHOLD MEMBERS
This item is to rate close relationships with significant mutual caring and sharing with immediate family or members of the subject's current household.

Suggested questions	Scoring
- Are you especially close with any of the people you currently live with or your immediate family?	0 - Virtually no intimacy 1 - 2 - Only sparse and intermittent intimate interactions
- Can you discuss personal matters with them?	3 -
- How much have you talked with them?	
- What are these relationships like?	4 - Some consistent intimate interactions but reduced in extent or intensity; or intimacy only present erratically
- Can they discuss personal matters with you?	
- What sorts of things have you done together?	
- When at home, have you spent much time around your family or were you generally alone?	5 - 6 - Adequate involvement in intimate relations with household members or immediate family

---

9 - Score here if lives alone and no
immediate family nearby

Note: (For Factor and Total Scores, prorate this item on the basis of Items 2 through 8.)

2. RATE INTIMATE RELATIONSHIPS
This item is to rate close relationships with significant mutual caring and sharing, with people other than immediate family or household members. Exclude relationships with mental health workers.

Suggested questions

- Do you have friends with whom you are especially close other than your immediate family or the people you live with?
- Can you discuss personal matters with them?
- How many friends do you have?
- How often have you spoken with them recently, in person or by phone?
- What have these relationships been like?
- Can they discuss personal matters with you?

Scoring

0 - Virtually absent

1 -

2 - Only sparse intermittent relations

3 -

4 - Some consistent intimate relations but reduced in number or intensity; or intimacy only present erratically

5 -

6 - Adequate involvement with intimate relationships with more than one other person

3. RATE ACTIVE ACQUAINTANCES

This item is to rate relationships with people based on liking one another and sharing common activities or interests but without the intimate emotional investment of the above item. Exclude relationships with mental-health workers and other household members.

Suggested questions

- Apart from close personal friends, are there people you know with whom you have enjoyed doing things?
- How many?
- How often have you gotten together with them?
- What things have you done together?
- Have you been with people as a part of clubs or organize activities?
- Have you had extra social contact with co-workers, such as going to lunch together or going out after work?

Scoring

0 - Virtually absent

1 -

2 - Few active acquaintances and

3 -

4 - Some ongoing active acquaintance but reduced contact and limited shared activity

5 -

6 - Adequate involvement with active acquaintances

4. RATE LEVEL OF SOCIAL ACTIVITY

This item is to rate involvement in activities with other people done for enjoyment.
Exclude social activity that is primarily instrumental for other goals, for example, work and school.
Exclude psychotherapy.

Suggested questions

- How often have you done things for enjoyment that involve other people?
- What sort of things?
- Have you participated in clubs or other organized social groups?

Scoring

0 - Virtually absent

1 -

2 - Occasional social activity but lack of regular pattern of such activity, or limited only to activity with immediate family or members of household

3 -

4 - Some regular social activity but reduced in frequency or diversity

5 -

6 - Adequate level of regular social activity

5. RATE INVOLVED SOCIAL NETWORK

This item is to rate the extent to which other people concern themselves with the person, care about his fortunes or know about his activities. Exclude mental-health workers.

Suggested questions

- Are there people who have been concerned about your happiness and well being?
- How many?
- How did they show it?
- If some important and exciting thing happened to you, who would you contact or inform?
- Are there people who often provided you emotional support or help in day-to-day matters such as food, transportation, and practical advice?
- Are there people you could turn to or depend on for help if anything happened?

Scoring

0 - Virtually absent

1 -

2 - Minimal in number or degree of involvement, and/or limited to immediate family

3 -

4 - Presence of some involved social network but reduced in number of degree of involvement

5 -

6 - Adequate involved social network in both extent and in degree of involvement

6. RATE SOCIAL INITIATIVES

This item is to rate the degree to which the person is active in directing his social interactions – what, how much, and with whom.

Suggested questions

- Have you often asked people to do something with you, or have you usually waited for others to ask you?
- When you have had an idea for a good time, have you sometimes missed out because it's hard to ask others to participate?
- Have you contacted people by phone?
- Have you tended to seek people out?
- Have you usually done things alone or with other people?

Scoring

0 - Social activity almost completely dependent on initiatives of others

1 -

2 - Occasional social initiative, but social life significantly impoverished due to his pattern of social passivity, or initiative limited to immediate family

3 -

4 - Evidence of some reduction of social initiative, but with only minimal adverse consequences on his social activity

5 -

6 - Adequate social initiative

7. RATE SOCIAL WITHDRAWAL

This item is to rate the degree to which the person actively avoids social interaction due to his discomfort or disinterest.

Suggested questions

- Have you felt uncomfortable with people?
- Have you turned down offers to do things with other people? Would you if you were asked?

Scoring

0 - Active avoidance of virtually all social contact

1 -

2 - Tolerates that social contact

- Have you done this even when you have had
  nothing to do?
- Have you avoided answering the phone?
- How has this interfered with your life?
- Have you dealt with people only when it's
  necessary to accomplish something you
  want?
- Have you stayed to yourself at home?
- Have you preferred to be alone?

required for meeting
other needs, but very little
social contact for its own
sake, or lack of withdrawal
only with immediate family
3 -
4 - Some satisfying and enjoyable
social engagement, but
reduced due to avoidance
5 -
6 - No evidence of significant social
withdrawal

8. RATE SOCIOSEXUAL RELATIONS

*This item is to rate the capacity for mature intimate relations with members of the opposite sex
and satisfying sexual activity. The wording assumes a heterosexual preference. In clear cases of
consistent homosexual preference, reword accordingly and rate these same capacities.*

Suggested questions if single:
- Have your social activities involved
  women (men)?
- Have you avoided them or found it too
  uncomfortable to deal with them?
- Have you dated?
- Did you have one or more girlfriends?
  (boyfriends?)
- Have the relationships been satisfying?
- Have emotionally involved were you?
- Were you in love?
- Were you having sexual activity?
- Was it satisfying?
- Did you show physical signs of affection,
  such as hugging and kissing?

Scoring
0 - No interest in opposite sex, or active
avoidance
1 -
2 - Some limited contact with opposite sex but
superficial with avoidance of intimacy; or
sexual activity as just physical release
without emotional involvement; or
relationships marked by severe and
chronic disruption, dissatisfaction or
affective chaos
3 -
4 - Relationships with some intimacy and
emotional investment, predominantly
satisfying, and perhaps some sexual
expression or physical signs of affection
5 -
6 - Usually has satisfying relationships,
emotionally rich and intimate and
appropriate sexual expression and physical
signs of expression

Suggested questions if married or living
with someone:
- Were you happy in your relationship with
  your partner?
- Have you done many things together?
- Did you talk together much?
- Did you discuss personal thoughts and
  feelings?
- Did you fight much?
- Has your sex life been satisfying?
- Did you show physical signs of affection
  such as hugging and kissing?
- Did you feel close to her (him)?

Scoring
0 - No interest in opposite sex, or active
avoidance
1 -
2 - Some limited contact with opposite sex
but superficial with avoidance of
intimacy; or sexual activity as just
physical release without emotional
involvement; or relationships marked
by severe and chronic disruption,
dissatisfaction or affective chaos
3 -
4 - Relationships with some intimacy and
emotional investment,

predominantly satisfying, and perhaps some sexual expression or physical signs of affection

5 -

6 - Usually has satisfying relationships, emotionally rich and intimate and appropriate sexual expression and physical signs of expression

9. RATE EXTENT OF OCCUPATIONAL ROLE FUNCTIONING

This item is to rate the amount of role functioning the person is attempting, not how well nor how completely he is succeeding. For homemakers, consider whether for a person with normal efficiency the responsibilities would represent a full-time job seeking activity.

Suggested questions
- Have you had a job?
- How many hours a week did you work?
- Were you involved in school in addition to work?

Suggested questions
- What sort of education program were you pursuing?
- How many classes were you taking?
- How much time did school take per week?
- Were you also working, caring for children or responsible for housekeeping?

Suggested questions for homemakers

- How much was involved in taking care of your home and family?
- Were you raising children?
- What were your responsibilities in the home?
- How much did other people help with these responsibilities?

0 - Virtually no role functioning

1 -

2 - Less than half-time

3 -

4 - Half-time or more, but less than full-time

5 -

6 - Full-time or more

10. RATE LEVEL OF ACCOMPLISHMENT

This item is to rate the level of success and achievement in fulfilling the particular role the person has chosen to attempt.

Question the subject regarding salary and raises, the challenge and responsibility of the job, praise or reprimands from employer, adequacy of interaction with co-workers, absenteeism, promotions or demotions. For students, question regarding grades, the difficulty of the curriculum, praise or criticism from teachers, adequacy of interaction with other classmates, class attendance, completion of assigned work, and extracurricular activities. For homemakers, question regarding the

Scoring

0 - Attempting no role function or performing at level so poor as to imminently threaten the ability to continue in that role

1 -

2 - Functioning just well enough to keep position with very low level of accomplishment

3 -

adequate performance of required tasks such as cooking, shopping, washing dishes, cleaning, dusting, laundry, management of household budget, physical care of children, and meeting the emotional needs of children. Question further regarding praise or criticism by family members about either housekeeping or child raising.

4 - Generally adequate functioning

5 -

6 - Very good functioning with evidence of new or progressive accomplishments and/or very good functioning in some areas

11. RATE DEGREE OF UNDEREMPLOYMENT
This item is to rate the degree to which the existing extent of and accomplishment in occupational role functioning reflects full utilization of the potentiality and opportunities available to the person. Consider innate abilities, physical handicaps, education, economic, and social culture factors. Obviously, limitations directly reflecting any mental illness or personality disorder should not be considered in estimating the person's potential.

Suggested questions
This item requires a complex judgment. Ask any further questions needed to clarify the abilities and opportunities of this individual.

Scoring
0 - Almost complete failure to actualize potentials

1 -

2 - Significant underemployment of abilities or unemployed but looking for work actively.

3 -

4 - Somewhat below the person's capacity

5 -

6 - Role functioning commensurate with person's abilities and opportunities

12. RATE SATISFACTION WITH OCCUPATIONAL ROLE FUNCTIONING
This item is to rate the extent to which the person is comfortable with his choice of role, the performance of it, and the situation in which he performs it. It also is to rate the extent to which it provides a sense of satisfaction, pleasure, and fulfillment to him.

Suggested questions
- Did you like your work or schooling?
- Would you have preferred to be doing something else?
- Do you plan a change? Why?
- Did you get good feelings from doing your work - pleasure, fulfillment, etc.
- Did your work or school make you feel good about yourself?
- Are you enthusiastic about your job?
- Do you look forward to going to work?

Scoring
0 - Pervasive unhappiness and dissatisfaction with occupational role

1 -

2 - Little or no definite evidence of unhappiness or dissatisfaction, but role does not provide any positive pleasure or fulfillment. Perhaps boredom is evident.

3 -

4 - Little or no discontent and some limited pleasure in work

5 -

6 - Rather consistent sense of fulfillment and satisfaction, perhaps in spite of some limited complaints

9 - Not applicable if patient not involved in any occupational role functioning

Note: (This item should be rated 2 if item #9 is rated less than 3. For Factor and Total scores, prorate this item on the basis if items 9 through 11.)

13. RATE SENSE OF PURPOSE

This item is to rate the degree to which the person posits realistic, integrated goals for his life. If the person's current life reflects such goals, it is not necessary that he (she) be planning a change in order to be judged to have a good sense of purpose.

Suggested questions
- What makes life worth living for you?
- Do you think much about the future?
- Have you set any goals for yourself?
- What do you anticipate your living and working situation to be a few months from now?
- What plans do you have for your life over the next year or so - personal as well as job related ones?

Scoring
0 - No plans, or plans are bizarre, delusional, or grossly unrealistic
1 -
2 - Has plans, but they are vague, somewhat unrealistic, poorly integrated with one another, or of little consequence to the person's life
3 -
4 - Realistic and concise plans for next year or so but little integration into long-range life plan
5 -
6 - Realistic, concise, and integrated plans, both short- and long-range

14. RATE DEGREE OF MOTIVATION

This item is to rate the extent to which the person is unable to initiate or sustain goal-directed activity due to inadequate drive.

Suggested questions
- How have you been going about accomplishing your goals?
- What other things have you worked on or accomplished recently?
- Have there been tasks in any area that you wanted to do but didn't because you somehow didn't get around to it?
- Has this experience of just not getting around to it interfered with your regular daily activities?
- How motivated have you been?
- Have you had much enthusiasm, energy, and drive?
- Have you tended to get into a rut?
- Have you tended to put things off?

Scoring
0 - Lack of motivation significantly interferes with basic routine
1 -
2 - Able to meet basic maintenance demands of life, but lack of motivation significantly impairs any progress or new accomplishments
3 -
4 - Able to meet routine demands of life and some new accomplishments, but lack of motivation results in significant underachievement in some areas
5 -
6 - No evidence of significant lack of motivation

15. RATE CURIOSITY

This item is to rate the degree to which the person is interested in his surroundings and questions those things he doesn't understand. Exclude interest in hallucinations or delusions or other psychotic products. However, pathological preoccupation with psychotic products or other themes may limit curiosity or interest in other things.

Suggested questions
- How often have you seen or heard about
  something that you wanted to know more
  about or understand better?
- What sorts of things?
- Have you done anything to learn more about
  them? Please specify.
- Have you read the newspapers, or listened to
  thenews on TV or radio?
- Were you interested in any issues in current
  events or sports?
- How curious about things have you been?

Scoring
0 - Very little curiosity or interest in
    new topics or events
1 -
2 - Some sporadic curiosity, but not
    pursued in thought or action
3 -
4 - Some curiosity and time spent
    thinking about topics or
    interest and some actual
    effort to learn more
    about them
5 -
6 - Curiosity about a number of topics
    and some effort to learn
    more about some of them
    such as reading, asking questions
    and planned observation

16. RATE ANHEDONIA

This item is to rate the person's capacity to experience pleasure and humor. Do not rate anhedonia that presents as the result of a clear and observable depressive syndrome, e.g., agitation, crying, marked feelings of wickedness and worthlessness, etc. However, anhedonia accompanied by apathy and withdrawal from which depression may be inferred should be rated. Ask any questions necessary to determine the presence of depression and its effect on hedonic capacity. This is to be distinguished from the capacity to display affect, which is not rated here.

Suggested questions
- Have you been able to enjoy yourself?
- How often have you really enjoyed or gotten
  satisfaction from something you were
  doing?
- How often did you choose to do something
  that struck you as amusing or made you feel
  like laughing?
- Did you have trouble getting enjoyment from
  things that seemed like they should be fun?
- Do other people seem to get more enjoyment
  in things than you do?
- Did you often spend the better part of the day
  bored or disinterested in things?

Scoring
0 - Nearly complete inability to
    experience pleasure
    or humor
1 -
2 - Some sporadic and limited
    experiences of pleasure or
    humor but a predominant
    lacking of these capacities
3 -
4 - Some regular experiences of
    pleasure and humor but
    reduced in extent and
    intensity
5 -
6 - No evidence of anhedonia or
    can be explained completely
    by concurrent depression
    or anxiety

17. RATE TIME UTILIZATION

This item is to rate the amount of time passed in aimless inactivity – sleeping during the day, lying in bed, sitting around doing nothing or in front of the TV or radio when not particularly interested.

Suggested questions
- Did you spend much time doing nothing just sitting around or in bed?
- Did you spend much time watching TV or listening to music - were you really interested or just had nothing better to do?
- Did you sleep much during the day?
- How much of your days were spent in these ways?
- How have you utilized your time?
- Did you tend to waste time?

Scoring
0 - Spends the vast majority of his day in aimless activity
1 -
2 - Spends about half of his days in aimless activity
3 -
4 - Some excessive aimless inactivity but less than half his day
5 -
6 - No excessive aimless inactivity beyond the normal amount required for relaxation

18. RATE COMMONPLACE OBJECTS

This item assumes that basic participation in living in this culture nearly always requires a person to possess certain objects.

Suggested questions
For this question, inquire about each of the 12 items listed below.

Are you wearing or carrying the following?
(1) a wallet or purse
(2) keys
(3) a driver's license
(4) a watch
(5) a credit card
(6) a Social Security or Medical Assistance card

Do you have with you at your place of residence the following?
(1) a map of the city or area
(2) your own alarm clock
(3) a comb or hair brush
(4) an overnight bag
(5) a library card
(6) postage stamps

Scoring
0 - Absence of nearly all commonplace objects (0 items)
1 -
2 - Major deficit of commonplace objects (3-4 items)
3 -
4 - Moderate deficit (7-8 items)
5 -
6 - Little or no deficit (11-12 items)

19. RATE COMMONPLACE ACTIVITIES
This item assumes that basic participation in living in this culture nearly always requires a person to engage in certain activities.

Suggested questions

For this item inquire about each of the eight items listed below. Which of the following have you done in the past 2 weeks?: (1) read a newspaper, (2) paid a bill, (3) wrote a letter, (4) gone to a movie or play, (5) driven a car or ridden public transportation alone, (6) shopped for food, (7) shopped for other than food, (8) eaten in a restaurant, (9) taken a book or record out of the library, (10) participated in a public gathering, (11) attended a sporting event, (12) visited a public park or other recreational facility.

Scoring

0 - Absence of nearly all activities (0 items)
1 -
2 - Major deficit (3-4 items)
3 -
4 - Moderate deficit (7-8 items)
5 -
6 - Little or no deficit

20. RATE CAPACITY FOR EMPATHY
This item is to rate the person's capacity to regard and appreciate the other person's situation as different from his own – to appreciate different perspectives, affective states and points of view. It is reflected in the person's description of interactions with other people and how he views such interactions. Specific probing to elicit the person's description and assessment of relevant situations can be done at this time if sufficient data has not emerged thus far in the interview.

Suggested questions

- Consider someone you are close to or spend a lot of time with:
- What about them irritates or annoys you?
- What about you irritates or annoys them?
- What things do they like? What things that you do please them?
- If they appear upset, how do you usually react?
- If you have an argument or difference of opinion with them, how do you handle it?
- Are you usually sensitive to the feelings of others?
- Are you affected very much by how other people feel?

Scoring

0 - Shows no capacity to consider the views and feelings of others
1 -
2 - Shows little capacity to consider the views and feelings of others
3 -
4 - He can consider other people's views and feelings but tends to be caught up in his own world.
5 -
6 - He spontaneously considers the other person's situation in most instances, can intuit the other person's affective responses, and uses this knowledge to adjust his own responses.

21. RATE CAPACITY FOR ENGAGEMENT AND EMOTIONAL INTERACTION WITH INTERVIEWER
This item is to rate the person's ability to engage the interviewer, to make him feel affectively in touch and acknowledge him as a participant individual in the encounter, and to react in a give and take way.

This is a global judgment based on the entire interview.

<u>Scoring</u>
0 - Interviewer feels virtually ignored with essentially no sense of engagement, with very little reactivity
1 -
2 - Very limited engagement
3 -
4 - Engagement somewhat limited or present erratically
5 -
6 - Consistently good engagement and reactivity

Scoring of Quality of Life Scale

Mean scores of the following subscales and total (prorate items 1 and 12 for missing data as indicated in the manual).

Subscale Scores:

I. Interpersonal Relations (1–8): _____
II. Instrumental Role (9–12): _____
III. Intrapsychic Foundations (13–17, 20, 21): _____
IV. Common Objects and Activities (18, 19):___
III plus IV (13–20): _____
Total Score (Items 1–21): _____

ABNORMAL INVOLUNTARY MOVEMENT SCALE (AIMS)

Patient's Name (Please print) _____   Patient's ID Information _____

Examiner's Name _____

CURRENT MEDICATIONS AND TOTAL MG/DAY

Medication #1 _____Total mg/Day _____   Medication #2 _____Total mg/Day _____

INSTRUCTIONS: COMPLETE THE EXAMINATION PROCEDURE BEFORE ENTERING THESE RATINGS.

	None, normal	Minimal (may be extreme normal)	Mild	Moderate	Severe
Facial and Oral Movements					
1. Muscles of Facial Expression eg, movements of forehead, eyebrows, periorbital area, cheeks; include frowning, blinking, smiling, grimacing	☐₀	☐₁	☐₂	☐₃	☐₄
2. Lips and Perioral Area eg, puckering, pouting, smacking	☐₀	☐₁	☐₂	☐₃	☐₄
3. Jaw eg, biting, clenching, chewing, mouth opening, lateral movement	☐₀	☐₁	☐₂	☐₃	☐₄
4. Tongue Rate only increases in movement both in and out of mouth. NOT inability to sustain movement	☐₀	☐₁	☐₂	☐₃	☐₄
Extremity Movements					
5. Upper (arms, wrists, hands, fingers) Include choreic movements (ie, rapid, objectively purposeless, irregular, spontaneous); athetoid movements (ie, slow, irregular, complex, serpentine). DO NOT include tremor (ie, repetitive, regular, rhythmic).	☐₀	☐₁	☐₂	☐₃	☐₄
6. Lower (legs, knees, ankles, toes) eg, lateral knee movement, foot tapping, heel dropping, foot squirming, inversion and eversion of foot	☐₀	☐₁	☐₂	☐₃	☐₄
Trunk Movements					
7. Neck, shoulders, hips eg, rocking, twisting, squirming, pelvic gyrations	☐₀	☐₁	☐₂	☐₃	☐₄

SCORING:
- Score the highest amplitude or frequency in a movement on the 0-4 scale, not the average;
- Score Activated Movements the same way; do not lower those numbers as was proposed at one time;
- A POSITIVE AIMS EXAMINATION IS A SCORE OF 2 IN TWO OR MORE MOVEMENTS or a SCORE OF 3 OR 4 IN A SINGLE MOVEMENT
- Do not sum the scores: e.g. a patient who has scores 1 in four movements DOES NOT have a positive AIMS score of 4.

Overall Severity					
8. Severity of abnormal movements	☐₀	☐₁	☐₂	☐₃	☐₄
9. Incapacitation due to abnormal movements	☐₀	☐₁	☐₂	☐₃	☐₄

	No awareness	Aware, no distress	Aware, mild distress	Aware, moderate distress	Aware, severe distress
10. Patient's awareness of abnormal movements (rate only patient's report)	☐₀	☐₁	☐₂	☐₃	☐₄

Dental Status	Yes	No
11. Current problems with teeth and/or dentures?	☐	☐
12. Does patient usually wear dentures?	☐	☐

Comments: _____

Examiner's Signature _____   Next Exam Date_____

Guy W. ECDEU Assessment Manual for Psychopharmacology - Revised DHEW Publ No ADM 76-338, US Department of Health, Education, and Welfare; 1976

Brief Psychiatric Rating Scale (BPRS)

Instructions: This form consists of 24 symptom constructs, each to be rated in a 7-point scale of severity ranging from 'not present' to 'extremely severe' If a specific symptom is not rated, mark 'NA' (not assessed). Circle the number headed by the term that best describes the patient's present condition.

Scoring Key:						
1	2	3	4	5	6	7
not present	very mild	mild	moderate	moderately severe	severe	extremely severe

1	Somatic concern	NA	1	2	3	4	5	6	7
2	Anxiety	NA	1	2	3	4	5	6	7
3	Depression	NA	1	2	3	4	5	6	7
4	Suicidality	NA	1	2	3	4	5	6	7
5	Guilt	NA	1	2	3	4	5	6	7
6	Hostility	NA	1	2	3	4	5	6	7
7	Elated Mood	NA	1	2	3	4	5	6	7
8	Grandiosity	NA	1	2	3	4	5	6	7
9	Suspiciousness	NA	1	2	3	4	5	6	7
10	Hallucinations	NA	1	2	3	4	5	6	7
11	Unusual thought content	NA	1	2	3	4	5	6	7
12	Bizarre behavior	NA	1	2	3	4	5	6	7
13	Self-neglect	NA	1	2	3	4	5	6	7
14	Disorientation	NA	1	2	3	4	5	6	7
15	Conceptual disorganization	NA	1	2	3	4	5	6	7
16	Blunted affect	NA	1	2	3	4	5	6	7
17	Emotional withdrawal	NA	1	2	3	4	5	6	7
18	Motor retardation	NA	1	2	3	4	5	6	7
19	Tension	NA	1	2	3	4	5	6	7
20	Uncooperativeness	NA	1	2	3	4	5	6	7
21	Excitement	NA	1	2	3	4	5	6	7
22	Distractibility	NA	1	2	3	4	5	6	7
23	Motor hyperactivity	NA	1	2	3	4	5	6	7
24	Mannerisms and posturing	NA	1	2	3	4	5	6	7

TOTAL SCORE (Total of circled responses): _____

(From Ventura, Green, Shaner & Liberman (1993) Training and quality assurance with the brief psychiatric rating scale: "The drift buster" International Journal of Methods in Psychiatric Research.)

Chapter 11
Brief Rating Scales for the Assessment of Cognitive and Neuropsychological Status

Matthew R. Baity

Abstract The use of brief rating scales to assess cognitive/neuropsychological status has been studied in the field of psychology for several decades. While some scales like the Mini-Mental Status Exam (Folstein M, Folstein S, McHugh P. *Journal of Psychiatric Research* 12: 189–198, 1975) (MMSE) have been used and even accepted as the gold standard in medical and mental health areas, advances in knowledge and scale design have allowed for the introduction of a more sensitive and abbreviated measure. In the current environment of shorter hospital stays and circumscribed treatments, the need to quickly and accurately assess a patient's mental status has become paramount. Additionally, the comorbidity of cognitive dysfunction in psychiatric populations is being increasingly recognized and studied. Brief rating scales can allow clinicians to assess and make recommendations for follow-up treatment in populations that may have increased difficulty tolerating a full neuropsychological battery. This chapter is designed to provide both empirical and clinical information to assist the reader make informed decisions about the scales to choose and how that data might be applied in a variety of clinical settings.

Keywords Cognitive testing · Neuropsychological testing · Screening · Rating scales · Assessment · Psychiatry

In recent years the use of brief rating scales in the field of mental health has received an increased amount of attention as the health-care system has encouraged practitioners to not only be more accountable for their services, but also to provide faster results. Given that most comprehensive neuropsychological batteries can take upwards of 6 h to complete, the need for brief measures of cognitive status is becoming apparent. This need has become particularly relevant in the field of psychiatry

M.R. Baity (✉)
Alliant International University, California School of Professional Psychology – Sacramento, 2030 West El Camino Ave, Sacramento, CA 95833
e-mail: mbaity@alliant.edu

L. Baer, M.A. Blais (eds.), *Handbook of Clinical Rating Scales and Assessment in Psychiatry and Mental Health*, Current Clinical Psychiatry, DOI 10.1007/978-1-59745-387-5_11, © Humana Press, a part of Springer Science+Business Media, LLC 2010

where the value of brief objective cognitive screening tools for treatment planning is becoming increasingly common [2].

Recent reports have elaborated on the extent of cognitive problems that are comorbid with many psychiatric disorders [3, 4]. In many situations, cognitive impairment takes the form of an interruption in functional capacity as has been found in patients with schizophrenia [5]. Several studies examining cognitive functioning in psychiatric patients have found that those patients with greater functional impairment have less positive outcomes [5, 6] and are more likely to require structured treatment following hospital discharge than psychiatric patients without cognitive impairment [6]. Such patients are also more likely to be hospitalized after being seen in the emergency room [7]. Depression is a very common psychiatric disorder and repeated links between this syndrome and cognitive impairment have been made in the literature. In some cases, the level of temporal (memory) and executive dysfunction seen in depressed patients may be similar to that of a demented patient [8]. Needless to say, the impact of cognitive status on the treatment of psychiatric disorders is a widespread, and often underappreciated, complication. Cognitive impairment presents an obstacle to providing effective treatment in that clinicians are often required to alter their explanations or adjust their approach to better match patients' levels of comprehension. Furthermore, patients with cognitive difficulties may be limited in their ability to participate meaningfully in their own treatment. Therefore, it is imperative that decisions made about mental status are quick *and* accurate. This is especially true on inpatient services where providers often have to work rapidly to develop treatment plans and initiate care. In these situations, cognitive screening not only serves the function of making broad estimations of current cognitive ability, but also indicates the need for more extensive testing. In short, the purpose of having brief rating scales is to reliably assess gross cognitive functioning, to quickly identify general areas of impairment, and to make recommendations for follow-up treatment or additional evaluation.

Mini-Mental State Exam (MMSE)

By far, the standard for assessing gross cognitive status has been the Mini-Mental Status Exam [1] (MMSE, not reproduced in this chapter because the scale is copyrighted by PAR, Inc, and is available at their website: www.parinc.com). The MMSE is a 30-item test covering a broad range of cognitive abilities. The MMSE's popularity comes from its ease of use, quick administration, and sensitivity to dementia in the moderate to severe range [9]. In general, the recommended cutoff for the MMSE is 23, where patients who obtain a score below this point are often referred for follow-up testing or other evaluation procedures. However, this cutoff has proved unsatisfactory in many research studies utilizing a variety of patient samples. As a result several different cutoff points for the MMSE have been recommended depending on the age and educational level of the population being studied [10]. The resulting multiple cutoff scores places a burden upon the clinician attempting to employ the MMSE and achieve adequate sensitivity and specificity across diverse patient populations.

In the words of Lopez et al. [10], "At best the MMSE should have only two possible conclusions: 'needs no further evaluation' or 'needs a more extensive examination to determine if cognitive deficits exist'" (p. 143). In a meta-analysis on the MMSE, Tombaugh and McIntyre reported that while this measure seems to have some sensitivity to more severe levels of cognitive dysfunction, it lacks sensitivity to milder impairment resulting in an increased number of false negatives and is subject to education effects [11]. The lack of sensitivity of this measure is most apparent on inpatient units where, ironically, the MMSE is used most often. From a strict clinical observational perspective, patients who score below the MMSE cutoff of 23 (the generally accepted cut off score for the MMSE) are often impaired enough in casual interactions that administration of the MMSE is almost unnecessary. Despite the popularity of the MMSE, there clearly is need for a broader yet brief and sensitive measure of cognitive impairment suitable for psychiatric patients.

Modified Mini-Mental State Exam (3MS)

Efforts to address the limitations of the MMSE have produced numerous modified versions of the scale. Teng and Chui [12] undertook an extensive modification of the MMSE in developing the Modified MMSE (3MS). Like the MMSE, the 3MS is based on an interview-style administration that takes about 5 min to complete. The 3MS is a 15-item test and incorporates all of the components of the original MMSE plus four additional subtests (Date and Place of Birth, Word Generation, Similarities and a second Delayed Recall). In addition, the scoring of the 3MS items was expanded to include partial credit, thus increasing the range of possible scores from 0–30 (for the MMSE) to 0–100 for the 3MS. For example, an item that requires individuals to copy interlocking pentagons is scored as 0 (incorrect) or 1 (correct) on the MMSE, but is given a 0–10 point range on the 3MS. The 3MS was chosen as the measure to define gross cognitive functioning in two large, multisite prospective studies on dementia and aging in Canada [13, 14]. An initial cutoff score of 78 or higher was identified in the first of these studies as it had the most optimal diagnostic efficiency statistics for identifying individuals with dementia. This cutoff score has also been routinely used in other 3MS research. However, only one study has produced 3MS norms with an inpatient psychiatric population [6].

According to its authors, the 3MS represents an improvement over the MMSE in that it has more quantitative scoring, a broader sampling of cognitive domains, and a greater range of item difficulty. The initial report on the 3MS has been encouraging. Teng et al. [15] reported that the 3MS was more reliable and more sensitive to detecting dementia than the MMSE. Several other groups of researchers have examined the psychometrics of the 3MS in a variety of clinical and community settings [6, 16–21]. In a study that used patients from one of the multisite projects mentioned above

[21], researchers compared the 3MS with the MMSE in an effort to identify which instrument was more sensitive to detecting cognitive impairment. Results showed that both measures had comparable psychometric properties (internal consistency) and performed equally well at detecting dementia in the elderly [18]. Internal consistency (coefficient alpha) for the 3MS was 0.82 in the non-cognitively impaired group and 0.88 in a group of patients with probable Alzheimer's disease. Receiver operator characteristic (ROC) curves showed that neither the MMSE nor the 3MS was better able to identify patients with dementia. However, the researchers did note that any differences between the tests might be due to the animal naming task (word generation) that is only found on the 3MS. The advantage of word generation in detecting cognitive impairment is consistent with a large body of research showing that semantic fluency tasks are highly sensitive to frontal lobe dysfunction [22].

In a follow-up to the MMSE/3MS comparison study [18], Blais and Baity examined the utility of the 3MS to detect cognitive impairment in a sample of psychiatric patients hospitalized on an acute inpatient unit [6]. While much of the research with the 3MS to date has been with geriatric populations or with patients known to have a cognitive disorder, the use of a younger psychiatric population helped extend the utility of the 3MS. To evaluate clinical value, these authors explored the relationship of admission 3MS and MMSE scores to two treatment outcome variables: length of stay (LOS) and the need for placement or additional services (i.e., partial hospital, day treatment) at discharge. To expand on previous findings from the MMSE/3MS comparison study, they also explored the incremental utility of the four new subtests included in the 3MS (Date and Place of Birth, Word Generation, Similarities, and Delayed Recall).

The mean score for the 3MS in this sample was 88.68 (SD = 9.04, range 61–100) and the mean MMSE score was 26.18 (SD = 3.27, range 15–30). As would be expected, the 3MS and MMSE were highly correlated ($r = 0.83, p < 0.001$). On both the 3MS and the MMSE, psychotic patients (those with a diagnosis of schizophrenia or schizoaffective disorder [$n=18$]) scored significantly lower than non-psychotic patients. The mean 3MS scores for the psychotic patients were 82.27 (SD = 10.46), while scores for the non-psychotic patients were 89.72 (SD = 8.42). MMSE mean scores were 23.36 (SD = 3.69) and 26.66 (SD = 2.98) for the psychotic and non-psychotic patients, respectively. In terms of a ceiling effect, 22 patients scored 29 or 30 on the MMSE (30%), while only five patients (7%) scored 99 or 100 on the 3MS. In fact, the modal score on the MMSE was 29 with 17 patients (23% of the sample) obtaining this score, while the modal score on the 3MS was 93 obtained by only seven patients (9.5% of the sample). These findings highlight the susceptibility of the MMSE to ceiling effects in non-demented samples.

Multivariate analyses found that the 3MS total score was negatively related to LOS above and beyond variance accounted for by demographic and treatment variables. In other words, lower scores on the 3MS (greater impairment) were related to longer hospital stays independent of other factors. The finding that the 3MS total score was able to account for unique variance after the removal of the demographic and treatment variables was an impressive finding and demonstrated the power of this simple screening test. The second multivariate analysis looked at the prediction of need for post-hospital services. The raw number of Axis III disorders (medical conditions) and the total 3MS score were the only significant contributors to the regression equation. When the four new 3MS items (Date and Place of Birth, Word Generation, Similarities and Delayed Recall) were evaluated independently, word generation made a significant contribution to the overall model. This finding is consistent with previous research that found word generation to be especially sensitive to mild cognitive impairment [20]. A recent meta-analysis of verbal fluency studies indicated that while both phonemic and semantic tasks were sensitive to executive dysfunction, semantic tasks were dependent on semantic memory, thus making them more sensitive to a broader range of cerebral dysfunction. Taken together, the findings help highlight the added utility of the 3MS as a potential screening instrument for gross cognitive impairment in psychiatric patients.

All in all, it appears that the 3MS holds a great deal of promise as a screening tool for cognitive impairment in psychiatric samples. However, additional empirical research and broader clinical applications are needed before this measure can reach its potential. Obviously, the lower a patient scores on the 3MS, the greater confidence one can have in the presence of gross cognitive impairment. In general (non-geriatric) psychiatric populations, any patient who scores below the established 77/78 cutoff on the 3MS and graduated high school should likely need further testing. These cases are typically easy to pick out, and like the patient who scores below a 23 on the MMSE, you almost do not need to give a screening instrument to appreciate their cognitive troubles. What is more challenging, and where the 3MS is at an advantage over the MMSE, is being able to detect milder forms of impairment. One downside to the 3MS is that the published normative data are in populations aged 65 and over, leaving those working with patients below this age level to develop our own norms. The 3MS has been given at the MGH psychiatric inpatient facility for over 5 years to nearly every new admission, where the average age is 45 and level of education is about 12 years. The mean 3MS scores are 91.92 for patients 18–45 years old (SD= 9.35), 90.38 for patients 46–65 years old (SD= 7.29), and 80.15 for patients 66 and older (SD=12.77). Using these local "norms," we are better able to classify our younger patients' performance as either "within the expected range" or "needs additional evaluation." We encourage the collection of local norms no matter what screening instrument you employ [6]. Despite the benefits of the 3MS over the MMSE, questions about impairment can still be present even with a 3MS score in the 90s. This is especially true with younger patients who have greater than a high school education. Typically, 3MS scores below 95 can raise suspicion of cognitive impairment in more highly educated populations and may require further screening or inquiry.

Supplemental Tests

The review above suggests that no single instrument is likely to be adequate for all cognitive screenings across a wide range of patient populations and clinical settings; therefore, a utilizing standard screening battery may have greater utility. A basic inpatient cognitive screening battery could consist of the 3MS, The Clock Drawing Test (CDT), and Trail Making Test A and B (TMT). Such a battery would continue to be low burden, while applying multiple screening measures and increasing the sensitivity as a positive finding on any of the three tests would produce the "further evaluation needed" verdict.

Clock Drawing Test (CDT)

The CDT (reproduced in the appendix to this chapter) is a basic "command and copy" task where the patient is either asked to draw a clock face with the numbers in the correct places or is given a pre-drawn circle and asked to fill in the numbers. Then, the patient is asked to make the clock read a certain time. One pitfall of this task is that it suffers from "too many cooks in the kitchen," as there is wide variation on how this test is administered and scored [23, 24]. Some clinicians feel that providing a pre-drawn circle is a missed opportunity to see how an individual initially organizes and executes a task, while others feel that the numbers and clock hands are more important. Most administrations require patients to draw some time so that one clock hand is on each vertical hemisphere of the circle (11:10, 10:50, 10:20, etc.) as a quick screen for visual neglect. We recommend giving the patient a blank sheet of paper and asking them to "draw a clock face with all the numbers on it and set the hands to 10 past 11." Patients who ask to have directions repeated or seem confused by the task may be showing signs of inattention, carelessness, or verbal processing difficulties. Incorrect drawings can indicate deficits in visual-spatial processing and/or executive dysfunction including planning and organization. Setting the hands to 10 and 11 (as opposed to 11 and 2) can be a sign that the patient is "stimulus bound" and may indicate executive dysfunction. Despite its simplicity, the CDT has been shown to be sensitive to mild impairment even when MMSE scores given to the same patients were in the normal range (> 23) [25], as well as identifying dementia and delirium in a sample of medical inpatients [26].

While many people who administer the CDT go by clinical judgment alone, it recommended that readers interested in this test seriously consider adopting a scoring method both to allow for test measurement error as well as flexibility in interpretation. One such scoring system exists based on patients diagnosed with Alzheimer's and Huntington's Diseases and can be found in the appendix to this chapter [27]. Points are divided between the accuracy of the clock face and the placement of numbers and clock hands with lower scores resulting from greater distortions or errors. Patient drawings typically fall into one of three categories: no errors, some errors, or major distortions. The scoring system will likely be of most use for those drawings that fall in the "some errors" category where the level of impairment is not easily classifiable. The authors of the scale recommend that scores of 9–10 do not suggest any difficulties, 8 = borderline impairment, 6–7 = mild impairment, 4–5 = moderate impairment, and 0–3 = major impairment.

Table 11.1 Description of scoring system for Clock Drawing Test

Clock face accuracy	
0–2 points	2 = no errors
	1 = minor errors (e.g., elliptical clock face)
	0 = major errors in clock face drawing (e.g., distorted circle, tick marks outside circle)
Clock numbers	
0–4 points	4 = no errors
	3 = slight spacing errors
	2 = major spacing errors or numbers outside the clock
	1 = gross distortion or added/missing numbers
	0 = no numbers or undecipherable characters
Clock hands	
0-4 points	4 = no errors
	3 = no difference in hand length
	2 = major clock hand placement error
	1 = one clock hand
	0 = no hands or errors in drawing (e.g., drawing lines between numbers instead of from center of clock)

Note. Adopted from original source [33].

Trail Making Test (TMT)

Like the CDT, the TMT [28] (reproduced in the appendix to this chapter) has a long history in neuropsychological assessment. Several expansions of the TMT exist, but the standard administration includes the Trails A and B test. The basic procedure for the test includes the patient drawing a line between stimuli in a predetermined sequential order. For Trails A, the patient is asked to draw a line connecting circled numbers from 1 to 25 as quickly as they can without making errors. This test is thought to primarily be an estimate of attention though other faculties such as visual-spatial processing and motor skill also contribute to completing this task. Recent research has suggested that in combination with several other neuropsychological tests, Trails A can help distinguish among patients with normal aging, dementia with Lewy bodies, and Alzheimer's disease [30]. Trails B requires patients to draw a line alternately connecting numbers and letters in ascending order. It is thought to be a measure of executive functioning beyond what is needed for Trails A. Patients' scores are based on the time to complete each task with longer times suggesting more impairment. On average, an unimpaired individual should be able to complete Trails A in about 30 s and Trails B in 60 s. Performances that fall within one standard deviation of the mean typically do not indicate significant impairment. Some debate has circulated about the nature of executive functioning required for the Trails B task with the two most discussed abilities being cognitive flexibility and response set maintenance [31]. Some research suggests that Trails B may have more to do with cognitive flexibility due to its unique relationship with the number of perseverative errors from the Wisconsin Cart Sorting Task [29].

Clinical Application

Using data from the 3MS, CDT, and TMT can provide the clinician with a range of information about a patient's functioning in areas of attention, memory, language, visual spatial, and executive skills. All three tests can yield a total score giving a general sense about a patient's gross cognitive structure, and the individual tasks can highlight more specific areas of concern. Although the 3MS does have several tasks that measure executive functioning (e.g., semantic fluency, pentagon drawing), it represents a small subset of higher order reasoning skills. With their quick administration time and ease of interpretation, the CDT and TMT can improve measurement of this important cognitive function. On medical floors, the 3MS can be an invaluable tool in detecting mild cognitive impairment. However, the addition of the TMT and CDT can often help the assessor identify problem areas even when patients are able to "pass" the MMSE. However, there are times when even the 3MS and the supplemental tests CDT and TMT are not sufficient to detect impairment.

Beyond Screening Instruments: Med-range Neuro-cognitive Assessment Tools

A correlation exists between a patient's level of functioning and the difficulty level of tests they should be administered. In other words, patients who are unable to properly execute their activities of daily living (e.g., showering, dressing, eating, taking medications) will likely struggle a great deal with more complex tests such as the Wisconsin Card Sorting Task or Wechsler Adult Intelligence Scales. However, such patients may perform well on very brief screening battery. Fortunately, there are brief measures that are more comprehensive that the MMSE or 3MS but take less time than a full neuropsychological assessment. The Repeatable Battery for the Assessment of Neuropsychological Status (RBANS) is a five-factor, 12-subtest instrument that measures Immediate and Delayed Memory, Visual spatial, Language, and Attention. The factors are transformed to standard scores (M = 100, SD = 15) and are summed to create a total index score. Total administration time is around 20–30 min. Unlike most other instruments, the RBANS has a counterbalanced alternate form to allow for ongoing monitoring of a patient's cognitive status. The RBANS has gained a great deal of clinical acceptability due to its quick administration, comprehensive coverage of cognitive domains, and psychometric foundation. Some distinctive features of the RBANS that makes it popular for comprehensive brief screenings are a word list and story recall (similar to the Wechsler Memory Scales), complex figure drawing (similar to Rey Complex Figure), and a word generation task. In many hospital settings, questions will arise about intellectual capacity either to assist in treatment planning or when seeking services from government agencies (i.e., Department of Mental Retardation). At 2–3 h administration time alone, most intelligence tests are too cumbersome for inpatient hospital work. The Wechsler Abbreviated Scales of Intelligence (WASI) was created, in part, to fill the role of needing a quick estimation of intellectual functioning [30]. The full version of the WASI contains the four subtests (Vocabulary, Similarities, Block Design, Matrix Reasoning) that have the strongest correlation to the VIQ and PIQ of the WAIS-III. While the items of the subtests are different from the WAIS-III to address practice effects, the rules of administration are identical. A four-subtest WASI takes about 30 min to complete and provides an estimation of VIQ, PIQ, and a FSIQ. A two-subtest WASI may also be given in about 15 min but only a FSIQ is provided. An estimated IQ score can add a great deal to a brief cognitive evaluation, as it may indicate that a patient's higher order cognitive abilities remain generally intact, despite the presence of neuropsychological deficits [32]. Tests such as the RBANS and WASI represent a step up in length and complexity from ultra brief measures such as the 3MS or CDT but do not have to act as replacement tests. For example, the 3MS and RBANS can complement each other and provide a more complete evaluation of their shared domains.

Summary

The purpose of this chapter was to provide the reader with a resource for using brief cognitive assessment tools. While the most commonly used test, the MMSE, has a long history in the medical and mental-health fields, it suffers from a ceiling effect thus making it prone to a high rate of false negatives. The 3MS was presented as an alternative to the MMSE along with a growing body of research showing that the 3MS is more sensitive to mild cognitive impairment, as well as being related to important treatment outcome variables (length of hospital stay, need for post-hospitalization services) within a psychiatric population. Adding other brief measures such as the CDT and TMT to the 3MS creates a standard brief screening test battery that can be used in a variety of clinical settings (inpatient unit, emergency room, clinical interview). Additional measures were also discussed that can be added to any assessment when a more thorough, yet relatively short, evaluation of cognitive (RBANS) or intellectual (WASI) status is necessary. The decision to use brief measures in any psychological assessment reflects a cost benefit analysis of time, necessity, and the level of information needed to clarify the clinical question. The information presented in this chapter was intended to help clinicians make informed and thoughtful choices when confronted with these challenging treatment situations.

References

1. Folstein M, Folstein S, McHugh P. Mini-mental state: A practical method for grading the cognitive state of patients for the clinician. *Journal of Psychiatric Research* 12: 189–198, 1975.
2. Roffman J, Stern T. Diagnostic rating scales and laboratory test. In Stern T, Fricchione G, Cassem N, Jellinek M, Rosenbaum J (Eds.) *Handbook of General Hospital Psychiatry*. (5th Ed), Philadelphia, 2004, Mosby Inc.

3. Jaeger J, Berns S. Neuropsychological management, treatment and rehabilitation of psychiatric patients, In Calev A (Ed.) *Assessment of Neuropsychological Functions in Psychiatric Disorders*. Washington, 1999, American Psychiatry Press.
4. Keefe R. The contribution of neuropsychology to psychiatry. *American Journal of Psychiatry*152: 6–14, 1995.
5. Harvey P, Howanitz E, Parrella M, White L, Davidson M, Mohs R, Hoblyn J, Davis K. Symptom, cognitive functioning, and adaptive skills in geriatric patients with lifelong schizophrenia: A comparison across treatment sites. *American Journal of Psychiatry* 155: 1080–1086, 1998.
6. Blais MA, Baity, MR. A comparison of mental status examinations in an inpatient psychiatric sample. *Assessment* 12: 455–461, 2005.
7. Galynker I, Harvey, P. Neuropsychological screening in the psychiatric emergency room. *Comprehensive Psychiatry* 33: 291–295, 1992.
8. Brown RG, Scott LC, Bench CJ, Dolan, RJ. Cognitive function in depression: Its relationship to the presence and severity of intellectual decline. *Psychological Medicine* 24: 829–847, 1994.
9. Folstein MF, Folstein SE, McHugh PR, Fanjang, G. *Mini-mental status* exam *user's guide*. Odessa, 2001, Psychological Assessment Resources.
10. Lopez MN, Charter, RA, Mostafavi, B, Nibut, LP, Smith, WE. Psychometric propertied of the Folstein Mini-Mental State Examination. *Assessment* 12: 137–144, 2005.
11. Tombaugh TN, McIntyre NJ. The Mini-Mental State Examination: A comprehensive review. *Journal of the American Geriatrics Society* 40: 922–935, 1992.
12. Teng EL, Chui HC. The Modified Mini-Mental State (3MS) Examination. *Journal of Clinical Psychiatry* 48: 314–318, 1987.
13. Candian Study of Health and Aging. The Canadian study of health and aging: Study methods and prevalence of dementia. *Canadian Medical Association Journal* 159: 899–913, 1994.
14. Sambrook R, Herrmann N, Hebert R, McCraken P, Robillard A, Luong D, Yu A. Canadian outcomes study in dementia: Study methods and patient characteristics. *Canadian Journal of Psychiatry* 49: 417–427, 2004.
15. Teng EL, Chui, HC, Gong A. Comparison between the Mini-Mental State Exam (MMSE) and its modified version – the 3MS test. *Psychogeriatrics: Biomedical and Social Advances*. Tokyo, 1990, Excerpta Media.
16. Lamarre CJ, Patten SB. Evaluation of the Modified Mini-Mental State Examination in a general psychiatric population. *Canadian Journal of Psychiatry*36: 507–511, 1991.
17. Grace J, Nadler JD, White DA, Guilmette TJ, Giuliano, AJ, Monsch AU, Snow MG. Folstein vs Modified Mini-Mental State Examination in geriatric stroke: Stability, validity, and screening utility. *Archives of Neurology* 52: 477–484, 1995.
18. Abraham IL, Manning CA, Boyd, MR, Neese JB, Newman MC, Plowfield LA, Reel SJ. Cognitive screening of nursing home patients: Factor structure of the Modified Mini-Mental State (3MS) Examination. *International Journal of Geriatric Psychiatry* 8: 133–138, 1993.
19. Bland RC, Newman SC. Mild dementia of cognitive impairment: The Modified Mini-Mental State Examination (3MS) as a screen for dementia. *Canadian Journal of Psychiatry* 46: 506–510, 2001.
20. Tombaugh TN, McDowell I, Kristjansson B, Hublet AM. Mini-Mental State Examination (MMSE) and the Modified MMSE (3MS): A Psychometric comparison and normative data. *Psychological Assessment*8: 48–59, 1996.
21. Rapp SR, Espeland MA, Hogan P, Jones BN, Dugan E. Baseline experience with the Modified Mini-Mental State Exam: The Women's Health Initiative Memory Study (WHIMS). *Aging & Mental Health* 7: 217–223, 2003.
22. Henry J, Crawford J. A meta-analytic review of verbal fluency performance following focal cortical lesions. *Neuropsychology* 18: 284–295, 2004.

23. Manos PJ, Wu R. The ten-point clock test: A quick screen and grading method for cognitive impairment in medical and surgical patients. *International Journal of Psychiatric Medicine* 24: 229–244, 1994.

24. Freedman M, Leach L, Kaplan E, Winocur G, Shullman KI, Delis DC. *Clock drawing: A neuropsychological analysis*. New York, 1994, Oxford University Press.

25. Manos PJ. Ten-point clock test sensitivity for Alzheimer's Disease in patients with MMSE scores greater than 23. *International Journal of Geriatric Psychiatry* 14: 454–458, 1999.

26. Manos PJ. The utility of the ten-point clock test as a screen for cognitive impairment in general hospital patients. *General Hospital Psychiatry* 19: 439–444, 1997.

27. Reitan RM. *Trail Making Test: Manual for Administration and Scoring*. Tucson, 1986, Reitan Neuropsychological Laboratory.

28. Ferman TJ, Smith GE, Boeve BF, Graff-Radford NR, Lucas JA, Knopman DS, Petersen RC, Ivnik RJ, Wszolek Z, Uitti R, Dickson DW. Neuoropsychological differentiation of dementia with Lewy bodies from normal aging and Alzheimer's disease.*Clinical Neuropsychologist* 20: 623–636, 2006.

29. Randolph C. *Repeatable Battery for the Assessment of Neuropsychological Status (RBANS)*. San Antonio, 1998, Psychological Corporation.

30. Wechsler D. *Wechsler Abbreviated Scales of Intelligence*. San Antontio, 1999, Psychological Corporation.

31. Kortte KB, Horner MD, Windham WK. The Trail Making Test Part B: Cognitive flexibility or failure to maintain set. *Applied Neuropsychology* 9: 106–109, 2002.

32. Axelrod BN, Validity of the Wechsler Abbreviated Scale of Intelligence and other very short forms of estimating intellectual functioning. *Assessment* 9: 17–23, 2002.

33. Rouleau I, Salmon DP, Butters N, Kennedy C, McGuire K. Quantitative and qualitative analyses of clock drawings in Alzheimer's and Huntington's Disease. *Brain and Cognition* 18: 70–87, 1992.

Clock Drawing Test

Patient's Name: _____   Date: _____

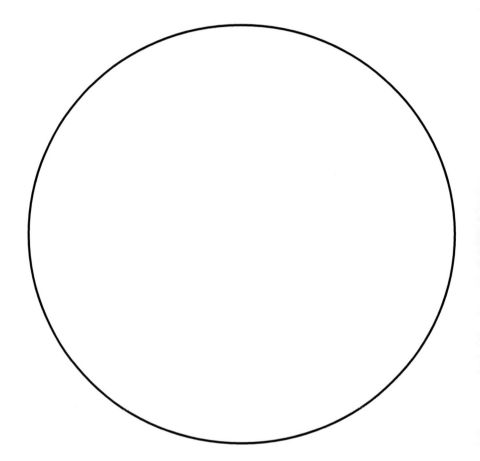

Instructions for the Clock Drawing Test:

Step 1:   Give patient a sheet of paper with a large (relative to the size of handwritten numbers) predrawn circle on it. Indicate the top of the page.

Step 2:   Instruct patient to draw numbers in the circle to make the circle look like the face of a clock and then draw the hands of the clock to read "10 after 11."

Scoring:

Score the clock based on the following six-point scoring system:

Score	Error(s)	Examples
1	"Perfect"	No errors in the task
2	Minor visuospatial errors	(a) Mildly impaired spacing of times (b) Draws times outside circle (c) Turns page while writing so that some numbers appear upside down (d) Draws in lines (spokes) to orient spacing
3	Inaccurate representation of 10 after 11 when visuospatial organization is perfect or shows only minor deviations	(a) Minute hand points to 10 (b) Writes "10 after 11" (c) Unable to make any denotation of time
4	Moderate visuospatial disorganization of times such that accurate denotation of 10 after 11 is impossible	(a) Moderately poor spacing (b) Omits numbers (c) Perseveration: repeats circle or continues on past 12–15, etc. (d) Right-left reversal: numbers drawn counterclockwise (e) Dysgraphia: unable to write numbers accurately
5	Severe level of disorganization as described in scoring of 4	See examples for scoring of 4
6	No reasonable representation of a clock	(a) No attempt at all (b) No semblance of a clock at all (c) Writes a word or name

Higher scores reflect a greater number of errors and more impairment. A score of   3 represents a cognitive deficit.

Trail Making Test (TMT) Parts A and B

Instructions:

Both parts of the Trail Making Test consist of 25 circles distributed over a sheet of paper. In Part A, the circles are numbered 1–25, and the patient should draw lines to connect the numbers in ascending order. In Part B, the circles include both numbers (1–13) and letters (A–L); as in Part A, the patient draws lines to connect the circles in an ascending pattern, but with the added task of alternating between the numbers and letters (i.e., 1-A-2-B-3-C, etc.). The patient should be instructed to connect the circles as quickly as possible, without lifting the pen or pencil from the paper. Time the patient as he or she connects the "trail." If the patient makes an error, point it out immediately and allow the patient to correct it. Errors affect the patient's score only in that the correction of errors is included in the completion time for the task. It is unnecessary to continue the test if the patient has not completed both parts after 5 minutes have elapsed.

Step 1:   Give the patient a copy of the Trail Making Test Part A worksheet and a pen or pencil.

Step 2:   Demonstrate the test to the patient using the sample sheet (Trail Making Part A – *SAMPLE*).

Step 3:   Time the patient as he or she follows the "trail" made by the numbers on the test.

Step 4:   Record the time.

Step 5:   Repeat the procedure for Trail Making Test Part B.

Scoring:

Results for both TMT A and B are reported as the number of seconds required to complete the task; therefore, higher scores reveal greater impairment.

	Average	Deficient	Rule of Thumb
Trail A	29 seconds	> 78 seconds	Most in 90 seconds
Trail B	75 seconds	> 273 seconds	Most in 3 minutes

Trail Making Test Part A

Patient's Name: _____   Date: _____

Trail Making Test Part A – *Sample*

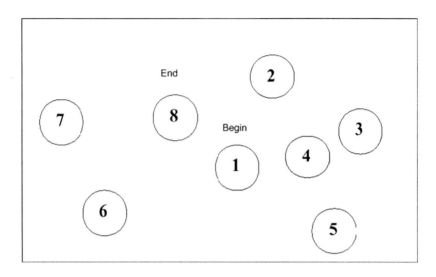

Trail Making Test Part B

Patient's Name: _____   Date: _____

Trail Making Test Part B – *Sample*

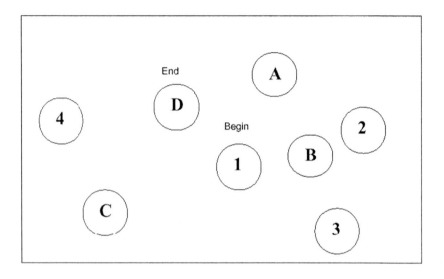

Chapter 12
Rating Scales in Psychotherapy Practice

Jesse Owen and Zac Imel

Abstract Therapists can gain invaluable information by administering rating scales to clients throughout the therapy process. Indeed, research has demonstrated therapists who utilize client feedback can improve their clients' outcomes. We provide an overview of the research of using rating scales in therapy. Next, we describe some practical considerations in the selection of rating scales; specifically, we highlight the benefits and feasibility of using global outcome and working alliance scales. Finally, we provide examples of brief, psychometrically sound, rating scales that can be integrated into practice.

Keywords Psychotherapy · Psychology · Rating scales · Questionnaires · Assessment · Psychiatry

Medical practitioners often rely on specific diagnostic tests to provide feedback on the progress of treatment and inform future decision making. Beyond diagnosis, the use of formalized assessment protocols to guide clinical decision making is decidedly less common in mental care. Feedback on the progress of treatment is often ambiguous and "maybe try" is a common collegial response to struggling clinicians in need of direction. Taking psychotherapists to task for this lack of specificity, Dawes [1] claimed:

> Two conditions are important for experiential learning: one, a clear understanding of what constitutes an incorrect response or error in judgment, and two, immediate, unambiguous feedback when such errors are made. In the mental health professions, neither of these conditions is satisfied (p. 111).

Although Dawes may go too far in his critique, it is fair to suggest that clinical experience does not often provide the stipulated conditions for learning (unlike surgery for example) from experience. Indeed, negotiating the confusion that accompanies

J. Owen (✉)
Licensed Psychologist, Assistant Professor, Department of Educational and Counseling Psychology, College of Education and Human Development University of Louisville, Louisville ky-40292
e-mail: owen002@gannon.edu

L. Baer, M.A. Blais (eds.), *Handbook of Clinical Rating Scales and Assessment in Psychiatry and Mental Health*, Current Clinical Psychiatry, DOI 10.1007/978-1-59745-387-5_12,
© Humana Press, a part of Springer Science+Business Media, LLC 2010

therapeutic work is a large part of the art of psychotherapy. Supervision has been the traditional avenue for instilling a reflective orientation in psychotherapy trainees [2]. However, supervised experience is less common after training and therapists can often be left without the resources to facilitate ongoing feedback on the progress of treatment. In the current chapter, we provide a rationale, based on a brief review of the therapy process and outcome literature, for why utilizing rating scales may help augment the clinical practice of therapists. First, we note that therapists are commonly more potent predictors of outcome in psychotherapy than is the type of treatment. Second, we note the therapeutic alliance as one potential source of this therapist variability and highlight the evidence that suggests providing therapists with feedback from patient-rated scales can enhance therapy outcomes. After a description of several rating scales, we focus on practical ways that therapists can incorporate rating scales into their practice.

Therapy Process and Outcome: What Do We Know?

After the claim of Eysenck [3] that psychotherapy is, at best, ineffective and at worst harmful, psychotherapy researchers have sought to demonstrate that psychotherapeutic treatments are beneficial to patients. Often, researchers compare various approaches of psychotherapy (e.g., cognitive-behavioral, interpersonal, psychodynamic) to determine if certain treatments are more effective than others. After a half century and hundreds of clinical trials, there is little support that any therapy is better than another in the treatment of most clinical disorders [4, 5]. Perhaps the most robust conclusion to be drawn from psychotherapy research is that treatment is more effective than no treatment and that bonafide psychotherapies [i.e., treatments that (a) are intended to be therapeutic (b) include a psychological rationale and the provision of some specific techniques, and (c) also include an emotionally-charged confiding relationship with a trained professional] are more effective than control or supportive interventions that are not intended to be therapeutic. For instance, Wampold et al. [6] meta-analyzed the effects of cognitive therapy as compared to other therapies for depression. They found that cognitive therapy was no more effective than other bonafide therapies; however, cognitive therapy did better than supportive interventions that were intended as control groups. Accordingly, the preponderance of evidence suggests that the differences between psychotherapies may not be nearly as important as what they have in common [7].

In contrast to treatment type, therapists account for a meaningful percentage of therapy outcomes [8, 9]. For instance, McKay et al. [10] reanalyzed the findings from the large NIMH treatment of depression collaborative research program [11] to examine the effects of psychiatrists who were providing either the imipramine hydrochloride or placebo on patient's rating of depression. They found that both psychiatrists and treatment accounted for variability in outcomes. However, psychiatrist effects were "at least as large, and probably larger, than medication effects" [10]. This finding appears to be generalizable to psychotherapy as well [12]. However, there is still limited understanding about why some therapists do better than others. For instance, therapists' years of experience, level of education (e.g., PhD., Masters'), or type of education (e.g., clinical, counseling, psychiatry) appear to have little relation to therapy outcome [13].

One major common factor across psychotherapies and a potential source of therapist differences is *therapeutic alliance* [14]. Indeed, the therapeutic alliance is among the most consistent predicts of outcome in psychotherapy [15]. For instance, patient ratings of poor therapeutic alliance early in therapy is an indicator of therapy drop out [16]. The therapeutic alliance has been generally defined as (a) the relational or emotional bond between patient and therapist, (b) agreement on the goals of therapy, and (c) the methods to reach those goals [17]. As noted by Hatcher and Barends [18], the alliance construct is not reducible to the bond between a therapist and patient but may capture the extent to which the dyad is involved in collaborative and meaningful work. Although therapist and client collaboration are likely involved in the formation of a solid alliance, it may also be that more effective therapists are better at developing strong alliances with their patients. One way for therapists to gain reliable information on how their patients have experienced the work of therapy is the regular use of process and outcome rating scales.

The Case for Rating Scales in Psychotherapy

Although the general trajectory of change in the psychotherapy process is well known and predictable, nearly 4–8% of patients deteriorate and approximately 25–50% of patients show no change in functioning at the time they leave therapy [19–24]. Early positive gains in therapy and the therapeutic alliance are two of the most valuable predictors of therapy outcome [25, 26]. Thus, providing therapists with this information may serve to enhance clinical judgments and warn of possible treatment failures.

To make judgments about clinical progress, many therapists rely on informal clinical decisions predicated on the wisdom of clinical experience. However, clinical experience lacks any clear relationship to enhanced clinical judgments or therapy outcome [27]. In fact, therapists are not particularly good at identifying patients who are deteriorating [25, 28]. However, research indicates that therapists who receive feedback on the progress of their patients are more effective than those who do not [26, 29–33]. In a large and diverse sample of psychotherapy patients ($N > 6{,}000$), Miller et al. [26] found that providing therapists with patients' ratings of therapy outcome and alliance nearly doubled therapists' effectiveness and reduced patients' dropout. Furthermore, Lambert [19], in a summary of his research program investigating the use of feedback to improve patient outcomes, concluded that feedback is particularly useful in helping therapists identify patients who are not improving in therapy. Consequently, therapists receiving feedback appear better equipped to make mid-treatment corrections and to provide better care for their more challenging patients.

More broadly, the use of rating scales may provide a feedback loop to thera-pists such that they may intervene with deteriorating patients before the treatment becomes a failure, or so that ruptures in the therapeutic alliance may be addressed. Accordingly, feedback can be seen as an on-going intervention. That is, the feed-back is a chance to *join or realign* with the patient throughout the course of therapy. These findings and clinical implications provide a clear justification for the use of feedback to enhance clinical practice.

Scale Selection Considerations

Due to the sheer number of scales in existence, scale selection can be a daunt-ing task. In addition to traditional psychometric issues, we suggest that therapists should consider both the purpose of the assessment and its logistical considerations when choosing a scale that will be integrated into clinical practice. These issues will be discussed with some practical suggestions to help guide the decision-making process.

Purpose of the Scales

Scales can be examined based on both their domain and scope. The two primary domains that should be assessed are therapy outcome and therapeutic alliance. Addi-tionally, therapists should consider the scope or the specificity (versus generality) of the scale. The scope of the therapy outcome scale(s) selected depends on patient need and the goals for therapy. Some patients have very specific goals (e.g., over-coming a major depressive episode) where more specific symptom-based scales might be warranted (e.g., Beck's Depression Inventory). However, many patients have multiple stressors or diagnoses and their gains in therapy are more global and would not be as easily captured by a specific disorder-based scale. In our experience, it can become burdensome for therapists to find a measure that fits each patient's symptoms. Moreover, patients with the same DSM-IV diagnosis might present very differently based on their specific symptomology, cultural background, personality factors, or other issues. However, the impact of most presenting problems can be captured in patients' perceptions of their overall psychological well-being. Accord-ingly, we suggest that therapists should, at minimum, assess overall psychological well-being.

In regards to therapeutic alliance, the other major domain, many scales are based on Bordin's [17] trans-theoretical model of the alliance (e.g., goals, methods, and bond). Some alliance scales have subscales for the three dimensions noted earlier (e.g., Working Alliance Inventory) while others assess therapeutic alliance more globally (e.g., Session Rating Scale [34]; Inpatient Therapeutic Alliance Scale [35]). Furthermore, the selection of a specific alliance scale may depend on the therapeutic modality. For instance, many alliance scales are designed to assess the relation-ship between the patient and therapist (i.e., individual therapy). In contrast, couples therapy involves multiple therapeutic relationships and alliances, which therapists might want to assess (e.g., couples alliance with each other, a patient's perception of his/her partner's alliance with the therapist, etc; see [36]). Regardless of the therapeutic approach, therapists can immediately use the information about the therapeutic alliance more directly in session, which is a notable advantage of these scales.

Logistical Considerations

Like most scholars, we agree that multiple sources of reporting (e.g., therapist, client, observer) are necessary to fully understand therapy process and outcome [37, 38]. However, given a choice, a patient's experience of process and outcome is perhaps the most valuable to track. There are many brief patient-rated scales (50 items or less [39]), which can be completed in a relatively short time (e.g., 5–10 min). Yet, with over two-thirds of psychologists not using any type of ratings scales in their practice [40], it begs the question: why not? One contributing factor could be that therapists feel that scales that take more than 5 min are impractical for use in weekly therapy [41]. In contrast, four to ten item scales have been developed that have clinical value, can be done in a matter of minutes, and have been found to be generally embraced by clinicians [42]. From a clinical perspective, a therapist can easily glance at four to ten items to determine how the patient is progressing or feeling about the therapeutic relationship. This is more challenging when the scales are longer. In our experience, scales that are easy for the patients to complete and for the therapists to score are more likely to be filled out each week. The ultimate value of the scales is through their consistent use, so the simplicity of the administration and scoring is vital.

Examples of Brief Scales for Therapy Practice

We highlight three scales that can be easily integrated into therapy practice: the Outcome Rating Scale (ORS [42]) and the Schwartz Outcome Scale (SOS-10 [43]) to assess therapy outcome and the Session Rating Scale (SRS [34]) to assess therapeutic alliance. Each of these scales is used extensively in clinics and provide useful information to clinicians, but is quick and easy to administer. In our description of these scales, we will focus on the psychometric properties of the scales and how to administer, score, and interpret the scales.

Generally, therapists can have more confidence in scales that have adequate psychometric properties (e.g., reliability and validity; see Chapter 1 and [44] for a discussion of psychometrics). Reliability describes the overall consistency of scores. While there are many indicators of reliability, the most commonly reported index is internal consistency (referred to as Cronbach's alpha). This index describes the commonality or relatedness between items. However, a reliable scale that provides irrelevant information is hardly useful. Thus, validity estimates provide information regarding the degree to which scores on a scale adequately reflect the construct of interest. Validity estimates are typically provided by correlations with other established scales and/or other outcomes (e.g., no hospitalizations, obtaining a job, etc).

Although estimates of psychometric properties are essential to determining the utility of a scale, the validity and reliability of a scale are products of the assessment environment and not completely of the measure itself. Specifically, if the patient does not feel safe providing the therapist feedback about the therapeutic alliance, any information obtained from a scale will be of limited utility. Thus, we encourage therapists to not be overly dogmatic about absolute scale scores. Rather, scales should be seen as therapeutic tools used in concert with clinical judgments and patient input.

Schwartz Outcome Scale-10

The SOS-10 [43] is a measure of psychological well-being, normed with patients from inpatient, outpatient, and college counseling settings as well as non-patient community and college samples. The purpose of the scale is to measure general well-being, not specific psychological symptoms. The SOS-10 is atheoretical, which enables practitioners from various disciplines (e.g., psychiatrists, social workers, psychologists, etc) and theoretical orientations (e.g., CBT, interpersonal, psychodynamic, integrative) to use the scale. The SOS-10 has 10 items that are rated on a seven-point Likert scale (*range* 0–6) where higher scores indicate better functioning (see appendix to this chapter).

Across studies, the SOS-10 has exhibited strong internal consistency; Cronbach's alpha (α) *range*= 0.90–0.96 [43, 45]. Cronbach's alpha should be in the high range for outcome and alliance scales (e.g., α =0.80–0.90). The SOS-10 is highly correlated with the longer Outcome Questionnaire-45 [46], a popular clinical outcome measure, at $r = -0.84$, which provides support for the validity of the scale [47]. Furthermore, validity evidence has been shown through correlations, in the predicted direction, with a variety of clinical and psychological well-being scales (e.g., Beck's Hopelessness Scale, PANAS, and Personality Assessment Inventory; see [45] for a review).

The SOS-10 should be given prior to the start of each session (possibly while the patient is in the waiting room). The scoring of the scale consists of summing the items of the scale (*range* 0–60). Scales that have more than two items missing are considered an invalid administration; however, for two or less missing items, mean replacement is suggested [45].

There are two main ways of using the scores obtained from the SOS-10. First, therapists can compare the scores to the norming sample as a frame of reference. In the norming sample, on average non-patients ($n = 2336$) scored 45.3, outpatients ($n = 1598$) 33.28, and inpatients ($n = 5119$) 25.57 [45]. Based on the distribution of scores, a *reliable cutoff score* between non-patient and patient sample is 41. This score reliably differentiates between clinical outpatients and non-clinical patients.

Second, therapists can monitor the gains in therapy on a weekly basis. Accordingly, scales should be sensitive to changes that occur on a weekly basis. The scale's sensitivity to change is typically described by the *reliable change index*.

In general, this score is based on the standard error of the scale. Consider the example of weighing yourself every morning. If you know the scale is accurate give or take two pounds, then when the scale goes up or down by more than two pounds you can be more confident that the scale reflects a change in your "true" weight and is not due to random fluctuation in the scale (error). Likewise, the reliable change index score enables therapists to detect meaningful changes over the course of therapy (versus error associated with the scale). For the SOS-10, the *reliable change index score* is calculated at 8.27 or simply 8 [45]. In other words, therapists can have confidence that changes in scores of 8 or more are not due to chance.

Outcome Rating Scale

The ORS was developed specifically to monitor therapy outcome [42]. The ORS has four items that assess global functioning (e.g., individual well-being, relationships, work/school, overall functioning [42]). It differs in format from the SOS-10. The ORS is a visual analog rating scale. That is, patients indicate their response by placing a mark (X) on a 10-cm line (see appendix to this chapter). Cronbach's alphas, for the ORS, have ranged from 0.79 to 0.93 [42, 48]. These scores are quite acceptable, especially considering the length of the scale. In terms of validity, the ORS has shown repeated correlations with the OQ-45, a widely used measure of symptom change in psychotherapy, average $r = 0.58$ [42].

The ORS should be administered prior to starting the session. To score the ORS, therapists measure the mark on the scale by using a ruler. Therapists should be sure that the line is 10 cm in length, so that the score reflects 0–10, with the millimeters used for a finite level of detail. The scores from the four items are added for a total score (*range* 0–40). Similar to the SOS-10, therapists can compare their patients' scores to the norming sample or the reliable change index. For instance, the ORS norming sample non-clinical patients typically score 28.0, clinical patients score 19.6, and the *reliable clinical cutoff score* is 25 [48]. In other words, patients who are generally distressed typically score 25 or below on the ORS. Furthermore, the reliable change index score is 4.3 [48]. As such, therapists can be confident that a change of five points is not due to chance. For example, if a patient had an initial ORS score of 7 and a fifth-session ORS score of 20, then the therapist can speculate that the client is still somewhat distressed, but has made significant change from intake that is not likely due to chance.

Session Rating Scale

The purpose of SRS is to measure the therapeutic alliance based on Bordin's concept of alliance and Duncan and Miller's (2000) client's theory of change [34]. The four-item scale focuses on therapeutic bond, goals, method, and general impression of the therapy process (see appendix to this chapter). Cronbach's alphas have been high ($\alpha = 0.88$–0.96) [48]. Furthermore, correlations with the Helping Alliance Questionnaire-II ($r = 0.48$) and a measure of therapy outcome ($r = 0.29$) demonstrate some validity for the SRS [34].

In contrast to the therapy outcome measures, the SRS should be given at the end of the session. The SRS shares the same format as the ORS and is scored similarly (*range* 0–40). The *reliable clinical cutoff score* for the SRS is 36. This cutoff indicates the likelihood of a patient having a negative therapy outcome or dropping out of therapy [48]. It is noteworthy that some patients might score very high because they do not want to hurt the feelings of the therapist. In these cases, therapists should process how the patients are interpreting the alliance scale, provide a safe environment for an honest discussion about the alliance, and address discrepancies between therapists' clinical impressions and patients' ratings if they emerge.

How to Use Rating Scales: From Intake to Termination

Therapists should be prepared for potential changes that may occur when starting to use rating scales in therapy. Enlisting patients in providing corrective feedback about the therapy process may begin a shift towards a more egalitarian approach to therapy. Additionally, patients and therapists may become more directly aware of progress (or lack thereof) and feelings about the therapeutic alliance. Consequently, therapists should be prepared for these possibilities and think about how they will address these issues with patients. In fact, it may be a willingness to discuss these issues that mediates the benefit of feedback in psychotherapy.

At intake, patients will need to be oriented to the purpose and procedure of completing the scales. This discussion is compatible (and can occur concomitantly) with therapists' general discussion about their approach to therapy and the therapeutic frame (e.g., length of treatment, options for treatment) that occurs in the initial session. The initial score will serve as a baseline level of functioning to compare with future ratings. After the intake session, the rating scales can be thought of as an ongoing intervention that addresses the questions: "are we making progress in therapy" and "are we working well together"?

The degree to which therapists use this information in session is dependent on their style and the scores. Some therapists discuss the scales and the meaning behind the scales each session. At minimum, we recommend that a discussion about the scales occurs often enough that the purpose of filling out the scales is not lost for the patients (e.g., once every three sessions). Furthermore, the feedback is most helpful for patients who are at risk for a negative outcome in therapy. Thus, it is important to address these issues immediately with these patients. For instance, if a patient was to score the SRS very low at the end of the session, therapists should address the disconnection in order to help prevent drop out.

Summary

The research examining the impact of using rating scales in practice has shown that patients benefit from providing the therapist with feedback. The use of rating scales, like the ORS, SRS, and SOS-10, which are easy to administer and score, allows a convenient transition to incorporating feedback into therapy practice. These rating scales can provide a systematic and reliable way to generate useful feedback about therapy outcome and the therapeutic relationship. We encourage therapists to empower themselves and their patients with feedback.

References

1. Dawes, R. M. (1994). *House of cards: Psychology and psychotherapy built on myth.* New York: Free Press.
2. Bernard, J. M., & Goodyear, R. K. (2004). *Fundamentals of clinical supervision* (3rd ed.). New York: Allyn & Bacon.
3. Eysneck, H. J. (1952). The effects of psychotherapy: An evaluation. *Journal of Consulting Psychology, 16,* 319–324.
4. Smith, M. A., & Glass, G. V. (1977). Meta-analysis of psychotherapy outcome studies. *American Psychologist, 32,* 752–760.
5. Wampold, B. E., Mondin, G. W., Moody, M., Stich, F., Benson, K., & Ahn, H. (1997). A meta-analysis of outcome studies comparing bona fide psychotherapies: Empirically, 'all must have prizes'. *Psychological Bulletin, 122:* 203–215.
6. Wampold, B. E., Minami, T., Baskin, T. W., Tierney, S. C. (2002). A meta – (re) analysis of the effects of cognitive therapy versus "other" therapists' for depression. *Journal of Affective Disorders, 68:* 159–165.
7. Imel, Z. E., & Wampold, B. E. (2008). The importance of treatment and the science of common factors in psychotherapy. In S. Brown, & R. W. Lent (Eds.), *The handbook of counseling psychology* (4th ed.) (pp. 249–266). New York: Wiley.
8. Okiishi, J. C., Lambert, M. J., Eggett, D., Nielsen, L., Dayton, D. D., Vermeersch, D. A. (2006). An analysis of therapist treatment effects: Toward providing feedback to individual therapists on their patients' psychotherapy outcome. *Journal of Clinical Psychology, 62:* 1157–1172.
9. Crits-Christoph, P., & Mintz, J. (1991). Implications of therapist effects for the design and analysis of comparative studies of psychotherapies. *Journal of Consulting and Clinical Psychology, 59:* 20–26.
10. McKay, K. M., Imel, Z. E., & Wampold, B. E. (2006). Psychiatrist effects in the psychopharmacological treatment of depression. *Journal of Affective Disorders, 92:* 287–290.
11. Elkin, I., Shea, M., Watkins, J., Imber, S., Sotsky, S., & Collins, J., et al., (1989). NIMH treatment of depression collaborative research program: General effectiveness of treatments. *Archives of General Psychiatry, 46:* 971–982.
12. Kim, D., Wampold, B. E., & Bolt, D. M. (2006). Therapist effects in psychotherapy: A random-effects modeling of the national institute of mental health treatment of depression collaborative research program data. *Psychotherapy Research, 16,* 161–172.
13. Beutler, L. E., Machado, P. P. P., & Neufeldt, S. A. (1994). Therapist variables. In A. E. Bergin & S. L. Garfield (Eds.) pp. 229–269. Handbook of psychotherapy and behavior change (4th ed.). New York: Wiley.
14. Orlinsky, D. E., Ronnestad, M. H., & Willutzki, U. (2004). Fifty years of process-outcome research: Continuity and change. In M. J. Lambert (Ed.), *Bergin and Garfield's handbook of psychotherapy.*
15. Horvath, A. O., & Bedi, R. P. (2002). The alliance. In J. C. Norcross (Ed.), *Psychotherapy relationships that work: Therapist contributions and responsiveness to patients.* (pp. 37–69). Oxford: Oxford University Press.
16. Miller, S. D., Duncan, B. L., & Hubble, M. A. (2004). Beyond integration: The triumph of outcome over process in clinical practice. *Psychotherapy in Australia, 10*(2), 2–19.

17. Bordin, E. S. (1979). The generalizability of the psychoanalytic concept of the working alliance. *Psychotherapy: Theory, Research, and Practice, 16,* 252–260.
18. Hatcher, R. L., & Barends, A. W. (2006). How a return to theory could help alliance research. *Psychotherapy: Theory, research, practice, training,* 43, 292–299.
19. Lambert, M. J. (2007). Presidential address: What we have learned from a decade of research aimed at improving psychotherapy outcome in routine care. *Psychotherapy Research, 17:* 1–14.
20. Haas, E., Hill, R., Lambert, M. J., & Morrell, B. (2002). Do early responders to psychotherapy maintain treatment gains? *Journal of Clinical Psychology, 58,* 1157–1172.
21. Whipple, J. L., Lambert, M. J., Vermeersch, D. A., Smart, D. W., Nielson, S. L., & Hawkins, E. J. (2003). Improving the effects of psychotherapy: The use of early identification of treatment failure and problem solving strategies in routine practice. *Journal of Counseling Psychology, 58,* 59–68.
22. Howard, K. I., Kopta, S. M., Krause, M. S., & Orlinsky, D. E. (1986). The dose-effect relationship in psychotherapy. *American Psychologist, 41,* 159–164.
23. Draper, M. R., Jennings, J., Baron, A., Erdur, O., Shankar, L. (2002). Time-limited counseling outcome in a nationwide college counseling center sample. *Journal of College Counseling, 5*(1), 26–38.
24. Nielsen, S. L., Smart, D. W., Isakson, R. L., Worthen, V. E., Gregersen, A. T., & Lambert, M. J. (2004). The consumer reports effectiveness score: What did consumers report? *Journal of Counseling Psychology, 51*(1), 25–37.
25. Hannan, C., Lambert, M. J., Harmon, C., Nielson, S. L., Smart, D. W., Shimokawa, K., & Sutton, S. W. (2005). A lab test and algorithms for identifying patients at risk for treatment failure. *Journal of Clinical Psychology: In Session, 61,* 155–163.
26. Miller, S. D., Duncan, B. L., Brown, J., Sorrell, R., & Chalk, M. B. (nd.). Using formal client feedback to improve retention and outcome: Making ongoing, real-time assessment feasible. Unpublished manuscript.
27. Garb, H. N. (1998). *Studying the clinician: Judgment research and psychological assessment.* Washington, D.C.: American Psychological Association.
28. Norcross, J.C. (2003). Empirically supported therapy relationships. In J. C. Norcross (Ed.), Psychotherapy relationships that work (pp. 3–16). New York: Oxford University Press.
29. Hawkins, E. J., Lambert, M. J., Vermeersch, D. A., Slade, K., & Tuttle, K. (2004). The effects of providing patient progress information to therapists and patients. *Psychotherapy Research, 14,* 308–327.
30. Lambert, M. J., Whipple, J. L., Smart, D. W., Vermeersch, D. A., Nielsen, S. L., & Hawkins, E. J. (2001). The effects of providing therapists with feedback on patient progress during psychotherapy: Are outcomes enhanced? *Psychotherapy Research, 11,* 49–68.
31. Lambert, M. J., Whipple, J. L., Vermeersch, D. A., Smart, D. W., Hawkins, E. J., Nielson, S. L., & Goates, M. K. (2002). Enhancing psychotherapy outcomes via providing feedback on patient progress: A replication. *Clinical Psychology and Psychotherapy, 9,* 91–103.
32. Harmon, S. C., Lambert, M. J., Smart, D. W., Hawkins, E. J., Nielson, S. L., Slade, K., & Lutz, W. (2007). Enhancing outcome for potential treatment failures: Therapist/patient feedback and clinical support tools. *Psychotherapy Research, 17,* 379–392.
33. Lambert, M. J., Whipple, J. L., Hawkins, E. J., Vermeersch, D. A., Nielson, S. L., & Smart, D. W. (2003). Is it time for clinicians to routinely track patient outcome? A meta-analysis. *Clinical Psychology: Science & Practice, 10:* 288–201.
34. Duncan, B. L., Miller, S. D., Sparks, J. A., Claud, D. A., Reynolds, L. R., Brown, J., & Johnson, L. D. (2003). The session rating scale: Preliminary psychometric properties of a working alliance measure. *Journal of Brief Therapy, 3,* 3–12.
35. Blais, M. A. (2004). Development of an inpatient treatment alliance scale. *Journal of Nervous and Mental Disease, 192*(7), 487–493.
36. Pinsoff, W. M. (1994). An integrative systems perspective on the therapeutic alliance: Theoretical, clinical, and research implications (pp. 173–195). In A. O. Horvath & L. S.

Greenberg (Eds.), The Working Alliance: Theory, Research, and Practice. New York: John Wiley & Sons.

37. Lambert, M. J., & Ogles, B. M. (2004). The efficacy and effectiveness of psychotherapy. In M. J. Lambert (Ed.), Bergin and Garfield's handbook of psychotherapy and behavior change (5th ed., pp. 139–193). Oxford: Wiley.

38. Lambert, M. J. & Hawkins, E. J. (2004). Measuring outcome in professional practice: Considerations in selecting and using brief outcome instruments. *Professional Psychology: Research and Practice, 35*(5), 492–499.

39. Fisher, J.& Corcoran, K. (2007). *Measures for Clinical Practice and Research: A Source Book* (4th ed., vol. 2), pp. 661–662. Oxford Publishing.

40. Phelps, R., Eisman, E. J., & Kohout, J. (1998). Psychological practice and managed care: Results of the CAPP practitioner survey. *Professional Psychology: Research and Practice, 29,* 31–36.

41. Brown, J., Dreis, S., & Nace, D. (1999). What really makes a difference in psychotherapy outcome? Why does managed care want to know? In M. A. Hubble, B. L. Duncan, & S. D. Miller (Eds.) The Heat and Soul of Change: What works in therapy (pp. 389–406). Washington D.C.: APA Press.

42. Miller, S. D., Duncan, B. L., Brown, J., Sparks, J. A., & Claud, D. A. (2003). The outcome rating scale: A preliminary study of the reliability, validity, and feasibility of a brief visual analog measure. *Journal of Brief Therapy, 2,* 91–100.

43. Blais, M. A., Lenderking, W. R., Baer, L., deLorell, A., Peets, K., Leahy, L., & Burns, C. (1999). Development and initial validation of a brief mental health outcome measure. *Journal of Personality Assessment, 73,* 359–373.

44. Clark, L. A. & Watson, D. (1995). Constructing validity: Basic issues in objective scale development. Psychological Assessment, 7(3), 309–319.

45. Blais, M. A. & Baity, M. R. (2005). *Administration and scoring manual for the Schwartz Outcome Scale-10 (SOS-10).* Department of Psychiatry Massachusetts General Hospital Harvard Medical School.

46. Lambert, M. J., Burlingame, G. M., Umphress, V. J., Hansen, N. B., Vermeersch, D., Clouse, G., & Yanchar, S. (1996). The reliability and validity of the Outcome Questionnaire. *Clinical Psychology and Psychotherapy, 3,* 106–116.

47. Young, J. L., Waehler, C. A., Laux, J. M., McDaniel, P. S., & Hilsenroth, M. J. (2003). Four studies extending the utility of the Schwartz outcome scale (SOS-10). *Journal of Personality Assessment, 80,* 130–138.

48. Miller, S. D. & Duncan, B. L. (2004). The outcome and session rating scales: administration and scoring manual. Institute for the Study of Therapeutic Change.

Schwartz Outcome Scale – 10 Item Version (SOS-10)

Name: _____ .   **Date:**

SOS-10 ™

Instructions: Below are 10 statements about you and your life that help us see how you feel you are doing. Please respond to each statement by circling the response number that best fits how you have generally been over the last seven days (1 week). There are no right or wrong responses, but it is important that your response reflect how you feel you are doing. Please be sure to respond to each statement.

1) **Given my current physical condition, I am satisfied with what I can do.**
    Never   0   1   2   3   4   5   6   All or nearly all of the time

2) **I have confidence in my ability to sustain important relationships.**
    Never   0   1   2   3   4   5   6   All or nearly all of the time

3) **I feel hopeful about my future.**
    Never   0   1   2   3   4   5   6   All or nearly all of the time

4) **I am often interested and excited about things in my life.**
    Never   0   1   2   3   4   5   6   All or nearly all of the time

5) **I am able to have fun.**
    Never   0   1   2   3   4   5   6   All or nearly all of the time

6) **I am generally satisfied with my psychological health.**
    Never   0   1   2   3   4   5   6   All or nearly all of the time

7) **I am able to forgive myself for my failures.**
    Never   0   1   2   3   4   5   6   All or nearly all of the time

8) **My life is progressing according to my expectations.**
    Never   0   1   2   3   4   5   6   All or nearly all of the time

9) **I am able to handle conflicts with others.**
    Never   0   1   2   3   4   5   6   All or nearly all of the time

10) **I have peace of mind.**
    Never   0   1   2   3   4   5   6   All or nearly all of the time

Outcome Rating Scale (ORS)

Name _____ Age (Yrs):____
ID# _____ Sex: M / F
Session # ____ Date: _____

Looking back over the last week, including today, help us understand how you have been
doing in the following areas of your life, where marks to the left represent low levels and
marks to the right indicate high levels.

Individually:
(Personal well-being)

_____

Interpersonally:
(Family, close relationships)

_____

Socially:
(Work, School, Friendships)

_____

Overall:
(General sense of well-being)

_____

Institute for the Study of Therapeutic Change
_____

(For individual use only after signed agreement – download copies from this website
www.talkingcure.com)

© 2000, Scott D. Miller and Barry L. Duncan

Session Rating Scale Version 3.0 (SRS V.3.0)

Name _____	Age (Yrs):____
ID# _____	Sex: M / F
Session # ____ Date: _____	

Please rate today's session by placing a hash mark on the line nearest to the description that best fits your experience.

Relationship:

I did not feel heard, understood, and respected	———————————————————————	I felt heard, understood, and respected
We did not work on or talk about what I wanted to work on and talk about	———————————————————————	We worked on and talked about what I wanted to work on and talk about
The therapist's approach is not a good fit for me.	———————————————————————	The therapist's approach is a good fit for me.
There was something missing in the session today	———————————————————————	Overall, today's session was right for me

Institute for the Study of Therapeutic Change

(For individual use only after signed agreement – download copies from this website www.talkingcure.com)

Chapter 13
Assessing the Ongoing Psychological Impact of Terrorism

Samuel J. Sinclair and Alice LoCicero

> *At present the psychological science needed to provide proper and effective treatment for victims of horrendous events such as September 11... simply does not exist.*
>
> *Bruce Bongar [1]*

Abstract The terror attacks of 9/11/2001 dealt a serious blow to the sense of security, well-being, and economic stability of Americans, and altered the mental health landscape for those within the United States and other parts of the world. Paralleling this, new threats to emotional and psychological well-being have materialized in the form of anticipatory, prospective fears of future terrorist attacks. In light of this evolving environment, the present chapter seeks to augment the current science by presenting an assessment paradigm relevant to terrorist events specifically. This approach to psychological assessment expands on current models which focus on the impact of discrete events by also evaluating the impact of prospective fears of future attacks. Reflecting this paradigm shift, we introduce the *Terrorism Catastrophizing Scale (TCS)* as a means of evaluating the ongoing impact of terrorism on psychological functioning.

Keywords Terrorism catastrophizing scale · TCS · Pre-traumatic stress syndrome · Anticipatory fear · Terrorism · Trauma

Introduction

Since the horrific events of 9/11, the socio-political environment has been radically changed and new threats to emotional and psychological well-being have emerged. The purpose of this chapter is to present an assessment paradigm suitable for use

S.J. Sinclair (✉)
Massachusetts General Hospital and Harvard Medical School, Department of Psychiatry, Psychological Evaluation and Research Laboratory (the PEaRL), One Bowdoin Square 7th floor, Boston, MA 02114, USA
e-mail: jsincl@post.harvard.edu

L. Baer, M.A. Blais (eds.), *Handbook of Clinical Rating Scales and Assessment in Psychiatry and Mental Health*, Current Clinical Psychiatry, DOI 10.1007/978-1-59745-387-5_13, © Humana Press, a part of Springer Science+Business Media, LLC 2010

following terrorist events. This approach to assessment is not simply limited to the immediate effects of the discrete attacks, themselves, but begins to address the need for more comprehensive assessment outlined below. In addition, we introduce the Terrorism Catastrophizing Scale (TCS, reproduced in the appendix to this chapter), a recently developed instrument designed to evaluate the ongoing impact of terrorism on psychological functioning.

As Bongar points out, the infrastructure for assessing and treating people in the wake of mass-casualty terrorist attacks is only now being developed, as a function of the new urgency to understand and plan for such contingencies in light of the events over the last 8 years [1]. We must create a body of scientific knowledge in the following three areas before effective response models are able to be developed:

1) The specific and unique aspects of reactions to terrorism as differentiated from reactions to other man-made or natural disasters.
2) The range of reactions, including but not limited to PTSD, that adversely impact those affected.
3) The effects of anticipating future attacks, including variations that may manifest following (a) reports of distant terrorist attacks and (b) changes in the perceived immediacy of the threat of a local attack.

Anticipation of Future Terrorism

Part of the challenge in developing this science has been that traditional measurement systems have not always translated well to the issue of terrorism. For example, research has shown that population rates for disorders such as post-traumatic stress disorder (PTSD) specific to terrorist attacks like 9/11/2001 generally returned to baseline in the general population after a few months [2–5]. Despite this, the terrorist threat against countries such as the United States continues, potentially affecting people's health and functioning in negative ways. The impact of these ongoing threats is supported both by preliminary research [6–7] and by polling evidence [8]. In relation to the US government's color-coded terror alert system, Zimbardo has characterized this psychological phenomenon as a "pre-traumatic stress syndrome," and he is careful to differentiate between reactions to discrete past events (retrospective reactions) and fearing future devastating attacks (prospective reactions) [9].

In general, research has focused almost exclusively on assessing rates of psychopathology *in response* to discrete attacks such as 9/11, without much attention paid to ongoing reactions and fears, and specifically how anticipating future attacks impacts people's functioning moving forward. Ruzek et al. recently noted, "Although some interventions exist to help individuals cope with the aftermath of trauma and terrorism, there is scarce information about how people deal with the ongoing and potential threat of terrorism, especially in communities at risk" [10]. They make recommendations for interventions that are extrapolated from the existing literature on disaster mental health, given that no research has been available on terrorism impact specifically. Despite this, experts have pointed out that there are emerging problems with this method, including evidence that traditional treatments and assessment methodologies do not translate well to victims of terrorist attacks [11].

Unique Reactions to Terrorism

There are several reasons why terrorism is a special case of disaster, needing specific attention. First and foremost, as noted by the International Society for Traumatic Stress Studies (ISTSS), terrorism poses an ongoing sense of "exposure to, or threat of danger" [12]. This ongoing sense of threat is apt to have all the intended and unintended consequences of fear, anxiety, and stress. Second, for the community, the terrorists who perished in the 9/11 attacks represent an unknown, but presumed large number of others who are at large and who are willing and interested in harming us. This causes a decrease in general trust, a tendency to apply strict ingroup–outgroup distinctions, and thus limits openness to experience. Third, the planful destruction by terrorists, along with the threat of future terrorist attacks, forces members of the community to consider the potential of humans for destruction. While consigning them to an outgroup status, often colloquially called "evil doers," may help dissociate victim from perpetrator, this does not always work completely and leaves many pondering the human potential for hatred, violence, and destruction.

Gold Standard Scales

Perhaps in future editions of this volume, this chapter will cite multiple measures designed to assess the ongoing psychological impact of terrorism. However, as of yet, there exists no *Gold Standard* assessment tools in this area. Only recently has the paradigm shifted towards assessing the impact of prospective fears about terrorism, as opposed to the existing tools that are designed to measure "traumatic event exposure and post-traumatic effects," as discussed by Elhai et al. [13]. This chapter proposes a new measurement paradigm for understanding the ongoing psychological impact of terrorism that addresses a unique feature of terrorism in comparison with most other disasters: the likelihood of it happening again. It proposes a framework that is prospective, as opposed to the current paradigm that is retrospective. The Terrorism Catastrophizing Scale (TCS) [7] represents the first known tool rooted in this new paradigm.

Empirical and Theoretical Bases of the TCS

The development of the *Terrorism Catastrophizing Scale* (*TCS*) is a reaction to the recent call to academia to develop the "psychological science" necessary to provide proper and effective mental-health treatment for victims and others suffering as a result of terrorist attacks [7]. Since effective treatment must begin with valid and reliable assessment, we developed the TCS to measure the effects of ongoing fear of future terrorism. Rather than importing assessment methodologies from general disaster mental health, a methodology that has not always translated well, we have developed a tool to assess prospective fears of terrorism directly and specifically. This reflects our agreement with Flynn [11], who noted, "research [on terrorism response] is not nearly as extensive and complete as it needs to be and we are far too dependent on extrapolation from other types of traumatic events."

The TCS specifically measures the extent to which people experience antici-patory fears, or "catastrophize" about, future terrorism. Terror management [13] (TMT) and cognitive-behavioral [14–15] theories were used as theoretical frame-works, and are helpful in terms of framing *how* people function under the constant threat of annihilation by terrorism. TMT provides a conceptual framework for why people become so fearful of dying in a terrorist attack following events such as 9/11, and how people psychologically manage the inevitability of death, also referred to as "mortality salience." For many, particularly those proximal to the attacks, mass-casualty terrorism invokes anxiety and fear rooted in the recognition of the reality, and perceived greater likelihood, of death. Two variables have been shown to moderate these fears: (1) culture as providing a meaningful, stable, and perma-nent reality and (2) the belief that self is a meaningful and significant contributor to this reality [13].

Beck's cognitive model of psychopathology addresses how people develop pat-terned and generally consistent thought processes based on their experiences. Specific patterns of cognitive disorganization (also known as cognitive distortions) have been shown to predispose one to various forms of psychopathology [14]. The literature on cognitive distortions has shown that "catastrophizing" is a primary, underlying cognitive process fueling disorders of mood and anxiety [16–19].

A Cognitive-Behavioral Model of the Impact of Terrorism

A cognitive-behavioral model specific to the impact of terrorism is presented in Fig. 13.1, and outlines the cycle of terrorism-related fears, beginning with the cognitive process at the top of the figure.

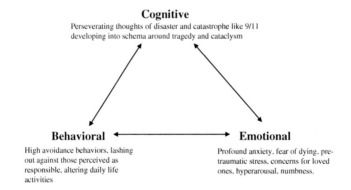

Fig. 13.1 A cognitive-behavioral model of the psychological impact of terrorism

Upon experiencing a terrorist event, it is hypothesized that people's schemas and ways of knowing around safety and security are challenged. As time passes, fears of further attacks persist. Often, such as following the attacks of 9/11/2001, the national debate on terrorism expands to include the probable use of biological, chemical, radiological, and nuclear weapons, which only serves to exacerbate existing fears [20–21]. This new sense of threat fuels the reorganization of existing schema (e.g., "My family and loved ones and I are safe") and the development of new schema (e.g., "The world is an extremely unsafe place" and "It is likely I will die in a terrorist attack"), especially for those close to New York City and Washington D.C. [5]. Faced with a constant sense of impending threat, some feel they are unable to do anything to minimize new threats and are unable to stop thinking about them. These problematic reactions map onto the underlying constructs identified by Sullivan et al., as being central to the process of catastrophizing: rumination, magnification, and helplessness [19].

Magnification. Magnification is defined as always thinking the worst will happen, despite evidence to the contrary [14–15, 22]. In terms of the terrorism threat, it is the notion that despite evidence to the contrary, catastrophic terrorism will continue and get worse. It also will likely involve the person believing that he or she will be a future victim of terrorism, despite the actual odds of this happening being very low.

Helplessness. Building on the work of Beck [23], Abramson et al. [24] proposed the learned hopelessness model of depression. This model assumes that various types of emotional disorders, and specifically hopeless depression, results as a consequence of two factors: (1) a negative-outcome expectancy and (2) a helplessness expectancy [25]. The former is conceptualized as being similar in nature to catastrophizing, or the notion that extremely unfavorable outcomes will continue and favorable outcomes will not. The latter construct (helplessness) relates to a person's belief that there is nothing he or she can do to change the likelihood of these outcomes. With respect to terrorism, helplessness has to do with the notion that there is nothing one can do to escape the threat, leaving oneself constantly vulnerable.

Rumination. In addition to the specific ways in which people distort their interpretation of events, which is more content focused, the notion of how people respond to having these distortions and to what extent they ruminate about these interpretations is important [26]. Nolen-Hoeksema has argued that the variability in severity and duration of depression and anxiety is directly related to how people respond to their mood states [27–28]. Those who ruminate over the mood states have a tendency to exacerbate their moods, whereas those who are easily able to distract themselves from their mood states are able to feel greater relief. A ruminative response style is one where individuals focus their attention on their symptoms, and on the potential causes and effects of those symptoms. According to Nolen-Hoeksema et al., ruminating may exacerbate mood in three different ways: (1) in negatively biasing how people think about and appraise events, (2) interfering with basic activities involving attention and concentration, which may lead to greater complications, and (c) interfering with more complex problems which impede the ability to attend to and problem-solve life's problems [26].

Development and Psychometric Testing of the TCS

After a thorough evaluation of psychometric properties and scaling assumptions, we developed a final 13-item version of the TCS from a larger item pool to measure: rumination ($k=5$), magnification ($k=3$), and helplessness ($k=5$). This process involved evaluating the scaling assumptions underlying the TCS scales, and included assessing item convergent and discriminant validity, internal consistency reliability, floor and ceiling effects, evaluation of the underlying factor structure, and the predictive validity of the scales and catastrophizing summary measure (Fig. 13.2).

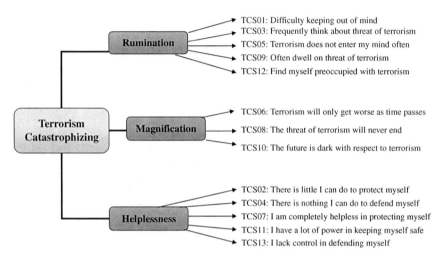

Fig. 13.2 The terrorism catastrophizing scale

A sample of adults ($N = 503$) representative of the general US population was used to evaluate the scaling assumptions and factor structure of the TCS, and to generate the norms used in scoring the scales and overall summary measure. Instructions for scoring are presented below.

Application and Method/Timing of TCS Administration

The TCS is a self-report questionnaire, where respondents are given a copy of the tool and are asked to answer the 13 items as best as they can. The TCS can also be administered by interview, where a clinician reads the questions followed by the response categories, and asks the respondent to select their answer to each question. However, current norms are based on self-administration, and mode effects should be considered if administered by interview. Administration time lasts somewhere between 3 and 6 minutes.

Scoring the TCS Scales and Summary Measure

Scoring instructions for the TCS scales and summary measure are provided here. Three scales (rumination, magnification, and helplessness) are scored to have a mean of 50 and standard deviation of 10 in the general US population. Using the principal components analysis scoring coefficients for these three scales (presented below), an overall catastrophizing summary measure is then aggregated. TCS items, scales, and overall summary measure are scored such that a higher score is indicative of greater magnitude of the construct. For example, someone scoring higher on the rumination scale would be thinking about and preoccupied with the threat of terrorism to a greater extent, whereas someone scoring lower would be thinking about terrorism less. Table 13.1 provides a brief summary of the content for the three TCS scales.

Table 13.1 Scoring the terrorism catastrophizing scale

Scale	Sum final item values (after recoding)	Lowest, highest possible raw score	Possible raw score range	Population Mean[a]	Population Standard Deviation[a]
Rumination	TCS01+TCS03+ TCS05+TCS09+ TCS12	5,25	20	33.3301924	22.0691549
Magnification	TCS06+TCS08+ TCS10	3,15	12	46.6563541	23.4780115
Helplessness	TCS02+TCS04+ TCS07+TCS11+ TCS13	5,25	20	45.3901830	21.7938409

[a]Population means (0–100 scoring) and standard deviations are derived from the US general population sample (Sinclair & LoCicero, in review).

Step 1: Item Recoding
   All out-of-range values, if unverifiable, should first be set to missing. Second, 11 items need to be reverse scored (TCS01, TCS02, TCS03, TCS04, TCS06, TCS07, TCS08, TCS09, TCS10, TCS12, and TCS13). Recoding can be done using the following formula:

$$\text{Recoded Value} = 6 - \text{original Value}$$

Step 2: Calculating 0–100 Scores for the Three TCS Scales
   The three TCS scales (rumination, magnification, and helplessness) are scored if half of the scale items or greater have been answered. When at least

half but not all of the items comprising a scale have been answered, a mean item value is calculated based on those items that have been answered. This value is imputed for those items with missing data. Second, items within a scale are then summed after recoding to derive the simple "sum-score." This score is then converted to a 0–100 metric, such that the score represents the percentage of the total possible score achieved, where higher values indicate a greater degree of the construct. See the following formula for the 0–100 transformation:

$$\text{Transformed scale} = \frac{(\text{actual raw score} - \text{lowest possible raw score})}{\text{possible raw score range}}$$

Step 3: Calculating Norm-Based (50/10) Scores for the Three TCS Scales

Using the normative means and standard deviations for the three scales (0–100 scores) presented in Table 13.1, scores are then transformed using a linear Z-score transformation to have a mean of 50 and standard deviation of 10 in the general US population to assist with interpretation. The following formulas are used to derive norm-based (50/10) scores:

Rumination:
RUMINATION Z SCORE=(RAW SCORE–33.3301924)/22.0691549;
RUMINATION SCALE SCORE=(Z SCORE∗10)+50;

Magnification:
MAGNIFICATION Z SCORE=(RAW SCORE–46.6563541)/23.4780115;
MAGNIFICATION SCALE SCORE=(Z SCORE∗10)+50;

Helplessness:
HELPLESSNESS Z SCORE=(RAW SCORE–45.3901830)/21.7938409;
HELPLESSNESS SCALE SCORE=(Z SCORE∗10)+50;

Step 4: Scoring the Terrorism Catastrophizing Summary Measure

The final step involves scoring the Terrorism Catastrophizing Summary Measure. After a Z-score has been computed for each scale (see above), they are aggregated using the Principal Components Analysis scoring coefficients for the normative sample ($N = 503$). Each Z score is multiplied by its respective factor score coefficient, summed, and transformed to have a mean of 50 and standard deviation of 10 in the general US population.

The following formula and scoring coefficients are used:
CATASTROPHIZING Z SCORE = (RUMINATION Z SCORE ∗ **0.46288**) +
(MAGNIFICATION Z SCORE∗ **0.54382**) +
(HELPLESSNESS Z SCORE ∗ **0.32517**);
CATASTROPHIZING SUMMARY SCORE = (CATASTROPHIZING Z SCORE∗10) + 50;

Please contact Samuel Sinclair at jsincl@post.harvard.edu for a TCS scoring program written in SAS.

Interpretation

The TCS profile and summary scores are calculated using norm-based scoring methods, and are referenced against a representative sample of adults living within the United States. The primary advantage of using the norm-based scoring methodology (T scores) is the added interpretation that comes with the scores, and knowledge about where they fall in the normal distribution. For example, someone with a T score of 60 on the three scales (rumination, magnification, and helplessness) and/or the Catastrophizing summary measure means that this person is 1 SD above the mean and in roughly the 84th percentile, and someone with a T score of 70 means they are 2 SD above the mean and in roughly the 96th percentile. Those scoring within this latter range are actively engaged in thinking about and magnifying the threat of terrorism, and are experiencing a significant amount of helplessness with respect to this threat. People with T scores above 70 for the overall catastrophizing summary measure are likely to report elevated symptoms of depression, anxiety, and stress, and are more likely to have changed their lives and behaviors as a result of this threat. In our norming sample, people scoring at 70 or above have also been shown to score at levels consistent with major depressive disorder using instruments such as the SF-8 Health Survey and Depression, Anxiety, and Stress Scales [30–31].

In addition to psychopathology, TCS scores have been found to be significantly related to behavioral change. That is, those scoring higher on the TCS scales and summary measure were more likely to reduce their behavior in, or completely avoid one or more of the following: (1) flying, (2) using public transportation, such as buses or trains, (3) traveling into public places, such as a mall or stadium, (4) voting in national or local elections, (5) interacting with other people from different racial and ethnic groups, (6) vacationing in certain areas thought to be targets, (7) working, going to school, or living in certain areas thought to be high-risk, such as in cities or skyscrapers, and (8) consuming terrorism-related media. In general, T scores at or above 55 corresponded with some degree of behavioral change. T scores below 55 did not reflect the likelihood that the individual was altering their lives in meaningful ways [7].

The TCS is interpreted in a two-step process, following the scoring of the profile scales and overall summary measure. First, the Catastrophizing summary measure is evaluated to see the degree to which it deviates from the norm (T score of 50). A T score of 70 or greater indicates a degree of symptoms and problems that is extremely unusual in the general population and likely reflects a clinically significant issue meriting attention. The second step involves evaluating the three sub-scales (rumination, magnification, and helplessness) to better clarify the meaning of elevations of the overall summary measure. For example, one person may elevate all three sub-scales into the clinical range, indicating a significant amount of time spent thinking about this threat, the belief that this threat is catastrophic, and a substantial amount of helplessness experienced as a result. In contrast, someone else may elevate the magnification and helplessness sub-scales, but not rumination, which might suggest substantial concerns about the terrorist threat, but more of an avoidant style

Table 13.2 Score ranges for mild, moderate, sub-clinical, and clinically significant severity

T-score range	Severity	Summary
0–49	Mild	Reflects minor amount of rumination, magnification, helplessness, and overall catastrophizing. The threat of terrorism does not impact the individual in a significant manner. This person will likely be experiencing no symptoms of depression, anxiety, or stress related to the terrorism threat, and will likely not be modifying their life routine to reduce perceived threat.
50–59	Moderate	Reflects somewhat elevated amount of rumination, magnification, helplessness, and overall catastrophizing. The threat of terrorism impacts the individual in a moderate manner. This person will likely be experiencing mild symptoms of anxiety, stress, and depression related to the terrorism threat, and will likely be modifying their life routine to reduce perceived threat in minor ways.
60–69	Sub-clinical	Reflects sub-clinical elevations of rumination, magnification, helplessness, and overall catastrophizing. The threat of terrorism impacts the individual in a meaningful and substantial manner. This person will likely be experiencing substantial symptoms of anxiety, stress, and depression related to the terrorism threat, and will likely be modifying their life routine to reduce perceived threat in significant ways.
70+	Clinically significant	Reflects clinically significant elevations of rumination, magnification, helplessness, and overall catastrophizing. The threat of terrorism impacts the individual in an extreme manner. This person will likely be experiencing clinically significant symptoms of anxiety, stress, and depression related to the terrorism threat, and will be modifying their life routine to reduce perceived threat in extreme ways to reduce perceived threat, including outright avoidance of some behaviors (e.g., using public transportation, living/working in the city, flying, socializing with people from different racial and ethnic groups).

in terms of thinking about and focusing on it. See Table 13.2 for more details on interpretation across various score ranges.

What represents a clinically significant change on this scale?

Assessing clinical significance for the TCS can be approached in several ways. First, because the TCS profile and summary scores are norm-based, the extent to which any individual's score deviates from the norm is indicative of clinical significance. T scores of above 60 and 70, respectively, are proposed for sub-clinical and clinically significant deviations from the norm based on their respective distance from the population mean (50). Second, because the reliability for the TCS scales and summary measure are so high, and the standard error of measurement

(SEM) around these scores has been found to be so small (1 SEM is roughly 0.5 points, meaning that the 95% confidence intervals around any given score is 49–51 in the general population), other established norms for determining clinically significant change difference are proposed. For example, when evaluating an individual's or group's change over time (such as following some sort of intervention), change scores of at least 0.5 standard deviations should be used as a rule of thumb. Effect sizes should also be used to provide a standardized measure of the magnitude of difference between two groups. Effect sizes are calculated by deriving the difference in means (or change scores) between the two groups in question, and dividing by the standard deviation from the US general population. Suggested guidelines for effect sizes define values of 0.20 as small, 0.50 as moderate, and 0.80 or greater as larger [32].

Validity and Reliability

The TCS has undergone rigorous psychometric evaluation using data from the general US population, and was examined in terms of internal structure and external validity. Briefly, psychometric results indicate that the final 13-item version of the TCS presented here, measuring three interrelated sub-scales (rumination, magnification, and helplessness), optimized model fit in a confirmatory factor analysis, and met all tests of scaling assumptions (e.g., item convergent and discriminant validity). Item convergent validity was supported for the TCS scales, with all items correlating >0.40 with their hypothesized scales. Item discriminant validity was satisfied, with all items correlating significantly greater ($p < 0.05$) with their hypothesized scales than with other competing scales. Internal consistency reliability was generally acceptable ($\alpha = 0.89$, 0.80, 0.88, and 0.85 for rumination, magnification, helplessness, and overall catastrophizing, respectively). No significant floor or ceiling effects were noted, indicating the full range of the scale was being utilized. Confirmatory factor analysis of the items generally supported a three-factor structure. A principal components analysis of the three scales was also conducted to test whether the model supported the scoring of an overall Terrorism Catastrophizing Scale. As hypothesized, only one factor was extracted, with an eigenvalue greater than 1 (1.65). This factor accounted for 56% of the scale-level variance.

The predictive validity of the TCS was also supported. Consistent with terror management and cognitive-behavioral theories, respectfully, results also show that self-esteem and social connectedness are negatively associated ($p < 0.05$) with terrorism catastrophizing, and that terrorism catastrophizing is a significant predictor ($p < 0.05$) of behavioral change to reduce perceived threat, and depression, anxiety, and stress symptoms (using the Depression, Anxiety, and Stress scales – 21-item version as dependent measures). Plans are currently underway to assess the test–retest reliability and temporal stability of the TCS over time, as well as the clinical utility and normative data for various clinical populations.

Other Scales Available for This Disorder

With the exception of the Perceptions of Terrorism Questionnaire – Short-Form (PTQ-SF), also developed by these authors [33], the authors are aware of no other instruments that assess the extent to which people are affected and impacted by the ongoing threat of future terrorist attacks. The PTQ-SF includes two scales, which assess general fears of terrorism and the impact of terror alerts, although the tool is atheoretical and there exists no normative data (the tool was developed using a university sample). The TCS was developed to account for and improve upon these weaknesses.

The Utility of the TCS

There are several reasons new assessment tools and methodologies such as the TCS have become necessary. First, as Sinclair and LoCicero have shown, the general American public is still affected adversely by the ongoing threat of terrorism, despite research that has illustrated symptoms of psychopathology related to 9/11/2001 having returned to baseline. Second, as Somer et al. have recently illustrated in their research, individuals are starting to seek mental-health services in response to anticipated threat; this is now in addition to discrete terrorist attacks [29]. This shift necessitates new assessment and treatment paradigms.

Further, Somer et al. demonstrated in their quasi-random, controlled study that a brief phone-based cognitive-behavioral therapy (CBT) was superior in reducing psychological distress when compared to treatment as usual in a sample of Israeli citizens contacting a mental-health hotline due to fears of terrorist attacks. The TCS lends itself to this sort of psychological treatment for several reasons. First, it provides for a measurement system that is inherently related to the treatment, and a method to measure treatment outcomes. Second, it allows mental-health professionals to identify and understand the degree to which people catastrophize about terrorism in general, but also how they are affected in sub-domains such as rumination, magnification, and helplessness. Interventions could then be tailored to the individual based on impact within and across domains. For example, if someone were elevated in the degree to which ruminate and magnify the threat of terrorism, but were not that affected in terms of helplessness, the clinician could focus treatment in these areas.

Conclusion

The development of the Terrorism Catastrophizing Scale is in response to the emerging need to build the necessary infrastructure for assessing and treating people in the wake of mass-casualty terrorist attacks. The TCS is theoretically based and has been rigorously tested in terms of its underlying psychometric properties. It provides for a measurement system that assesses the ongoing, chronic toll that perceived threat takes against one's person, community, and country. As opposed to the preponderance of the research that has examined retrospective reactions to discrete terrorist events, the TCS measures prospective fears and the effects of anticipating future attacks. Future TCS work will include (1) developing norms for populations who are vulnerable in terms of psychiatric and physical illness, and more precisely evaluating the relationship between vulnerability and catastrophizing about terrorism; (2) assessing TCS change in relation to the raising and lowering of the national, color-coded alert system, as well as following actual attacks that occur in places over seas, such as Bali, Madrid, and London; and (3) identifying those groups who are at greater risk, how they are at risk (in terms of which cognitive processes are affected), and the degree to which they are at risk in such a way that will enable first responders to target treatments and maximize outcomes. Please feel free to contact Samuel Sinclair at jsincl@post.harvard.edu for any questions or comments relating to, or for permission to use, the Terrorism Catastrophizing Scale (TCS).

References

1. Bongar B. The psychology of terrorism: Describing the need and describing the goals. In B. Bongar, L. Brown, Beutler, L., J. Breckenridge, & P. Zimbardo (Eds.), The Psychology of Terrorism, 2006; pp. 3–12. Oxford: Oxford University Press.
2. Laugharne J, Janca A, & Widiger T. Posttraumatic stress disorder and terrorism: 5 years after 9/11. Current Opinion in Pschiatry 2007; 20: 36–40.
3. Schuster MA, Stein BD, Jaycox LH, Collins RL, Marshall GN, Elliott MN, et al. A national survey of stress reactions after the September 11, 2001 terrorist attacks. New England Journal of Medicine 2001; 345: 1507–1512.
4. Silver RC, Holman EA, McIntosh DN, Poulin M, & Gil-Rivas V. Nationwide longitudinal study of psychological responses to September 11. Journal of the American Medical Association 2002; 288: 1235–1244.
5. Galea S, Vlahov D, Resnick H, Ahern, Susser E, Gold J, et al. Trends of probable posttraumatic stress disorder in new york city after the September 11 terrorist attacks. American Journal of Epidemiology 2003; 158: 514–524.
6. Kramer ME, Brown A, Spielman L, Giosan C, & Rothrock M. Psychological reactions to the national terror alert system. Paper presented at the American Psychological Association's 2004 annual conference.
7. Sinclair SJ, & LoCicero A. Anticipatory Fear and Catastrophizing About Terrorism: Development, Validation, and Psychometric Testing of the Terrorism Catastrophizing Scale (TCS). In Review.
8. Polling Report. War on Terrorism Polling Reports. Retrieved July 12, 2005 from www.pollingreport.com/terror.
9. Zimbardo P. Overcoming terror. Retrieved February 2004 from http://www.psychologytoday.com/htdocs/prod/ptoarticle/pto-20030724-000000.asp.
10. Ruzek JI, Maguen S, & Litz BT. Evidenced based interventions for survivors of terrorism. In B. Bongar, L. Brown, Beutler, L., J. Breckenridge, & P. Zimbardo (Eds.), The Psychology of Terrorism 2006; pp. 3–12. Oxford: Oxford University Press.
11. Flynn B. Commentary on "A national longitudinal study of the psychological consequences of the September 11, 2001 terrorist attacks: Reactions, impairment, and help-seeking. Can we influence the trajectory of psychological consequences to terrorism?" Psychiatry 2004; 67, 164–166.

12. The International Society for Traumatic Stress Studies. Mass Disasters, Trauma, and Loss. Retrieved April 2007 from http://www.istss.org/resources/disaster_trauma_and_loss.cfm.
13. Pyszczynski T, Solomon S, & Greenberg J. In the wake of 9/11: The psychology of terror, 2003. Washington, DC: American Psychological Association.
14. Beck AT. Cognitive therapy of depression. 1979. New York: The Guilford Press.
15. Beck JS. Cognitive therapy: Basics and beyond. 1995. New York: Guilford.
16. Brown TA, Antony MM, & Barlow DH. Psychometric properties of the penn state worry questionnaire in a clinical anxiety disorders sample. Behaviour Research & Therapy, 1992; 30, 33–77.
17. Startup HM, & Davey CL. Mood as input and catastrophic worrying. Journal of Abnormal Psychology, 2001; 110, 83–96.
18. Garnefski N, Teerds J, Kraaij V, Legerstee J, & van den Kommer T. Cognitive emotion regulation strategies and depressive symptoms: Differences between males and females. Personality and Individual Differences, 2004; 36, 267–276.
19. Sullivan MJL, Bishop SR, & Pivik J. The pain catastrophizing scale: Development and validation. Psychological Assessment, 1995; 7, 524–532.
20. Allison G. Nuclear terrorism: The ultimate preventable catastrophe. 2004. New York: Times Books.
21. Williams PL. Al qaeda connection: International terrorism, organized crime, and the coming apocalypse. 2005; New York: Prometheus Books.
22. Young JE, Weinberger AD, & Beck AT. Cognitive therapy for depression. In D.H. Barlow (Ed.), Clinical Handbook of Psychological Disorders: A Step by Step Treatment Manual-Third Edition. 2001; New York: The Guilford Press.
23. Beck AT. Cognitive therapy and the emotional disorders. 1976; New York: Basic Books.
24. Abramson LY, Seligman MEP, & Teasdale JD. Learned helplessness in humans: Critique and reformulation. Journal of Abnormal Psychology, 1974; 87, 49–74.
25. Abramson LY, Metalsky GI, & Alloy LB. Hopelessness depression: A theory-based subtype of depression. Psychological Review 96, 1989; 358–372.
26. Nolen-Hoeksema S, Morrow J, & Fredrickson BL. Response style and the duration of episodes of depressed mood. Journal of Abnormal Psychology, 1993; 102, 20–28.
27. Nolen-Hoeksema S. Sex differences in unipolar depression: Evidence and theory. Psychological Bulletin, 1987; 101, 259–282.
28. Nolen-Hoeksema S. Responses to depression and their effects on the duration of depressive episodes. Journal of Abnormal Psychology, 1991; 100, 569–582.
29. Somer E, Tamir E, Maguen S, & Litz BT. Brief cognitive behavioral phone-based intervention targeting anxiety about the threat of an attack: A pilot study. Behaviour Research and Therapy, 2005; 43, 669–679.
30. Turner-Bowker DM, Bayliss MS, Ware JE, & Kosinski M. Usefulness of the SF-8 health survey for comparing then impact of migraine and other conditions. Quality of Life Research, 2003; 12:1003–1012.
31. Antony MM, Bieling PJ, Cox BJ, Enns MW, & Swinson RP. Psychometric properties of the 42-item and 21-item versions of the depression anxiety stress scales (DASS) in clinical groups and a community sample. Psychological Assessment, 1998; 10, 176–181.
32. Cohen, J. Statistical power analysis for the behavioral sciences. 1978; Academic Press: New York.
33. Sinclair SJ, & LoCicero A. Development and psychometric testing of the perceptions of terrorism questionnaire short-form (PTQ-SF). New School Psychology Bulletin, 2006; 4, 7–37.

The Terrorism Catastrophizing Scale (TCS)

Currently, how much do you agree or disagree with the following statements? *Please Mark One Box on Each Line*				
	Strongly Agree	Agree	Uncertain	Disagree	Strongly Disagree
1. I have difficulty keeping the threat of terrorism out of my mind.	□1	□2	□3	□4	□5
2. There is little I can do to protect myself from terrorism.	□1	□2	□3	□4	□5
3. I frequently think about the threat of future terrorism.	□1	□2	□3	□4	□5
4. There is nothing I can do to defend myself from future terrorist attacks.	□1	□2	□3	□4	□5
5. The threat of terrorism does not enter my mind that often.	□1	□2	□3	□4	□5
6. I worry that terrorism will only get worse as time passes.	□1	□2	□3	□4	□5
7. I think that I am completely helpless in protecting myself from future terrorism.	□1	□2	□3	□4	□5
8. I worry that the threat of terrorism will never end.	□1	□2	□3	□4	□5
9. I often dwell on the threat of future terrorism.	□1	□2	□3	□4	□5
10. I believe the future is dark with respect to the threat of terrorism.	□1	□2	□3	□4	□5
11. I have a lot of power in keeping myself safe from terrorism.	□1	□2	□3	□4	□5
12. I frequently find myself preoccupied with thinking about terrorism.	□1	□2	□3	□4	□5
13. I lack control in defending myself and my loved ones against terrorism.	□1	□2	□3	□4	□5

Chapter 14
The Comprehensive Psychological Assessment

**Steven R. Smith, Jessica A. Little, Lisa A. Nowinski,
and Sara J. Walker**

Abstract Although rating scales and checklists are useful and informative for some
clinical situations and settings, there are times when a more comprehensive psychological or neuropsychological assessment is called for. The present chapter outlines
the different forms of psychological assessment and how a more comprehensive
assessment might lead to improved diagnosis and treatment. Furthermore, the use
of psychological assessment as a therapeutic intervention will also be addressed and
explained. Finally, the specifics of how to ask a good referral question that might
result in a beneficial assessment will be discussed.

Keywords Psychological testing · Rating scales · Questionnaires · Assessment ·
Psychiatry

Methods for assessing psychiatric and neuropsychological functioning among
patients include clinical interviews, behavioral observations, bedside assessments,
brief screening tools, and lengthier standardized measures. Although each has a
range of benefits, they may be more or less suitable for different patient concerns.
For instance, brief screening tools for anxiety and depression [1] and for alcohol
abuse [2] have been shown to provide cost-effective detection of at-risk patients.
However, even considering the utility of such screening measures, there are times
when a more comprehensive psychological assessment is warranted. The current
chapter addresses the benefits of comprehensive psychological and neuropsychological assessment, including unique contributions to diagnosis, conceptualization,
and treatment planning.

Throughout this chapter, the costs and benefits of both psychological assessment
and briefer screening tools are discussed, as are different models of psychological
assessment (e.g., neuropsychological, personality, behavioral). The utility of comprehensive psychological assessment in terms of what it can contribute to diagnosis,

S.R. Smith (✉)
Department of Counseling, Clinical and School Psychology, University of California,
Santa Barbara
e-mail: ssmith@education.ucsb.edu

L. Baer, M.A. Blais (eds.), *Handbook of Clinical Rating Scales and Assessment in*   287
Psychiatry and Mental Health, Current Clinical Psychiatry, DOI 10.1007/978-1-59745-387-5_14,
© Humana Press, a part of Springer Science+Business Media, LLC 2010

prognosis, and informing therapy is also presented. The current chapter addresses current trends in research and practice that seek to determine how assessment can serve as a therapeutic intervention. Finally, suggestions for how to pose a referral question to be answered through psychological assessment and how to locate assessment psychologists are offered.

Forms of Psychological Assessment

There are several forms of psychological assessment that can be of help to health-service providers. Ideally, there should be overlap between these forms of assessment. In fact, Meyer [3] suggests that a more comprehensive assessment leads to increased validity of test findings and diagnoses. Given the complexity of patient functioning, it is reasonable to suggest that various forms of assessment be integrated and interpreted in a clinically relevant manner. However, traditionally speaking, there are two broad forms of assessment: neuropsychological assessment and personality (or psychological) assessment.

1. *Neuropsychological Assessment*
   Neuropsychological assessment concerns itself with the measurement of brain–behavior relationships. Neuropsychology is a specialty of psychology, and practitioners are required to have additional years of training in neuroanatomy and assessment beyond the doctorate. Neuropsychologists are often well-versed in neuroanatomy, neuropathology, and the cognitive markers of various pathological conditions including dementia, Parkinson's disease, strokes, seizure disorders, and the sequelae of traumatic brain injury. A comprehensive neuropsychological assessment can measure memory dysfunction, hemispheric deficits, reading and articulation difficulties, executive dysfunction, learning disabilities, and functional impairments. A neuropsychological assessment can make important recommendations about a patient's safety, ability to make medical decisions and manage finances, treatment for dementing conditions, academic accommodations, or further psychiatric consultation.

2. *Personality Assessment*
   Personality assessment (also known more generally as "psychological assessment") is the comprehensive evaluation of a patient's interpersonal, cognitive, affective, and subjective experience. The questions answered by personality assessment psychologists relate to what a patient expects in his or her environment, their coping strategies, their emotional state (including diagnoses of depression or anxiety), and the types of situations that will be most beneficial or detrimental to their functioning. Personality assessment can substantially aid in the assignment of psychiatric diagnosis, but such categorical distinctions are not the best use of this type of evaluation. Psychologists will use a variety of tests and measures including measures of cognitive ability (including IQ tests),

self-report measures (e.g., the MMPI-2), performance-based assessment (e.g., the Rorschach and TAT), and verbal reports of the patient and/or their significant others.

Rating Scales and Screening Tools Versus Psychological Assessment

Rating Scales and Screening Tools

Most mental-health practitioners are familiar with the use of ratings scales and screening tools, and the use of these measures has been discussed extensively in previous chapters. However, some research suggests that psychiatrists do not regularly employ screening or outcome measures in clinical practice [4]. This is especially noteworthy as monitoring of patient's progress may lead to a decrease in the number of psychiatric hospitalizations needed and reduced financial strain on the patient [5]. When psychiatrists use screening tools, it is often to assess patients who have been unable to fully participate in a clinical interview (such as patients presenting with cognitive difficulties, severe depression or psychotic disorder, or patients resistant to treatment). In such instances, rating scales and screening tools may not be the most descriptive tool when used alone, as the ability of the patient to accurately understand, describe, or verbalize their experience may be limited [6]. A patient's inability to respond to self-report checklists/questionnaires, or a significantly impaired result on cognitive or behavioral indicators (such as the Mini-Mental State Exam, MMSE [7]) may indicate the need for a multi-method psychological assessment that is tailored to the patient's level of functioning and utilizes a variety of assessment techniques to arrive at a well-informed description of a particular patient's functioning.

Psychological Assessment

One could argue that psychological assessment is somewhat of a "psychological form of art," much like prescribing medication is a "psychiatric form of art." For example, psychiatrists who are adept at medication management understand that skillful prescribing requires much more knowledge than can be acquired from the manufacturer's suggested applications for a particular medication. Similarly, a psychologist who is specifically trained in assessment is able to see far beyond the numbers, data points, cut-off scores, etc. that are derived from a test, and can craft a report that provides insight into how a patient thinks, feels, may react under pressure, views the world, or even views his/her relationship with treatment providers. Psychological assessment differs from the use of rating scales and screening tools, as it focuses on obtaining data from various assessments and combining this information with knowledge of a patient's biological, sociological, historical, and behavioral contexts to form the most descriptive picture of a patient as possible [8].

Rating Scales and Screening Tools Versus Psychological Assessment: Pros and Cons

There is a clear distinction between the use of rating scales/screening tools and psychological assessment. The clinical use of each method has distinct benefits and disadvantages. A few pros and cons of each method are listed below.

Rating Scales and Screening tools

Pros:

- Provide a relatively quick assessment of a specific construct.
- Have standardized administration procedures, uniform items, and specific scoring instructions.
- Most are easy to score and interpret.
- Are time efficient [9] and cost efficient.
- Can be used to monitor treatment outcomes. Many managed care providers and accreditation committees require documentation of patient progress. Rating scales can provide quantitative data related to beneficial (or detrimental) changes in treatment.
- Do not require advanced training to use and interpret test results, although basic knowledge of psychometrics is needed to accurately select a scale for use with a particular client [10].

Cons:

- Poor self-reporting ability of patients may limit results. Reading level, capacity for self-reflection, tendency to respond in a socially desirable manner, and intentional faking may all distort the results of rating scales and screening tools [11].
- Rating scales and screening tools are not intended to be used as diagnostic instruments, especially when screening for disorders that have a low base rate. The specificity and sensitivity of screening instruments are greatly reduced, and the predictive value of the test significantly decreases when the base rate of a disorder is low [12].
- Psychometric information for many scales is lacking, thus making it difficult for providers to make informed decisions about the use of a particular scale [13].

Psychological Assessment

Pros:

- Can be used to answer a variety of difficult questions related to a patient's functioning, such as capacity for insight, diagnostic indicators, coping style, competency, reasoning abilities etc [14].

- Multi-method assessment reduces chances for test bias based on clinician perceptions/rater reliability [15], cultural implications [16], and other common biases that can lead to inaccurate results [17].
- Can assist in promoting working alliance or engagement in treatment [18–20].

Cons:

- Potentially costly and time-consuming [21]. May be especially costly to the patient if managed care providers will not pay for psychological assessment [22].
- Most assessments used in a psychological battery require significant knowledge of psychometrics and testing. Interpretation of results should be performed by a trained assessment specialist [23].

Purposes of Psychological Assessment

"What is the problem?" Although stated quite simply, understanding the nature of a patient's presenting problem is often the first challenge psychiatrists and psychologists must resolve when meeting a patient for the first time. Later in treatment, challenges may include gaining insight into particularly perplexing questions about a patient's level of functioning [24] or tracking therapeutic outcomes [25]. Clinical interviews can yield a wealth of information, but often additional knowledge is needed to accurately evaluate a patient and make informed clinical decisions [26]. Anything that can help us "get into the heads" and understand the lives of our patients will be advantageous in developing a better understanding of the difficulties, dynamics, and barriers to optimal psychological functioning that may require intervention in order for psychiatric treatment to be successful.

Although different forms of psychological assessment are used in different settings, there are five primary reasons to refer a patient for a comprehensive assessment [27]. These include description of pathology, description of everyday functioning, providing information for treatment planning, and the monitoring of progress. The fifth purpose of assessment, namely the use of assessment as a therapeutic intervention, will be reviewed in its own section of the chapter.

Description of Psychopathology, Neuropathology, and Differential Diagnosis

From the very first assessment tools devised in the early to mid-1900s, psychologists have hoped to use tests and measures to diagnose psychopathology and neuropathology in their patients. Compared to unstructured diagnostic interviews, psychological tests have the benefit of normative bases from which to begin interpretation. This characteristic, coupled with standardized administration procedures, yields diagnostic information that is often more predictive and robust than that obtained by interview or simple checklist procedures alone.

Description and Prediction of Everyday Behavior

The goal of personality assessment is to describe what people are like [28]. Although often used to examine issues of pathological behavior and mental illnesses, a comprehensive personality assessment should not focus solely on these aspects of functioning. The quality of a patient's interactions, their expectations of relationships, their personal strengths and attributes, and their typical means of coping with stress are all components of everyday behavior that should be included in a comprehensive personality assessment.

Likewise, a full neuropsychological evaluation should be informative about the patient's cognitive strengths and weaknesses, memory, executive functioning, attention, and planning among other domains. More than just a diagnosis of a particular form of dementia or other neuropathology, a neuropsychological assessment should discover how a patient reasons, plans, and executes behaviors to meet the demands of their environment. Indeed, there should be full consideration of a patient's interaction with their current life situation, and a good neuropsychological evaluation will be able to make very specific recommendations about what types of changes, if any, should be implemented.

Inform Medical or Psychological Treatment

The interpersonal, intrapersonal, dispositional, and situational descriptors of a psychotherapy client yielded by personality assessment can be an immensely helpful and cost-effective way of planning mental-health treatment [29]. Given the diversity of psychological treatments available, including different modalities of psychotherapy and medication, personality assessment might offer some insights into which of these might be most effective. For example, if assessment indicates that a client is uncomfortable expressing emotion, they might be more appropriate for a cognitive form of psychotherapy. Furthermore, because of the impact of personality factors in treating Axis I disorders such as depression and anxiety, personality assessment might be particularly helpful in describing these important features that might call for a more complex treatment program. In addition to informing treatment, research indicates that personality assessment prior to psychotherapy can enhance alliance early in treatment [18,19].

Similarly, neuropsychological assessment can yield important information regarding the types of treatments that might be the most appropriate. Providing comprehensive information regarding patient functioning, limitations, and strengths helps neurologists and other medical professionals plan the next phase of medical or occupational treatment. Often, the early identification of a dementia or other condition can help inform or guide treatment as well as offer the patient and their families an opportunity to effectively prepare.

Monitoring of Treatment

Many tests were designed to be sensitive to the changes that clients experience in psychotherapy or as the result of medical and/or neurological treatment. Some measures, such as the Beck Depression Inventory (BDI [30]) and the Repeatable Battery of Neuropsychological Status (RBANS [31]), were specifically designed to be used as adjuncts to treatment by measuring change. Assessment results can be used as baseline measures, with changes reflected in periodic re-testing. Clinicians can use this information to modify or enhance their interventions based on test results.

Assessment as a Therapeutic Process

The fifth purpose of assessment is that the process of assessment can be a powerful therapeutic intervention for patients and their families. Assessment research has long focused on the utility, reliability, and validity of assessment measures. However, recent research in the field of personality and neuropsychological assessment has moved away from examining primarily the psychometric characteristics of tests toward examining the potential therapeutic benefits of the process of psychological assessment. The notion that psychological assessment can be used as a therapeutic tool is a relatively new idea. Only in the last two decades have psychologists looked beyond the traditional "information-gathering models" of assessment [32–34] toward more collaborative models of psychological assessment. Many assessment psychologists have clearly begun to understand the impact of providing feedback to patients. A therapeutic or collaborative model of assessment can be helpful in building a therapeutic alliance, setting goals for treatment, resolving an impasse in treatment, and helping the patient or their family to adjust or alter their own life narrative in accordance with assessment results, ultimately replacing negative narratives with more realistic, accurate, and self-compassionate views of themselves [35].

What Makes Psychological Assessment Therapeutic?

At its core, therapeutic or collaborative assessment is defined as an approach to psychological assessment wherein the process of the assessment is considered "transformative," similar to a therapeutic intervention, and test scores can be used to interpret real life events, and empower patients to be active participants in constructing their own reality [32, 34–38]. It is based on humanistic psychology [39], and it differs from traditional information-gathering assessment in that its specific intent is to produce positive change in the patient's life. Finn [35] suggests that people do not easily change their beliefs about themselves and that one of the best ways to help patients move toward positive change is to provide emotionally supportive and interpersonally connected assessment and feedback.

Specifically, therapeutic assessment is a model of assessment in which the "assessors are committed to (a) developing and maintaining empathic connections with clients, (b) working collaboratively with clients to define individualized assessment goals, and (c) sharing and exploring assessment results with clients" [36 (p378)]. Unlike traditional models of assessment that cast the patient as the "subject" and the assessor as the "expert," therapeutic models of assessment view the patient as an active collaborator in the assessment process, placing value on the patients' own knowledge and "self-expertise." In therapeutic models of assessment, the tests facilitate the collection of standardized information *and* allow for a therapeutic dialog, encouraging the *patient* to make connections between his/her test performance and his/her behavior in real-life situations. Throughout the assessment, attention is given to the subjective experience of both the patient and the assessor and their interactions. Similar to a psychotherapist, a therapeutic-assessment clinician is interpersonally skilled and knowledgeable about tests, personality, and psychopathology.

Empirical Support

Across the field of assessment, clinicians and researchers agree that establishing rapport is essential component of the evaluation process [40, 41]. Research has shown that improved alliance during assessment is linked to better compliance with therapy, improved treatment follow-through, and sustained levels of alliance throughout the course of treatment [18, 19].

In one study of therapeutic assessment as a pre-therapy intervention, participants who were given a 1-hour therapeutic feedback session reported diminished symptomatic distress, increased self-esteem, and were generally more hopeful about their problems as compared to participants who received an equal amount of supportive, non-directive psychotherapy [32]. Also, several therapist characteristics and therapy techniques have been found to positively impact therapeutic alliance between patient and therapist. [42] Specifically, therapeutic models of assessment are able to foster collaboration and facilitate non-threatening interactions between the patient and the assessor [43–45]. Therapeutic models of assessment have aimed to bridge the gap between therapy and traditional assessment, by using psychological assessments as therapeutic tools.

Making a Referral: How to Ask a Good Referral Question

All psychological assessments begin with the ever-important referral question. Based on a comprehensive knowledge of the research data and their own experience and training, each psychologist has his/her own preferences as to which tests to use with each patient, so there is no need to make suggestions concerning what tests should be used. Rather, focus should be placed on composing a referral question. The referral question serves as the starting point from which an assessment psychologist forms all clinical decisions regarding how to assess a patient, what tests to

Table 14.1 Examples of "Bad" and "Good" referral questions

"Bad" referral question	"Good" referral question
"My patient is resistant and doesn't seem to take therapy seriously. How can I get her to change?"	"I have noticed that I am frustrated with my patient and I am not sure how to be helpful to him/her. What factors may contribute to our lack of therapeutic alliance, and in what types of situations might my patient respond favorably, and when might he/she feel threatened? What approaches may be best suited for treatment with this patient?"
"What are my patient's main personality characteristics?"	"My patient is requesting to attend a residential alcohol treatment program. In this program he will have significant daily interaction with others. He is currently detoxing from alcohol, and seems to be somewhat forgetful as he has been unable to recall the content of several conversations we have had during treatment. I would like to know what interpersonal and/or cognitive limitations may contribute to his potential ability to tolerate a residential program, and if there are any possible cognitive and or/personality factors that may make it difficult for him to obtain benefit from the program. Specifically, what is his level of impulsivity, what are his views of relationships with others, and is he experiencing any notable memory deficits?"
"Is this a decline in functioning?"	"A recent CT scan of my patient's brain shows no notable abnormalities. However, the patients family and the patient endorse significant decline in functioning.
"Is this psychosomatic?"	"Specifically, the patient reports inability to concentrate and difficulty following conversations. Does this decline/represent early-onset dementia or depression?"
"IQ test needed."	"I would like a cognitive assessment to determine the level of intellectual functioning of my patient. The results will be used to determine the patient's eligibility for special education services in the schools."

use, and eventually what treatment recommendations to make. When constructing a referral question, specificity is a key component to consider. (See Table 14.1 for examples of "bad" and "good" referral questions.)

The Importance of Specificity

Research has shown that referral questions are often quite vague, such as general requests for "personality testing" or "intellectual assessment" [46]. These types of referral questions are more likely to lead to a vague and general psychological report, as the assessor does not have an adequate guideline (generated by the referral question) to answer important questions related to the patient's functioning. Vague referral questions also increase the likelihood that an assessor will need to use a large number of tests to assess a patient, which intensifies the burden on the patient completing the test and the probability of obtaining findings that are not truly indicative of a patient's functioning but are due to statistical chance. Also, assessment reports that do not appear to have a specific purpose can contribute to feelings of disappointment in the utility of psychological assessment [36] or disenchantment with testing [47]. Overall, the more specific a referral question, the better able an assessor will be able to tailor the assessment, and provide explicit, helpful recommendations. A recent study by Brenner [48] suggests that recommendations are seen by both patients and referral sources as the most useful section of the report and contribute to the highest levels of satisfaction with the assessment process.

Suggestions for How to Be Specific

Given that constructing a specific referral question is an important task that sets the foundation for a beneficial psychological assessment, there are several guiding questions that may be helpful to explore when attempting to conceptualize a referral question that will ultimately provide you with useful information about a patient.

Why Now?

When considering a psychological assessment, first ask "Why now?" Patients are often referred for assessment at different stages in the treatment process. Evaluate what stage in treatment you are with a patient, and what makes you believe assessment may be necessary. For example, if it is the beginning of treatment, a patient may have had a long history of difficulties with other providers or has had many unsuccessful medication trials. Or, perhaps the patient has been in therapy for some time and a therapeutic impasse has developed. Attempt to identify why this particular point in time seems to be crying out for a comprehensive psychological assessment.

How Am I Feeling About the Patient?

After the question of "why now" is defined, then explore the question of "How am I feeling about my patient?" Providers can have a range of emotions about their patients, and these can often be very helpful in pin-pointing potential questions to ask in a psychological assessment. For example, if therapy is at an impasse, the first step is to acknowledge any emotions related to the patient and pose a question that takes into account one's own subjective feelings and how the therapeutic relationship is constructed around these feelings [35].

Be Clear About How the Psychological Report Will Be Used

Providers can use the information contained in a report for a variety of reasons. One important consideration is if there is a decision that is going to be made about a patient based on the results of assessment. If so, the assessor should be informed as to what this decision may be.

Note Any Specific Hypotheses About a Patient

Once it is understood why assessment is being sought presently, subjective feelings toward the patient have been identified, and it is clear how the results will be used, then ask "What are my hypotheses about this patient?" This is an especially important question if diagnostic clarity is the primary reason for seeking assessment [49]. It may be helpful to let the assessor know what hypotheses have been already been established about a patient and what evidence supports or disconfirms them.

Enlist the Input of Others When Constructing a Referral Question

If formulating a specific referral question proves difficult, collaboration with the assessment psychologist may be helpful in discerning what type of information can be gained from a psychological report, and what an exact referral question may be [33]. Also, if a patient sees a different psychotherapist or treating physician, or works closely with a case manager or other mental-health worker, it may be helpful to ask them how they perceive the patient or if there are any particularly puzzling questions they have about the patient that can be addressed through psychological assessment.

Additionally, asking the patient what types of questions he/she may have about him/herself may be appropriate. From a humanistic standpoint, involving patients at all points in the assessment process (including composing the referral questions) can lead to increased feelings of trust, self-efficacy, and decrease in feelings of depersonalization or artificiality associated with the assessment process [50].

Finding an Assessment Psychologist

Your search for an assessment psychologist might differ as a function of your referral question. Using your referral question as a guide, narrow the scope of your search for an assessment psychologist. For example, if your question is predominantly neuropsychological in nature, you might search for a neuropsychologist; if your question has more to do with the emotional functioning of your patient, then a psychologist with expertise in personality assessment might provide a better fit.

When referring a patient for comprehensive psychological assessment, there are a number of ways one can locate a psychologist to meet the patient's needs. An initial step might include consulting with colleagues for known psychologists who see patients for assessment. If you are employed by a hospital or agency, there might be an in-house psychology service that will provide this function, if available. An insurance provider list for psychologists is another resource to which one can refer. If your patient is not insured, university training clinics in clinical psychology programs often offer assessment services at reduced rates.

Summary

Psychological assessment, in its many forms and varied uses, has the potential to provide valuable information regarding a patient's diagnosis, current level of functioning, future difficulties, and ability to engage and benefit from therapeutic intervention. Beginning with an appropriately designed referral question, and ending with a detailed psychological report, a multi-method psychological assessment process can improve a mental-health provider's ability to capture the complex nature of a patient's concerns [51].

Despite its potential benefits, the field of psychological assessment has been under scrutiny from practitioners, clients, and managed care companies [52] who have begun to reject psychological testing as being costly and potentially de-humanizing to patients [36]. However, by incorporating standardized and psychometrically sound measures of multiple areas of functioning, psychological tests have been shown to possess strong test validity, often comparable to that of medical tests [27]. Psychological assessment can also have a number of lasting effects that extend beyond aiding in treatment planning or clarifying diagnosis including promoting culturally congruent treatment [53], engaging mandated or resistant clients in the therapeutic process [43], or creating a strong working alliance between treatment providers and patients [18–20].

For all mental-health practitioners, it is valuable to think of psychological assessment as a willing ally and trusted helper that can highlight important aspects of a patient's psychological functioning and can assist in making knowledgeable, well-reasoned clinical decisions and interventions.

References

1. Mori D, Lambert J, Niles B, Orlander J, Grace M, LoCastro J. The BAI-PC as a screen for anxiety, depression, and PTSD in primary care. *J Clin Psychol Med S.* 2003;10(3): 187–192.
2. Cherpitel CJ. Screening for alcohol problems in the U.S. general population: comparison of the CAGE, RAPS4, and RAPS4-QF by gender, ethnicity, and service utilization. *Alcohol Clin Exp Res.* 2002; 26(11):1686–1691.
3. Meyer GJ. Implications of information-gathering methods for a refined taxonomy of psychopathology. In: LE Beutler, ML Malik, eds. *Rethinking the DSM: A Psychological Perspective.* Washington, DC: American Psychological Association; 2002: 69–105.
4. Gilbody S, House A, Sheldon T. Psychiatrists in the UK do not use outcome measures: A national survey. *Brit J Psychiat.* 2002;180(2):101–103.
5. Slade M, McCrone P, Kuipers E, et al. Use of standardized outcome measures in adult mental health services: randomized controlled trial. *Brit J Psychiat.* 2006;189(4):330–336.

6. Atkins M, Zibin S, Chuang H. Characterizing quality of life among patients with chronic mental illness: a critical examination of the self-report methodology. *Am J Psychiat.* 1997;154:99–105.
7. Folstein MF, Folstein SE, McHugh PR. "Mini-mental State": A practical method for grading the cognitive state of patients for the clinician. *J Psychiat Res.* 1975;12:189–198.
8. Handler L, Meyer GJ. The importance of teaching and learning personality assessment. In: L Handler, MJ Hilsenroth, eds. *Teaching and Learning Personality Assessment.* Mahwah, NJ: Lawrence Erlbaum Associates Inc; 1998.
9. Stanton J, Sinar E, Balzer W, Smith P. Issues and strategies for reducing the length of self-report scales. *Pers Psychol.* 2002;55(1):167–194.
10. Cicchetti DV. Guideline, criteria, and rules of thumb for evaluating normed and standardized assessment instruments in psychology. *Psychol Assessment.* 1994;6(4):284–290.
11. Piedmont R, McCrae R, Riemann R, Angleitner A. On the invalidity of validity scales: Evidence from self-reports and observer ratings in volunteer samples. *J Pers Soc Psychol.* 2002;78(3):582–593.
12. Clark A, Harrington R. On diagnosing rare disorders rarely: Appropriate use of screening instruments. *J Child Psychol Psyc.* 1999;40(2):287–290.
13. Schrauf R, Navarro E. Using existing tests and scales in the field. *Field Methods.* 2005;17(4): 373–393.
14. Camara W, Nathan J, Puente A. Psychological test usage: implications in professional psychology. *Prof Psychol-Res Pr.* 2000;31(2):141–154.
15. Garb HN. *Studying the Clinician: Judgment Research and Psychological Assessment.* Washington, DC: American Psychological Association; 1998.
16. Roysircar G. Culturally sensitive assessment, diagnosis, and guidelines. In: Constantine MG, Sue DW, eds. *Strategies for Building Multicultural Competence in Mental Health and Educational Settings.* Hoboken, NJ: John Wiley & Sons Inc; 2005.
17. Reynolds, C.R., & Ramsey, M. Bias in psychological assessment: An empirical review and recommendations. In: JR Graham, JA Naglieri, eds. *Handbook of Psychology: Assessment Psychology.* Hoboken NJ: John Wiley & Sons; 2003:10 67–93.
18. Ackerman SJ, Hilsenroth MJ, Baity MR, Blagys MD. Interaction of therapeutic process and alliance during psychological assessment. *J Pers Assess.* 2000;75(1):82–109.
19. Hilsenroth MJ, Peters EJ, Ackerman SJ. The development of therapeutic alliance during psychological assessment: Patient and therapist perspectives across treatment. *J Pers Assess.* 2004;83:331–344.
20. Ben-Porath D. Strategies for securing commitment to treatment from individuals diagnosed with borderline personality disorder. *J Contemp Psychother.* 2004;34(3):247–263.
21. Yates B, Taub J. Assessing the costs, benefits, cost-effectiveness, and cost-benefit of psychological assessment: We should, we can, and here's how. *Psychol Assess.* 2003;15(4): 478–495.
22. Piotrowski C. Assessment practices in the era of managed care: Current status and future directions. *J Clin Psychol.* 1999;55:787–796.
23. Matarazzo JD. Psychological assessment versus psychological testing: Validation from Binet to the school, clinic, and courtroom. *Am Psychol.* 1990;45:999–1017.
24. Carter A, Marakovitz D, Sparrow S. Comprehensive psychological assessment: A developmental psychopathology approach for clinical and applied research. In: Cicchetti D, Cohen DJ, eds. *Developmental Psychopathology, Theory and Method.* 2nd ed. Hoboken, NJ: John Wiley & Sons Inc; 2006:1181–1210.
25. Ogles B, Lambert M, Fields S. *Essentials of Outcome Assessment.* New York, NY: John Wiley &Sons; 2002.
26. Reed G, Kihlstron J, Messer S. What qualifies as evidence of effective practice? In: Norcross, JC Beutler, LE Levant RF, eds. *Evidence-based Practices in Mental Health: Debate and Dialogue on the Fundamental Questions.* Washington, DC: American Psychological Association; 2006:13–55.

27. Meyer GJ, Finn SE, Eyde LD, et al. Psychological testing and psychological assessment: A review of evidence and issues. *Am Psychol.* 2001;56(2):128–165.
28. Rorer LG. (1990). Personality assessment: A conceptual survey. In: LA Pervin ed. *Handbook of Personality: Theory and Research.* New York, NY: Guilford; 1990:693–720.
29. Miller TW, Spicer K, Kraus RF, Heister T, Bilyeu J. Cost effective assessment models in providing patient-matched psychotherapy. *J Contemp Psychother.*1999;29:143–154.
30. Beck AT, Steer RA. *Beck Depression Inventory Manual.* San Antonio, TX: The Psychological Corporation; 1987.
31. Randolph C, Tierney MC, Mohr E, Chase TN. The repeatable battery for the assessment of neuropsychological status (RBANS): Preliminary clinical validity. *J Clin Exp Neuropsychol.* 1998;20:310–319.
32. Finn SE, Tonsager ME. Therapeutic effects of providing MMPI-2 test feedback to college students awaiting therapy. *Psychol Assess.* 1992;4:278–287.
33. Fischer CT. *Individualizing Psychological Assessment.* Hillsdale, NJ: Lawrence Erlbaum Associates Inc; 1994.
34. Fischer CT. Collaborative, individualized assessment. *J Pers Assess.* 2000;74:2–14.
35. Finn SE. *In our Client's Shoes: Theory and Techniques of Therapeutic Assessment.* Mahwah, NJ: Lawrence Erlbaum Associates Inc; 2007.
36. Finn SE, Tonsager ME. Information-gathering and therapeutic models of assessment: Complementary paradigms. *Psychol Assess.* 1997;9:374–385.
37. Finn SE, Martin H. Therapeutic assessment with the MMPI-2 in managed health care. In: JN Butcher, ed. *Personality Assessment in Managed Health Care: Using the MMPI-2 in Treatment Planning.* New York, NY: Oxford University Press; 1997: 131–152.
38. Handler L. The use of therapeutic assessment in with children and adolescents. In: SR Smith, L Handler, eds. *Clinical Assessment of Children and Adolescents: A Practitioner's Handbook.* Mahwah, NJ: Lawrence Erlbaum Associates Inc; 2005:53–72.
39. Finn SE, Tonsager ME. How therapeutic assessment became humanistic. *Humanistic Psychologist.* 2002;30:10–22.
40. Baron IS. *Neuropsychological Evaluation of the Child.* New York, NY: Oxford University Press; 2004.
41. Freed DM. Consideration of neuropsychological factors in interviewing. In: M Hersen, SM Turner, eds. *Diagnostic Interviewing.* 3rd ed. New York, NY: Kluwer Academic/Plenum Publishers; 2003:67–82.
42. Ackerman SJ, Hilsenroth MJ. A review of therapist characteristics and techniques positively impacting the therapeutic alliance. *Clin Psychol Rev.* 2003;23:1–30.
43. Purves C. Collaborative assessment with involuntary populations: Foster children and their mothers. *Humanistic Psychologist.* 2002;30(1–2):164–174.
44. Finn SE. Therapeutic assessment of a man with "ADD". *J Pers Assess.* 2003;80:115–129.
45. Mutchnick MG, Handler L. Once upon a time : Therapeutic interactive stories. *Humanistic Psychologist.* 2002;30:75–84.
46. Lubin B, Larsen R, Matarazzo J, Seever M. Selected characteristics of psychologists and psychological assessment in five settings: 1959-1982. *Prof Psychol- Res Pr.* 1986;17(2): 155–157.
47. Berg M. Teaching psychological testing to psychiatric residents. *Prof Psychol- Res Pr.* 1984;15(3):343–352.
48. Brenner E. Consumer-focused psychological assessment. *Prof Psychol- Res Pr.* 2003;34(3):240–247.
49. Groth-Marnat G. *Handbook of Psychological Assessment.* 4th ed. Hoboken, NJ: John Wiley & Sons Inc; 2003.
50. Friedman HL, Macdonald DA. Humanistic testing and assessment. *J Humanist Psychol.* 2006;46(4):510–529.

51. Ganellen RJ. Assessing normal and abnormal personality functioning: strengths and weaknesses of self-report, observer, and performance-based methods. *J Pers Assess.* 2007;89(1):30–40.
52. Riddle B, Byers C, Grimsey J. Literature review of the research and practice in collaborative assessment. *Humanistic Psychologist.* 2002;30(1–2):33–48.
53. Allen J. Assessment training for practice in American Indian and Alaska native settings. *J Pers Assess.* 2002;79(2):216–225.

Chapter 15
The Role of Outcomes Assessment in Clinical Quality Improvement

Ilse R. Wiechers and Anthony Weiss

Abstract Although there has been a great deal of discussion about healthcare quality in recent years, the best way to identify high-quality healthcare remains a matter of some debate. Within the field of mental health, this debate is often focused on the optimal use of clinical rating scales and outcomes assessment tools. Much of the current thinking regarding the use of these scales is presented in this book. This chapter will provide the context for the use of these instruments as a core component of quality improvement efforts.

Keywords Outcomes · Assessment · Quality improvement · Quality control

Pressures to Improve Quality of Care

Healthcare quality is a multidimensional concept, perhaps best represented by Dr. Avedis Donabedian's Seven Pillars of Quality [1]:

1. **Efficacy:** The ability of the science and technology of healthcare to bring about improvements in health when used under the most favorable circumstances.
2. **Effectiveness:** The degree to which attainable improvements in health are attained.
3. **Efficiency:** The ability to lower cost of care without diminishing attainable improvements in healthcare.
4. **Optimality:** The balancing of improvements in health against the costs of such improvements.
5. **Acceptability:** Conformity to the wishes, desires, and expectations of patients and their families.
6. **Legitimacy:** Conformity to social preferences as expressed in ethical principles, values, norms, mores, laws, and regulations.

A. Weiss (✉)
Department of Psychiatry, Massachusetts General Hospital and Harvard Medical School, One Bowdoin Square, Room 734, Boston, MA 02114, USA
e-mail: aweiss@partners.org

L. Baer, M.A. Blais (eds.), *Handbook of Clinical Rating Scales and Assessment in Psychiatry and Mental Health*, Current Clinical Psychiatry, DOI 10.1007/978-1-59745-387-5_15, © Humana Press, a part of Springer Science+Business Media, LLC 2010

7. **Equity:** Conformity to a principle that determines what is just and fair in the distribution of healthcare and its benefits among members of the population.

Each of these pillars represents a high-level goal for the outcome of care. Outcomes measurement provides the tools with which we can determine our success in achieving these goals.

Despite incredible gains over the past century within medicine in general, and within psychiatry in specific, the current quality of healthcare still falls far short of its theoretical potential. Over the past decade, the Institute of Medicine (IOM) has carefully outlined these deficiencies with a series of reports, including *To Err is Human* [2], *Crossing the Quality Chasm* [3], and *Improving the Quality of Healthcare for Mental and Substance-Use Conditions* [4]. In these reports, the IOM brought to public attention the costs of medical errors and poor-quality care, recommended the adoption of quality aims to help guide quality improvement efforts, and addressed the unique challenges of quality improvement facing mental health and substance abuse care.

When coupled with the extraordinary growth in healthcare costs, the growing realization that healthcare is not as safe and effective as possible has led to increased pressure on clinicians to improve quality of care. There is a wide range of external forces involved, including accreditation and certification bodies, government agencies, third party payers, and even healthcare consumers. The common theme is a demand for more data, particularly outcomes data. For example, PacifiCare Behavioral Health (PBH) has a program called Honors for Outcomes, which assesses PBH practitioners' quality of care using patient-completed clinical outcomes questionnaires. PBH then reports its top quality providers on an Honor Roll list, which is accessible to plan members. PBH states that the Honors for Outcomes practitioner Honor Roll system was "developed in response to increasing consumer demand for meaningful information about healthcare practitioners to help guide their decisions about whom to select for the treatment of mental health and substance abuse problems" [5].

As illustrated by the Honors for Outcomes program, these pressures are becoming particularly intense in psychiatry, where data on the outcomes of care have historically been sparse. Increasingly, information on outcomes is being demanded in exchange for coverage of care. Although the specific instruments vary, each one attempts to collect information on improvements in distress, symptoms, or function in the context of known costs of care.

Outcomes Are Only One Aspect of Quality Improvement

Outcomes measurement is an important part of any quality improvement initiative, but it is only one aspect of the overall process. Quality improvement should start with a *patient-centered focus*, which identifies those aspects of care that need improvement from the perspective of a well-defined patient population (see

Fig. 15.1 Framework for
quality improvement

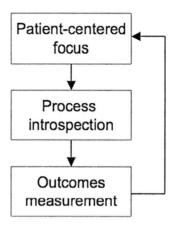

Fig. 15.1). This defining process includes the diagnostic aspects of the patient population as well as the particular microsystem in which they are receiving care [6]. For example, making improvements in the care of patients with depression requires different actions whether those patients are in the inpatient versus outpatient setting of care.

Once the population of interest is defined and their perspective considered, the next step is to evaluate the individual processes that form "healthcare" for this group. These processes include a broad range of activities including diagnosis, treatment, rehabilitation, prevention, and patient education. This evaluation requires intense *process introspection* in addition to an overarching sense of curiosity to take a fresh look at what we provide for patients as well as how and why we provide it. Identifying and systematically modifying these processes are at the heart of quality improvement. Indeed, as described by Dr. Brent James, Director of Healthcare Delivery Research at Intermountain Healthcare in Utah, quality improvement is best construed as the science of process management.

In this context, outcomes measures are tools for assessing whether process modifications have improved or worsened the quality of care along a number of dimensions (e.g., symptom severity, functionality, time to improvement, cost). Outcomes measurement is not the means to achieving this end, but rather a way to identify whether this end has been achieved. Choosing an appropriate outcomes measure requires understanding that disease progression, exacerbation, and treatment each occur within a particular time course. For example, the link between careful monitoring and control of blood glucose levels in patients with diabetes (process) and reduced likelihood of vascular complications (outcome) has now been well established. Yet evaluation of the retinal vasculature would be a poor outcome choice for any type of rapid cycle process improvement effort, given the substantial time delay between these events. Thus, measurement of hemoglobin A1c has become a popular and credible proxy (intermediate outcome) for determining the overall quality of diabetes care. Similarly, when considering quality improvement efforts for inpatients with severe major depression, we should consider measuring decrease in symptom severity rather than (or in addition to) functional outcomes since full resolution of function may not occur for several weeks to months after initiation of antidepressant medication.

Focusing on the patient, evaluating changes in process, and concluding with measurement are the framework not just for systems-level quality improvement but also for individual-level high-quality patient care. Nierenberg et al., in discussing their approach to measurement-based patient management, argue that the necessary dialog central to this type of collaborative care requires outcomes data [7]. Clinician and patient must make mutually acceptable decisions based on shared data. That data consist not only of basic psychoeducation materials regarding illness course and risks and benefits of a given treatment, but also the individual patient's response to treatment. It is the shared measurement of clinical response to treatment that allows the iterative process to continue to its next decision point.

Challenges of Implementation

The hard work of quality improvement lies in change management; that is, the management of human uncertainties associated with implementing change. There are significant organizational issues that must be addressed in order to effectively implement change in a clinical practice. First and foremost, the clinicians in a practice must support the implementation of outcomes measurement. Obtaining clinician support is made easier when clinicians have prior performance measurement experience, often through professional organizations or through state and local quality improvement collaboratives. Clinician support can also be garnered by providing them with ownership of the data or through use of pay-for-performance programs.

Other key components to transforming an organization are establishing a sense of urgency, forming a powerful guiding coalition, and creating a vision [8]. A sense of urgency provides the motivation needed to create change, but requires the discussion of potentially unpleasant facts. The guiding coalition requires not only the clinicians, as discussed above, but also leaders from a variety of support staff. Creating a vision helps to direct the change efforts. The vision in implementing outcomes measures relates to the goals for measurement and will facilitate creation of strategies for achieving those goals.

Leadership also needs to pay attention to establishing an infrastructure for change by obtaining the needed technological and human resources. For example, it may be necessary to purchase hardware and software to implement an electronic medical record or to create an outcomes database. Implementing a data structure may also require hiring a technician for data management or additional clinical staff for data collection. Determining the allocation of these resources requires close and careful consideration of the financial investment that may be necessary to implement quality improvement efforts. In addition to the direct costs of technological and human resources, there are significant time costs to implementing performance measures.

While certain efficiencies can be gained in the long run with such quality improvement efforts, in the short term, clinicians and support staff will require additional time for training and familiarizing with use of new systems.

It is important to think beyond making changes to *sustaining* changes, a process which quality guru Joseph Juran called "holding the gains." [9]. Once outcome measurement is implemented, annual review should be conducted to adjust the goals and metrics being used. A committee created by the initial leadership coalition should conduct this review. Part of the review process should assess need for continued updating of technology, for increased staff to complete internal quality improvement, and for provision of bonuses or rewards for meeting targets and goals.

Conclusion

There has been an extraordinary pace of change in assessing quality in healthcare over the past decade. Measurement of outcomes and quality improvement in mental healthcare has lagged behind the rest of medicine, but has recently gained the attention of both researchers and clinicians. Becoming involved with outcomes assessment now is in the interest of all psychiatric and mental-health clinicians. Making the necessary changes to implement outcomes assessment in clinical practice certainly requires significant effort and cost. However, to be proactive and ahead of the curve on these issues allows clinicians to help set the standards for measurement.

References

1. Donabedian A. The seven pillars of quality. Arch Pathol Lab Med 1990 Nov; 114(11): 1115–1118.
2. Institute of Medicine. To Err is Human: Building a Safer Healthcare System. Washington, DC: The National Academies Press, 2000.
3. Institute of Medicine. Crossing the Quality Chasm: A New Health System for the 21st Century. Washington, DC: The National Academies Press, 2001.
4. Institute of Medicine. Improving the Quality of Healthcare for Mental and Substance-Use Conditions. Washington, DC: The National Academies Press, 2006.
5. Honors for Outcomes Frequently Asked Questions. PacifiCare Behavioral Health, Inc., 2007. (Accessed March 7, 2007 at http://www.pbhi.com/Members_public/Shared_ Cust_Member/Provider_Directory/H4O_FAQ.asp).
6. Nelson EC, Batalden PB, Huber TP, Mohr JJ, Godfrey MM, Headrick LA, Wasson JH. Microsystems in health care: Part I. Learning from high-performing front-line clinical units. J Qual Improv, 28(9):472–493; September 2002.
7. Nierenberg AA, Ostacher MJ, Borelli D, et al. The integration of measurement and management for the treatment of bipolar disorder: A model of collaborative care in psychiatry. J Clin Psychiatry 2006: 67 Suppl 11: 3–7.
8. Kotter JP. Leading Change: Why Transformation Efforts Fail. Harvard Business Review 1995; March–April: 59–67.
9. Juran JM, and Godfrey AB (eds). Juran's Quality Handbook, 5th Edition. McGraw Hill, 1999.

Index

CPSIA information can be obtained at www.ICGtesting.com
Printed in the USA
LVOW101450280312

275091LV00005B/78/P